The Earthwise
HERBAL REPERTORY

Books by the Author

Seven Herbs: Plants as Teachers

Vitalism: The History of Homeopathy, Herbalism,
and Flower Essences

The Book of Herbal Wisdom: Using Plants as Medicines

The Practice of Traditional Western Herbalism:
Basic Doctrine, Energetics, and Classification

The Earthwise Herbal, Volume I:
A Complete Guide to Old World Traditional Plants

The Earthwise Herbal, Volume II:
A Complete Guide to New World Traditional Plants

Traditional Western Herbalism and Pulse Evaluation,
A Conversation (by Matthew Wood,
Francis Bonaldo Bégnoche, and Phyllis D. Light)

The Earthwise
HERBAL REPERTORY

The Definitive Practitioner's Guide

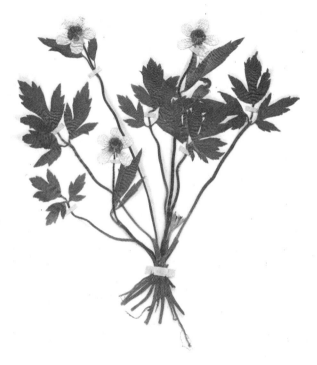

MATTHEW WOOD MSc (Herbal Medicine)
Registered Herbalist (American Herbalists Guild)

with **DAVID RYAN** CMT, C Ac

North Atlantic Books
Berkeley, California

Published by
North Atlantic Books
Huichin, unceded Ohlone land
Berkeley, California

Cover design by Nicole Hayward
Book design by Suzanne Albertson

Cover photo and interior photos by Frank Wood;
original plant pressings by Matthew Wood

Printed in the United States of America

The Earthwise Herbal Repertory: The Definitive Practitioner's Guide is sponsored and published by North Atlantic Books, an educational nonprofit based in the unceded Ohlone land Huichin (Berkeley, CA) that collaborates with partners to develop cross-cultural perspectives; nurture holistic views of art, science, the humanities, and healing; and seed personal and global transformation by publishing work on the relationship of body, spirit, and nature.

North Atlantic Books's publications are distributed to the US trade and internationally by Penguin Random House Publisher Services. For further information, visit our website at www.northatlanticbooks.com.

MEDICAL DISCLAIMER: The following information is intended for general information purposes only. Individuals should always see their health care provider before administering any suggestions made in this book. Any application of the material set forth in the following pages is at the reader's discretion and is their sole responsibility.

Library of Congress Cataloging-in-Publication Data

Names: Wood, Matthew, 1954– , author. | Ryan, David, CMT, author.
Title: *The earthwise herbal repertory : the definitive practitioner's guide* / Matthew Wood with David Ryan.
Description: Berkeley, California : North Atlantic Books, [2016] | Includes bibliographical references and index.
Identifiers: LCCN 2016005293| ISBN 9781623170776 (trade pbk.) | ISBN 9781623170783 (e-book)
Subjects: | MESH: Plants, Medicinal | Phytotherapy—methods |Homeopathy—methods
Classification: LCC RM666.H33 | NLM QV 766 | DDC 615.3/21—dc23
LC record available at http://lccn.loc.gov/2016005293

7 8 9 10 KPC 25 24 23

To the younger generation of herbalists. —Matthew

*To my long-suffering wife Sarah and children
Enrique, Helen, and Malachi, for enduring many hours
absent for study. —David*

Contents

PART I: ABOUT REPERTORIES

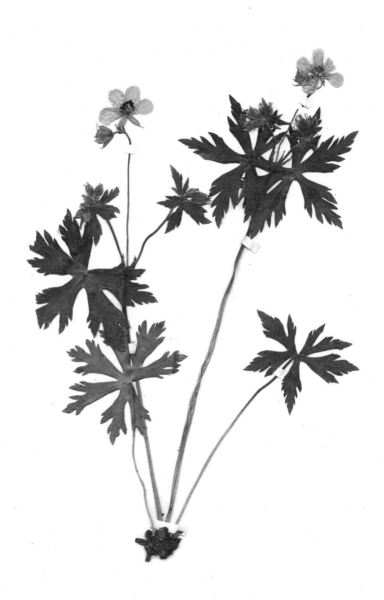

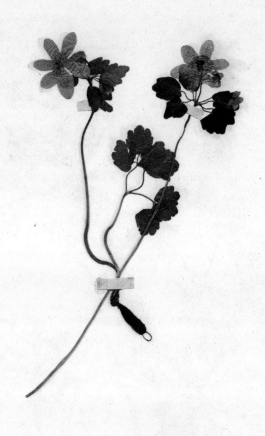

Introduction

> Such simples as the dandelion, celandine, worm-
> wood, comfrey, misseltoe, and holy thistle, taken
> in decoction, infusion, or tincture, will, if properly
> used, restore to health many who have been con-
> sidered incurable, and in most cases preserve the
> life of the patient for a considerable time, if they
> should fail in effecting a radical cure.
>
> —SAMUEL WESTCOTT TILKE (1844)

In traditional Western herbalism, the application of medicinal agents has often been very poorly defined. Dr. John M. Scudder (1829–93) described the situation as he found it at the end of the nineteenth century:

> In the past it was deemed sufficient to enumerate the remedies that might be employed in any given disease; as, for instance, in a case of pneumonia, you may give an emetic, cathartics, any of a dozen or more expectorants, diaphoretics, diuretics, narcotics, stimulants, tonics, etc. But the reasons for administering the one or the other, or the time or condition in which they would prove most available, was not, and could not, be designated. In a case of pneumonia, there was authority for the use of a hundred or more different medicines (Scudder 1898, 10).

Dr. Scudder was the "leading light" of the eclectic medical move-ment, a historically important school that used "whatever worked"—hence the name "eclectic" (Wood 2000). Among their characteristic approaches was a very strong emphasis on the use of medicinal herbs. Scudder tried to remedy the problem highlighted above by develop-ing a list of "specific indications"—precise symptoms indicating both a distinct pathological state and a corresponding single agent exactly suited to the problem.

Scudder matched the "specific medicine," as he called it, to the "specific indication"—a precise symptom complex that points to a pathological expression, not to the name of a disease. An example is the strong, hammering, driven pulse, which indicates the remedy *Veratrum viride*. This pulse also indicates that the heart is being driven or stressed by fever or high blood pressure. This "specific indication" can occur in any number of named diseases. It leads to a precise remedy, whereas the disease name leads (as Scudder shows above) to dozens or perhaps a hundred undifferentiated remedies. Scudder called both the remedy and the approach "specific medicine."

While *The Earthwise Herbal Repertory* does not follow Scudder's specific medicine exactly, it attempts to interject this kind of specificity into the application of herbal medicines. This is done through the use of specific indications (where known), "organ affinities" (when an herb acts on a particular organ or function), "energetics" (general tissue states, i.e., hot or cold, excess or deficient), and other known differentiating factors.

Despite Scudder's trenchant criticism, many herbal writers continued copying the old sources without improving the virtually useless "system" they had inherited. Herbs were still placed in long, undifferentiated lists under disease names or traditional "actions"— expectorant, diaphoretic, sedative, stimulant, etc. Since modern biomedicine had long ago moved some of these to the history books and generated new terminology. The focus on "action" puts an herb in a category that seldom relates to pathology or even modern biomedical diagnosis. "Actions" are essential herbal terminology, but not always a good basis for finding the right herb for the case.

The context for many actions died with Greek medicine, hundreds of years ago, and many new actions have been added to the traditional list through the adoption of new concepts such as antimicrobial, antibiotic, mucolytic, adaptogenic, etc. However, Scudder's criticism still goes unanswered: these actions do not tell us which case requires which mucolytic or adaptogen. This sort of poor description and classification—essentially, the lack of a system—is still found in Western herbal texts down to the present. Herbalism needed to be renewed.

The Herbal Renaissance

What were students to do without a system? Most figured out how to use Western herbs by applying other systems. These included Traditional Chinese Medicine (TCM), Ayurveda, and biomedicine. Here we particularly think of William LeSassier, Michael Tierra, Vasant Lad, Candace Canton, D. Winston, Michael Moore, Paul Bergner and other practitioners who first linked these old systems with Western herbs. In some families, the old ways of herbal medicine were not completely forgotten. Some herbalists such as Rosemary Gladstar, Phyllis Light, and Karyn Sanders learned herbalism from their elders.

My family were homeopaths, not herbalists. My Quaker grandfather was delivered by a Quaker homeopathic physician in 1900. In the little Quaker circles in which I grew up, the family physician was a cousin, and grandfather to one of my friends. On my mother's side, there were more recent converts to homeopathy; the late Julian Winston, longtime editor of *Homeopathy Today*, was my mother's first cousin. From him I learned the rudiments of homeopathy—but I was an herbalist at heart. So I applied homeopathic principles as best I could to herbal remedies. I also learned from the Bach flower essences; although Bach did not list physical indications, his little remedy descriptions for choosing a flower essence were quite complete and often worked for prescribing herbs as well.

From studying homeopathy and the Bach flower essences, I learned that each plant possesses an internal character that shows through disparate symptoms, properties, and uses, integrating them into a whole picture of a physiological function and its maladaption. Each plant also has a psychological profile that is related to the expression of the plant in physiological terms. Agrimony, for example, is useful for both psychological and physical tension. It turned out that most of the herbs used for homeopathy or flower essences have analogous uses in herbal tradition. Later I would discover Scudder's specific indications, which also emphasized the unique nature of each plant medicine.

Scudder and his eclectics were one of two major herbal medical movements in nineteenth century America. The other consisted of followers of the herbalist Samuel Thomson (1769–1843); they eventually called themselves "physiomedicalists." From them we learn the system of "six tissue states" used in this repertory. I have discussed both these herbal movements is my book *Vitalism* (2000).

The late Dorothy Hall of New South Wales, Australia also applied lessons from homeopathy and the Bach flower essences to the use of herbs. She also emphasized the unique psychological and physiological profile of each plant, and how they may be indicated by symptoms that are highly characteristic for each herb. I learned much from her, and I recommend her opus, usually entitled *Dorothy Hall's Herbal Medicine*.

Then, remarkably, Phyllis Light stepped forward to teach us a tradition that almost none of us had ever heard of—the folk medicine of the Southern United States.

The North American herbal renaissance was greatly assisted by herbalists trained in Great Britain, where herbalism still survived. David Hoffmann, Amanda McQuade Crawford, Jonathan Treasure, Anne McIntyre, and Mary Bove brought valuable contributions. David Hoffman's *Holistic Herbal* (in various editions from 1991 to the present) brought a breath of fresh herbal air to us from abroad, emphasizing organ systems and holism, and including one of our first herbal repertories. It turned out that physiomedicalism had survived in Britain. A. W. and L. R. Priest, in *Herbal Medication: A Clinical and Dispensary Handbook* (1983), contributed greatly to a more clearly defined use of herbs in the late twentieth century.

While I am recounting history, I would like the younger generation to appreciate some of the experiences we went through. The practice of herbal medicine was illegal in virtually every state—and all of us felt it. We feared arrest, and some of us were arrested—Dr.

John Christopher more than a dozen times. A friend of mine was arrested as late as 1998. She told an undercover investigator, posing as a client at her clinic, to go to the emergency room for a diagnosis: that was enough to be considered the unlicensed practice of medicine in Minnesota. But at least she wasn't firebombed, as was one herb store in Sonoma County, California in the 1970s. In that case it was rednecks showing their disapproval of hippies.

Most of the herb stores, health-food stores, and alternative restaurants I knew of in my area in the '80s were fronts for drug money. The herb store where I was employed was robbed at gunpoint more than once because—well, that's what happens in the drug trade. Occasionally we were also raided by the police. Those days are gone now, but I still value some of its lessons. I learned how to take a case history from a drug dealer: don't commit yourself to anything until you know the agenda of the person you are dealing with.

I've heard a lot of personal stories from herbalists about how tough it was in the old days. Phyllis Light told me how she dreaded becoming an herbalist because all the herbalists she knew "lived in shacks." But that was a step up from the late Tis Mal Crow, a Native American herbalist who started his career living under bridges. "Until I met you, Matthew," he told me, "I thought the only people interested in this kinda stuff were a bunch of little old people." The biographers of the late Tommie Bass (Crellin and Philpott 1990) noted that he never made more than five thousand dollars a year—and that amount was indeed about what I myself made for the first decade of my career.

There was an emotional toll to pay too. William LeSassier, the first in the younger generation of the "herbal renaissance," was saddened and tortured during the thirty-five years of his career by the long-term illegality, social ostracism, and just plain stress of being an herbalist. He didn't complain, but I could feel it in him. When he was young there were no prominent herbalists besides Dr. Christopher and himself. With real feeling, William once said to me, "If they're asking for volunteers to come back to this planet in the future, I'm sure not signing up." We miss you, William.

From Symptom List to Repertory

Whatever methods we adopt, competent practice, as Dr. Scudder foresaw, must be based on some degree of specificity in the relationship between a medicinal agent and the disordered physiological condition. Herbs are not suited to artificially imposed disease names but to naturally occurring and evolving processes within the body. To use herbs effectively, we need to educate ourselves to read pathological and physiological processes, not just parrot biomedical disease names. The former are the actual expressions of disease; names are invented for the convenience of doctors and patients.

Having said all this, we still need an "index" for looking up herbs when we need them. It needs to be more detailed than the lists Scudder criticized. Also, it needs to be suited to herbal medicine, specifically Western herbalism. It needs to include specific indications, organ affinities, energetics, and holistic thinking about physiological processes, as opposed to the reductionist approach of modern biomedicine. We also need to include input from our green-oriented friends from India, China, and elsewhere. And yes, sometimes we still need to list herbs by disease names.

Biomedicine is based on reductionism, which holds that the smallest particle operative in a system is the source or determining factor. For instance, disease is attributed to changes in molecular structure, and is to be treated by substances that change that structure. Modern drugs, therefore, are defined by their molecular structure. Holism, by contrast, views the largest tendencies or structures in the process or system as the governing powers and, if maladapted, the source of the problem. Treatment is therefore by holistic agents that act on the whole physiological process or whole person. These agents include homeopathy and herbalism.

The homeopaths long ago invented an index to suit their system. They called it a "repertory." Several prominent herbalists, including David Hoffman, Michael Moore, and Matthew Alfs have composed short "herbal repertories." I included a "repertory" in the back of *The*

Book of Herbal Wisdom (1997). Over the years I have wanted to expand this reference tool—and finally I have. Here it is.

The Homeopathic Repertory

All herbal repertories are based on the homeopathic prototype, and our study of the subject must begin with homeopathy. The repertory is a tool used by homeopaths to narrow down the number of possible remedies from many to several or one. It is arranged on a clear plan. It is not just a list of diseases and remedies, but contains tools to differentiate between remedies. That's the genius of a repertory.

Homeopathic repertories separate remedies based primarily on symptoms—not on disease names, or a physiological understanding of what is going on in the interior of the organism, nor even on an energetic or constitutional understanding of symptom patterns. In the oldest method, introduced by Baron Clemens Maria Franz von Boenninghausen, symptoms were broken down into location (region, not organ), sensation (burning, boring, itching, etc.), concomitants (symptoms occurring simultaneously), and modalities (aggravations and ameliorations). In many cases, looking up the main symptoms under location, sensation, concomitants, and modality pointed to only one choice of medicine. In others, it led to a few remedies, which (with further research) could be narrowed down to one.

The History and Use of the Herbal Repertory

Symptoms are of supreme importance in homeopathy, which largely ignores the pathological background behind them. They are of secondary significance in herbalism, and they are not used in the same way. Since they rarely describe physiological processes, symptoms in homeopathy are given without context. In herbalism, on the other hand, symptoms are almost always associated with their pathophysiological context: they refer to an organ, system, or function. This being the case, a repertory for herbalism has to be founded on a different set of variables.

The major traditions of herbal medicine in the old world are "humoral," or based on the idea of underlying fluids or "energies" controlling physiological function. This is true of Traditional Chinese Medicine, Ayurveda, Greek medicine, Scudder's specific medicine, physiomedicalism, and some American Indian practices. Therefore we find nearly universal agreement on basic principles; almost all herbalists tend to approach the organism from three or four primary directions.

Sometimes, the approach is **(1) symptomatic.** This is especially true when an herb is associated with a clear-cut, unique symptom. For instance, the ancient Greek physician Galen recorded the use of plantain *(Plantago major)* for "painless swelling of the tongue." It isn't for painful swelling, and it isn't for undifferentiated swelling, and it isn't for "the tongue" as such; there is a precise specificity in Galen's description.

A second method used by the herbalist is to determine the **(2) "energetic pattern"** or, in Greek medicine, the quality (whether hot, cold, damp, or dry). Galen specifies that plantain reduces an excess of "phlegm humor," or damp quality. This helps us know that plantain is for a swollen tongue caused by dampness. Also, phlegm may be present; the tongue is probably moist and possibly coated.

A third method used in herbal medicine is identifying **(3) organ affinity.** This was originally based on the "doctrine of signatures": the plant looks like the organ it treats. Later, this approach was based on increasing anatomical experience. The Greeks called this category "appropriation"—indicating that the herb was "appropriated" by a specific organ. Plantain has long been associated with the tongue because of its shape. The name used for plantain by Galen translates as "sheep's tongue."

A fourth method defines the **(4) "action" of the remedy:** plantain is astringent and mucilaginous, and therefore both drying and moistening, as well as contractive. This plant contains constituents that act oppositely: astringents are drying, while mucilage is moistening.

Galen tells of a patient with a painful, swollen tongue who refused to use plantain because he thought of it as a common weed that could not possibly have curative value. Later the patient had a dream about a sheep choking on its tongue. He then took the remedy with success, and apologized to Galen. This case history was described by the twelfth-century Spanish Arabic physician Ibn Zuhr, who confirms that both he and his father used the herb many times with success for this condition. (See Henry Azar's *The Sage of Seville*.)

Nicholas Culpeper's essay, "A Key to Galen's Method of Physick," found in most editions of *Culpeper's Complete Herbal*, describes the basic logic of herbal medicine as it was passed down to him from the ancient Greeks: first determine (1) the "temperature" (energetics), then (2) the "appropriation," or seat of the disease in the tissues, organs, or systems of the body, and then (3) the "action" required to alleviate the problem.

For the Greeks, the action was usually something like thinning, thickening, raising, or lowering. Today, actions describe energetic effects (stimulant, refrigerant, or relaxant, for example), organ affinities (stomachic, pulmonary, etc.), and functions (diuretic, emmenagogue, adaptogen, etc.), so they include the energetics and the organ affinities in one poorly defined, catch-all scheme.

To these three foundations of case-taking, I always add a fourth consideration: (4) the specific indication. This is used in traditional medicine, as we see from the example taken from Galen, but it was not thoroughly developed until the time of Scudder. Therefore, it does not appear in Culpeper's essay. Specific indications are extremely important because they are the most exact indicators for a remedy.

A fifth element — (5) taste — came to my attention as I was finishing this manuscript, so it is not well-developed in the repertory. Many skillful herbalists use taste as a guide to analyze the properties of a plant. They assess the pathophysiology of a case something like this: does the tissue need more tone (think astringent), stimulation (think pungent), cleansing (think bitter)? Then they start tasting their herbal supplies or running through their mental inventory of herbs and tastes. In this way the tastes act as a switchboard between the condition and the remedy. We can appreciate this as a simple, natural way of repertorizing each case.

I have watched herbalists practice in this way. Chinese and Ayurvedic medicine both classify by taste. This was one of the methods of the American Indian practitioners. Pioneers who watched them carefully noticed that they frequently looked over a case, then went into the woods and started tasting plants. The early nineteenth-century herbalist Samuel Thomson also practiced this way. See Virgil Vogel's *American Indian Medicine* (1970) and Thomson's *Narrative* accompanying his *Botanic Guide* (1835) for accounts of these practices.

If we weave these considerations together — energetics, organ affinity, actions, specific indications, and taste — they form an overarching organizational theme. I try to follow this model while taking a case history, and it is also the method used in the construction of this repertory.

Some will suggest that scientific documentation is needed to support these basic elements of the repertory. The problem, however, with research-driven information is that it is not useful until it has been proven in a clinical setting, and not all scientific information about herbs has been clearly proven in terms that are specific enough for our purposes. There is certainly room for future research in this area.

Now let's look at the five factors that help us choose the best remedy.

Energetics or Tissue States

The modern biomedical approach is reductionist: identify the smallest possible constituent peculiar to the disease. The holistic approach, by contrast, places the emphasis on broad patterns of dysfunction. This was the only option for premodern people, of course, as they lacked the technology to be reductionist. Does this mean they were incompetent, or that healing wasn't possible in their day and age? Modern biomedicine acts as if this were true, but healing works with the materials at hand. Using the naked eye, sound questions, and informed fingers, premodern medicine studied disease, medicines, and therapy in an effective if different fashion. These methods are still the ones we use today in herbal medicine because herbs are better suited to holistic processes, not fragmentary bits of process isolated by reductionism. They are themselves "whole processes" suiting to dealing with specific environmental imbalances – the "niches" in which they live.

Reductionism isolates an exact tissue lesion. This is defined by identifiable changes in the molecular structure of the tissue. The drug is then defined by molecular structure and how this modifies the molecular structure of the lesion. The results are legally definable in a courtroom. Holism, by contrast, looks for the "whole process" and the "whole person." These can only be described in terms of general tissue changes.

Holistic analysis of "general tissue changes" requires a specialized vocabulary. Throughout the world, such changes have been described as variations of the effects of "fire" and "water." Thus, we have "yang and yin" in Chinese herbalism, and "hot/cold, damp/dry" in ancient Greek medicine. A few additional values such as "wind" in TCM, or tension and relaxation in Greek practice, fill out the picture. Such terms describe about a half-dozen primal tissue changes in the body. I follow the method of the physiomedicalists (Cook 1869; Thurston 1900; Priest and Priest, 1983), who recognized four to six "tissue states."

The first thing we look for is the temperature or quality of tissues (hot, cold, damp, or dry), and the two tissue states (tense or relaxed), as described in ancient Greek medicine. These correspond to the sixfold-diagnostic method outlined by Thurston, the source for Priest and Priest's approach.

Heat	Excitation, irritation, overstimulation
Cold	Depression, understimulation
Dryness	Atrophy
Dampness	Torpor, stagnation
Tension	Tension, constriction, "wind" (TCM)
Relaxation	Relaxation

Relaxation keeps pores open, allowing for a continuous flux of fluids through tissues. Relaxation could thus also be considered "flowing dampness," as opposed to the "damp stagnation" of torpor, where the fluids build up because they are not flowing. Both would be considered a form of dampness in Greek or Chinese medicine; however, for simplicity, I usually identify torpor or stagnation with dampness, and relaxation with—well, relaxation.

There are also analogies to Ayurvedic medicine: the element of fire = heat; air = dryness; water = dampness; earth = cold; space = wind or tension (lack of space causes tension). Dampness is split into two categories—water and oil. The subdivisions of "excess" and "deficiency" are also used in all of these schools.

Ayurveda provides us with the three great categories of *vata* (air and wind), *pitta* (fire and oil), and *kapha* (water and earth). From a clinical standpoint, these three constitutional types are especially useful because they correlate with thin, medium, and thick types, respectively. People tend to fall sick according to these three variables. The thin *vata* people get dry and nervous, the thick *kapha* people under-exercise, overeat, and gain weight, while the medium *pitta* people get overheated. In the words of Brent Davis, DC, "Everybody either dries up, burns up, or melts."

There is a good correlation between the Ayurvedic elements and six major tissue states:

Fire	Excitation
Earth	Depression
Air	Atrophy
Oil	Stagnation
Space	Tension
Water	Relaxation

Organ Affinity

The ancients did not have a good understanding of anatomy or physiology, but from the location of the symptom and the impairment of function, along with a superficial knowledge of anatomy, they deduced the basic functions of organs and systems, and the remedies that suited them. This knowledge was greatly refined in the nineteenth century, when the organ was directly examined by palpation or dissection. This was a period when doctors could really visualize what was going on inside the organism.

Knowledge of the organ affinities of herbal and homeopathic remedies was developed by the English homeopath Dr. James Compton Burnett (1849-1900). He used herbs in material doses (containing actual plant substances) as well as homeopathic (extremely diluted), and his writings were influential in herbal as well as homeopathic circles. For instance, he was the first to introduce red root *(Ceanothus americanus)* into modern usage. Late in life, Scudder picked up this thread and wrote a series of articles arranging the eclectic *materia medica* by organ affinity, published posthumously in *The Eclectic Medical Journal.* The influence of these schools upon each other in the nineteenth century was continuous and important in the development of plant-knowledge.

In *Diseases of the Liver,* Burnett (1895, 3) observes, "the organ in the organism does indeed possess not only autonomy but hegemony, i.e., the organ is an independent state in itself and in and on the organism exerts an important [and, he might have added, an independent] influence." In consequence, "both a plus and a minus [an excess or deficiency] of a given organ results in diseases of the organism." In his informal style, he writes, "this idea has swam more or less before my mind for many years ... and its importance in my daily work increases with time."

The corresponding idea in herbal medicine is "trophorestorative," introduced by J. M. Thurston (1900). In the nineteenth century, it was more common for practitioners to describe spheres of function (or "trophisms") such as. . . . In the nineteenth century, it was more common for practitioners to describe spheres of function such as respiration, circulation, digestion, metabolism, elimination, nervous system, and locomotion. These were sometimes associated with the corresponding anatomical structures, and sometimes not. I have not used this term since Thurston tied it to the atrophic tissue state, which I thought was too narrow a definition.

In modern times, the immune, lymphatic, and endocrine systems would be included among the major organ systems and functions. More recently some, including myself, would include the extracellular matrix (ECM).

Altogether, we end up with about a dozen major body systems, or "spheres of activity." Listed by function and organ or system, these are:

Extracellular Matrix (includes Cells and the Fluids surrounding them)

Respiration (Lungs, Respiratory Tract)

Circulation (Cardiovascular System)

Digestion (Gastrointestinal System)

Assimilation (Lymphatics, Portal Vein)

Metabolism (including Liver, Gall bladder)

Elimination (Colon, Skin, Lungs, Kidneys)

Locomotion, (Muscular and Skeletal Systems)

Nervous, Central and Autonomic Nervous Systems

Endocrine System (Endocrine Cascade, Pancreas)

Lymph/Immune System (Spleen, Thymus, Bone Marrow, etc.)

Reproduction (Female and Male)

As we age, systems and organs naturally wear out, or may become overused and inflamed. One may be overworked to compensate for another that is worn out. Because of this, always look for organ compensation. Disease often starts in the organ system, which is why it is natural to base herbal teaching, practice, and repertory-making on organs, systems, and tissues.

Actions

In my experience, the energetics and organ affinities, plus the specific indications, are the necessary basis (three-legged stool) of a thorough case history. Culpeper also includes the category of "action."

Today the term "herbal action" would include everything: energetics (stimulants, sedatives, relaxants, astringents, mucilages, aromatics, etc.), organ affinities (stomachic, hepatic, diuretic, diaphoretic, laxative, etc.), the actions recognized by Culpeper (thinning, thickening, separating, conjoining, lifting, lowering, closing, opening, etc.), plus newly identified actions (antimicrobial, adaptogenic, etc.). I have included a few but not many actions in the repertory.

Specific Indications

The eclectics considered experience, or empiricism, to be an innate aspect of medical practice and an important plank upon which they constructed their medical knowledge. Scudder used this approach in the development of his system of specific medicine. Knowledge of specific indications and medicines were developed through experience, not experiment, as in the homeopathic provings or the biomedical randomized clinical trials (RCTs). Although modern herbalism now sometimes benefits from RCTs, the individual herbalist usually relies upon his or her experience. Herbalism as a whole is therefore more empirical than biomedicine.

The specific indication is a symptom complex or pattern that points to both a specific pathology and a specific remedy. These associations were discovered through clinical experience. The practitioner observed a symptom pattern that seemed to be characteristic in many different presentations. It possessed both detail and uniqueness, so that it could be noticed again in similar presentations in the sick. No matter what the name of the disease, the specific indication appeared again and again and was characteristic of a common pathophysiological expression. It could be defined as a characteristic pathology summed up in a precise symptom complex.

The next step involved finding a remedy for the specific indication. Scudder says that here the practitioner had to draw on his own clinical experience or established literature. Eventually a remedy was found that was specific to the indication. This was the "specific medicine." Sometimes, of course, learning occurred in the opposite direction: the practitioner understood the characteristic or specific symptoms treated by a medicine, and then began to see the pattern in the sick.

Let's study specificity through an example. Yarrow *(Achillea mille-folium)* is indicated by several very specific signs in the tongue—a carmine-red color, a pointed tip, a blue tinge in the center, a little dryness in the middle, and dampness towards the sides. I have used this indication scores of times—so many that I long ago gave up believing there is another herb suited to this precise but not uncommon presentation. When this symptom shows itself, even if only partially developed, yarrow always helps effect a cure.

A "specific indication" does not just indicate a specific remedy; it also indicates a condition of the tissues to which the plant is remedial. The above tongue condition indicates excessive heat (carmine-red color, pointed shape) with stagnant blood (blueness). Also, stagnant blood is less fluid, so the blue part of the tongue is drier. From another perspective, heat is burning off some of the fluids so that the center is drier and blood thicker as fluids are driven off through the periphery (causing moist sides). This condition is surprisingly common.

Another specific indication for yarrow is reddish skin with prominent blue (but not swollen) veins running through the redness. My interpretation would be that this shows that the veins are full and stagnant and block the capillaries from emptying as quickly as they should. This results in a congested capillary bed that causes redness on the skin. This is shown by the red periphery of the tongue with the blue in the center.

Yarrow is both a stimulant and an astringent, and it is thought that much of its healing power comes from its ability to stimulate and astringe (contract and tone) the veins, thus relieving capillary-blood stasis. British herbalist Christopher Hedley once explained in a lecture I attended that prickly ash *(Zanthoxylum)* is used in British herbalism in combination with yarrow because the former floods the capillaries with blood while the later drains them away through increased venous flow.

In addition to showing an organ affinity with the veins, capillaries, and circulation, these specific indications for yarrow also reveal the energetic condition: heat, or excess yang, is displayed in the red, pointed tongue, but this is combined with cold, depression, or yang deficiency (blue center).

Yarrow is an aromatic herb with a lot of volatile oils and a pungent, bitter, astringent taste. We associate the properties pungent, aromatic, and having volatile oils with stimulation, so it is probably through stimulating the veins and relieving stagnation that the capillaries are emptied. With no neuromuscular structure to speak of, veins are easily relaxed, and capillaries easily become engorged. These conditions respond to astringence. As a stimulating astringent, yarrow is a great remedy for severe, bright-red, hemorrhagic bleeding, an engorged endometrium, excessive menstrual bleeding, hemorrhoids, and varicose veins. The bitter elements in yarrow increase secretions to moisten the center of the body and tongue.

A further specific indication for yarrow comes from William LeSassier. He called it a "feathered tongue." This is one of the first facts I learned from William when I first met him. He considered yarrow specifically indicated when the center of the tongue shows a split or crack, especially if this opened up into dark-red tissue crisscrossed by little lines, so it looks like a "feather" in the center of the tongue. This indicates "heat attacking the blood" in TCM terminology. The expression refers to inflammation that severely irritates arterial vessels. The location in the center of the tongue refers us to the center of the body, especially the digestive tract, where the arterial vasculature is particularly inflamed. This extreme form of heat irritates the capillaries and tends to be associated with ulceration and hemorrhage. That was typical of William: the first time he met me he described my own tongue without seeing it.

Now let's say the reader does not know how to interpret the

tongue. It is still possible to understand yarrow in terms of symptomology alone, without reference to tongue evaluation. First of all, yarrow is indicated when a bruise is red and blue, showing inflammation and spilled blood. That is also an indication for arnica *(Arnica montana)* and safflower *(Carthamus tinctoria)*, but it differentiates from other remedies where the bruise colors are blue and gray, blue, green, yellow and gray, blue and yellow, or blue and black. Yarrow also is for prominent blue veins between reddish surfaces, as mentioned above.

Many herbalists know that yarrow is indicated in bright-red hemorrhaging—not without reason was it once named *"herba militaris."* These include cases of nosebleed, hemorrhages from accidents, bleeding from the lungs or GI, bleeding hemorrhoids, and especially in menstrual bleeding with bright-red hemorrhaging. Because herbs sometimes normalize two opposite states, it is also occasionally a remedy for amenorrhea. Yarrow is indicated in some cases of endometriosis, uterine fibroids, and excess menstrual conditions—but observe how we subordinate the name of the disease to the characteristic pathology.

Just as we compared the bruising of yarrow with other remedies, we also want to compare the hemorrhaging. Yarrow is indicated by bright-red bleeding, while shepherd's purse is indicated by dark, oozing blood, sumach by watery blood, goldenseal by clean cuts, and St. John's wort by pain. Yarrow also acts as a diaphoretic to promote sweating in fever. The bright-red hemorrhage has its analogy in strong fever brought on by exposure to the elements; we look for a fever with reddish skin.

These are examples of clear specific indications. By themselves, they offer an understanding of the pathology, energetics (capillary heat, venous relaxation, stagnation of the blood), organ location (capillaries, veins, circulation), and correspondence to the actions and tastes (aromatic, bitter, astringent). Yet they do not "name" the disease, which might be acute fever, enterocolitis, hepatitis, hemorrhoids, varicose veins, endometriosis, bleeding uterine fibroids, excessive menstrual bleeding, brain-surgery trauma, spinal injury, etc. I have used yarrow in all of these cases.

A "specific indication" is very different from what the homeopaths call a "characteristic," though it is more similar to the detailed "keynote" symptom. A "characteristic" symptom usually does not point out the pathological context, as a specific indication does. It may indicate a specific remedy or (like a specific indication) a few to pick among. A "keynote" is a complex of characteristic symptoms that very reliably points to a specific remedy, but also does not usually indicate the pathological context. A specific indication, by contrast, points to a specific remedy (or perhaps a few) as well as the pathological context.

A good example of a characteristic symptom is the classic homeopathic indication for *Bryonia alba* — "worse from motion." The person who needs *Bryonia* feels sharp pain on attempting movement of, for instance, chest, elbow, wrist, or muscles, or the passage of a bowel movement down the intestines. This almost always gives the answer away: use *Bryonia,* and chalk up another cure for homeopathy. However, the homeopathic literature does not appear to be interested in the pathophysiological meaning of this symptom.

We of the herbal persuasion, using *Bryonia,* would tend to think of this symptom as indicating drying-out of lubricating fluids — serous, synovial, or mucosal — so that parts are not lubricated when they move but instead catch against each other, causing sharp pain.

With the limited medical background of his era, Scudder laid out a simple approach to healing using indications. His method was more empirical (observational and pragmatic) than philosophical, dogmatic, or systemic. He relied largely on diagnosis from the general appearance and condition of the tongue, skin, pulse, and major symptoms revealed by the sick person. In the end, his system resembles Traditional Chinese Medicine — a method that similarly relies on the same sort of diagnosis and premodern understanding of anatomy, physiology, and pathology.

Scudder's approach is especially similar to the method taught by Huang Huang in *Ten Key Formula Families in Chinese Medicine (1994).* *Huang* lays out the profile of the herb. He says this is traditionally called the "presentation." He includes characteristic symptoms from the tongue, pulse, and other salient symptoms, the energetics, organ affinities, and major pathological observations. Many of his symptoms are actually specific indications that link one herb with one pathological presentation. He maximizes the description of the agent and its characteristics while minimalizing the "syndrome" or disease name to which it is traditionally linked in TCM. This is exactly what Scudder does.

Traditional Chinese Medicine is, of course, one of the most highly developed energetic systems in the world. However, it does not rely upon a single remedy, as Scudder often does. The profile of the remedy and the specific indications are usually not as highly developed. Huang Huang is an exception. He places less emphasis on TCM syndromes or "disease names" and more on specific indications from the pulse, tongue, appearance, and the tissues themselves. Thus, he speaks of the "rhubarb tongue" and its accompanying constitution. Though he doesn't use individual specifics, he uses the classic TCM formulas very specifically for each pathological presentation.

Specificity developed very slowly in Western herbalism. The Greeks were not great herbalists like the American Indians, but were good "food doctors," largely considering herbs to be specialized foods. Therefore, they associated them with the four qualities (hot, cold, damp, and dry), organ affinities, and actions, but did not fine-tune the indications. They used them in formulations, whereas the American Indians, as well as European peasants, often used specifics and developed specific indications as well as formulas. Specific indications were revived by David Winston, myself, and the late Australian herbalist Dorothy Hall. William LeSassier was another practitioner of specific medicine, but he did not publish much, so we are dependent on our memories of him, and his recorded lectures.

The most useful books on specific indications (in addition to those written by myself) are *Dorothy Hall's Herbal Medicine,* Dietrich Gümbel's *Herbal Essences and Aromatherapy,* anything by John Scudder or Finley Ellingwood, and Huang Huang's *Ten Key Formula Families in Chinese Medicine.* William Salmon's *The English Herbal, or Botanologia* (1710) is the best of the Renaissance herbals for specificity since he actually gives a "specifickation" for each herb.

The Magic of Specific Indications and Keynotes

These kinds of symptoms are not just important for precision in herbal practice; they are mneumonic devices. They may be seemingly forgotten, but when a patient presents with the symptom, the specific or keynote often pops into the mind of the practitioner. Only then, sometimes, does the logic of the indication reveal itself.

Our Native teacher, Tis Mal Crow, used these keynotes very consciously. He never explained what he was doing, but he would slow down his speech and ennunciate the symptom very clearly. It was always the same words, no matter how many times we heard him. For *Smilacina* he would slowly say "when the child cries without reason" or (less slowly) "the PMS psychobitch from hell." Who could forget such descriptions? (For both these applications use *Smilacina* as a smudge). Tis Mal was trained in Indian medicine, not only how to use plants, but how to influence the mind, and he took this type of education very seriously.

I recognized the technique when first I heard Tis Mal, because I had already observed it in the writings of the eclectic physicians and in the teaching of William LeSassier. He too was an esotericist trained to influence the mind, not just to "explain things." I have known educators who knew their material but didn't know how to plant these specific indications and keynotes in the memory. They were not as effective. I've known others who, hearing the method used once, immediately adopted it.

A keynote or specific indication always needs to be short, simple, and to the point. A good example is "tortured to capture the breath," a symptom for agrimony flower essence (or the herb) that goes back to one of Dr. Bach's protégés. It is not "tortured capture of the breath." That would indicate the person finally did catch the breath. But imagine the person who, for minutes, an hour, or longer, can't capture the breath; this person is "tortured to capture the breath." Once seen, it is not something forgotten, and there really is no other description. Yet if one had not seen such a terrible presenting symptom, one would think the exact words did not matter. One might read such a symptom and forget about it, but when a person presents the phrase flashes up from the memory into awareness. I know, because I had that experience with this exact symptom.

Specific indications and keynotes can be honed and refined to perfection through experience in the field. Usually, however, they simply pop up into the mind, from the experience at hand. The first keynote Tis Mal gave, "when the baby cries without reason," was an exact translation from the words of his teacher. The second was the product of experience.

Taste

I only added this category in the last phase of manuscript preparation but, as mentioned above, it is often an important part of the "internal repertory" a practitioner uses to analyze the case according to actions and energetics. The taste acts as the reference point for the actions, energetics, and properties of the herb, so that many practitioners will be thinking to themselves, "what taste is right for this condition?" Following are the major tastes, grouped by tissue state and followed by their actions and energetics.

Tissue State	Taste or Sensation	Action
Excitation	Sour (small doses)	cooling
	Bitter almond	cooling
	Citric acid (lime, lemon)	cooling
	Wet (cucumber, melon)	cooling
	Sweet narcotic	sedative
	Sweet aromatic	blood-thinning, cooling
Depression	Pungent, aromatic, spicy	warming
	Hot, burning	warming
	Piney, resinous	stimulating

Tissue State	Taste or Sensation	Action
	Diffusive (tingly)	stimulating
	Sweet aromatic	blood-thinning, stimulating
	Bitter aromatic	antiparasitic stimulating
Atrophy	Wet	moistening
	Mucilaginous (tacky)	moistening
	Emollient (salty)	softening
	Oily, nutty	moistening, nourishing
	Sweet	nourishing
	Meaty	nourishing
	Bitter	digestive
	Earthen (mineral taste)	mineralizing
Stagnation	Bitter	digestive
		metabolic
		laxative
	(Sometimes other flavors also act on this tissue state.)	
Tension	Acrid (bilious taste)	diaphoretic
		relaxant
		emetic
		entheogenic (spiritually mind-altering)
Relaxation	Astringent	closes pores
		stops flux
		tones tissue
		hardens

In Ayurvedic medicine, the sour flavor is considered warming, in large doses—acids burn. In small doses, or naturally occurring in fruits, however, it is cooling—illustrated by the fact that we eat fruits for their cooling effect in the hot summer.

What I have called the "sweet narcotic" flavor is found in *Papaver, Eschscholzia, Aesculus hippocastanum, Tilia,* and some other plants that are sedative and anodyne (pain-relieving).

Tastes operate by contraries, so that remedies address conditions with the opposite qualities: sour, cooling fruits (which are refrigerant, antifebrile, sedative, and sometimes anodyne) are used to reduce heat and excitation; damp mucilage remedies are moistening for dry conditions, and usually also nourishing or cooling. Pungent, hot, spicy herbs stimulate the circulation and are therefore used to warm and stimulate a cold, stagnant condition.

Formulary

At the end of most sections I have placed a short formulary. These are only advisory and not intended to be comprehensive; nor do they explain the logic behind the formulations as elegantly as Huang Huang does in *Ten Key Formula Families in Chinese Medicine.* Also, there is very little discussion of remedy preparation, which is widely available elsewhere.

For American herbalists, I recommend *Classical Formulas in the Western Herbal Tradition,* a beautiful formulary by Les Moore (2002). The author has collected many of the great formulas of Western herbalism and, even more significantly, has developed extensive indications for them. He treasures our history, and for this I highly appreciate and recommend his work.

For British herbalists, I recommend the *British Herbal Pharmacopeia 1983.* Fine, simple formulations are also given by A.W. and L.R. Priest in *Herbal Medication* (1984, 2001). Many of the great British formulas were directly borrowed from physiomedicalism, and are therefore influenced by American herbalism, but others are native to the United Kingdom.

Sources

The backbone of *The Earthwise Herbal Repertory* is the short repertory in my earlier *The Book of Herbal Wisdom* (1997), which drew on my own experiences, those of friends and acknowledged masters, and the great books they composed. My list of sources was very short (primarily David Hoffman's *Holistic Herbal*). The enlarged effort includes more sources, including Michael Moore's *Herbal Repertory in Clinical Practice* (1994); *Herbal Remedies* (2001) by Asa Hershoff and Andrea Rotelli; the *British Herbal Pharmacopoeia 1983;* Thomas Bartram's *Encyclopedia of Herbal Medicine* (1995); John Sherman's *The Complete Botanical Prescriber* (1993); William Boericke's *Pocket Manual of Homoeopathic Materia Medica* (1927), including a repertory by his brother, Oscar Boericke; and *Adaptogens: Herbs for Strength, Stamina, and Stress Relief* by David Winston and Steven Maimes (2007).

Ranking of Symptoms

The homeopathic repertory ranks symptoms into three or four grades, from less common to frequently encountered. Again, because we as herbalists focus less on symptoms than homeopaths do, we don't have a well-developed system for grading or ranking of symptoms. However, *Herbal Remedies* by Asa Hershoff and Andrea Rotelli (2001), and the *British Herbal Pharmacopoeia 1983,* rank remedies for us. I have used these books, plus my own experience and that of others, to grade remedies.

High-grade remedies—the most useful because they occur most frequently—are indicated in CAPITAL letters. Low-grade remedy names are not capitalized. While I have confidence that the high-grade remedies are very useful, many remedies listed as low-grade might also be considered high-grade as well. In the homeopathic repertory *italics* are used to indicate a middle grade; that is why the Latin herbs names in this repertory are not italicized, as would be customary in botanical literature.

Some herbalists will be surprised by the high grades assigned to some herbs. This may be because some of them are extensively used in some local region and less well known on a national or international scale. For instance, herbalists in Minnesota use *Polygonum persicaria* a great deal, so it ranks high for many fertility and sexual issues; yet it is comparatively unknown elsewhere. (This excellent remedy was introduced by Lise Wolff.)

Dosage

As I am a practitioner long known for recommending small doses, the reader might assume that I advocate small doses in the use of the herbs in this book. Nothing could be further from the truth; I frankly don't care what dosage my readers choose to use, unless the dosage is required to be small to minimize toxicity, or because the herb acts differently in small and large doses.

Readers may use the remedies in *The Earthwise Herbal Repertory* in any responsible dosage. However, "responsible dosages" are not often given in the text. That level has to be defined on a case-by-case basis, and may require further research. Generally, a *minute* dose means one drop or less, a *small* dose would be 1–10 drops, *medium* 10–25 drops, and *large* 20–35 drops. My preferred dose is 1–3 or 3–5 drops.

Contraindications and Safety

I have not included information about herbal contraindications, toxicities, drug interactions, side effects, or other problematic responses. I use small doses, and consequently encounter less of these effects, and I also do not consider myself an expert in this field. Therefore, I will leave this to others.

Please refer to other texts for information on this subject. Many fine books are available, as well as much information online—though a great deal of that may be untrue. A reliable source is Merrily A. Kuhn and David Winston's *Herbal Therapy and Supplements: A Scientific and Traditional Approach.*

Considerations on Two Sister Arts

Herbalism and homeopathy are "sister arts"—they share a common origin in Western alternative medicine, and use many of the same medicinal substances. Yet they are also quite different. Homeopathy is based on the "law of similars" (like treats like), while herbalism is primarily founded on the "law of contraries" (imbalances are addressed with opposing qualities), as we saw in the discussion of taste.

Herbalists may want to know whether indications in *The Earthwise Herbal Repertory* are different from those of other sources, since I use small doses: does the small dose make a remedy homeopathic? Homeopaths may want to know whether the *Herbal Repertory* can be applied in a homeopathic practice: if herbs act primarily by contraries, they must not be compatible with the homeopathic maxim.

These questions can be settled empirically. Almost all of the non-toxic herbs used in homeopathy (*Chamomilla, Eupatorium perfoliatum, Eupatorium purpureum, Sambucus, Hypericum, Calendula, Carduus* or *Silybum marianum, Cnicus benedictus, Arnica, Cimicifuga, Caulophyllum, Phytolacca, Urtica, Chimaphila, Solidago, Ceanothus, Chionanthus, Quercus, Valeriana*, etc.) are used essentially the same way by herbalists. I can think of only two exceptions, though there are undoubtedly others: *Rumex crispus* is used to treat cough in homeopathy but is primarily a mild laxative in herbalism, while *Gnaphalium obtusifolium* is used for sciatica in homeopathy and for respiratory problems in Southern folk medicine. Herbs have many uses, and different traditions overlap but also differ, so even the exceptions do not constitute a serious contradiction.

All the plants above were adopted into homeopathy from herbal medicine. A few that had been forgotten by herbalists, such as *Hypericum, Calendula, Arnica,* and *Ceanothus,* were picked up by homeopaths and then adopted back into herbalism. So we see an interplay between the two in terms of a common pharmacopeia. Still, a suspicion remains that these agents are being used differently. Therefore, to fully satisfy the questions of our readers, we will move beyond the study of these herbs and their properties into what can only be called the "pharmacological principles" of opposite reaction. While homeopaths and herbalists have been imagining differences, modern pharmacology has actually been studying this subject.

Similars and Contraries

Ancient and traditional medicine defined this debate in terms of "similars" and "contraries." By "similarity," the homeopath means that a substance causes the same symptoms it cures. In order to gain information about medicinal agents, therefore, substances are given to healthy people until they produce symptoms. This is called a "homeopathic proving." Many of the substances used in homeopathy are poisons, and need to be given in minute doses. Homeopaths observed that they produced one set of symptoms as they entered the body as a poison, and another set of symptoms as the body reacted against the poison and restored itself to health. These were named the "primary" and "secondary" symptoms. It has long been accepted in homeopathy that both types of symptoms can be used to select a remedy.

Homeopaths have long recognized that foods do not easily produce a proving. (If they did, the organism would get sick every time it consumed food.) Because foods have a low level of toxicity, "proving" them would require giving them in large and prolonged doses, or giving them to particularly food-sensitive people. Foods follow the law of contraries: when we are hungry, we eat.

What about the nontoxic herbs? In every major system of herbal medicine (Chinese, Ayurvedic, Greek, Tibetan, and some Native American) these are defined by tastes, as foods are; many herbs are even used as foods. Only a few herbal powerhouses such as *Lobelia*, *Phytolacca*, *Convallaria*, and *Podophyllum* are strong enough to be considered toxic. These are easily "proven" or, in the case of

Lobelia (and *Valeriana*), readily produce contrary actions even in herbal use.

What this means is that the homeopathic model is better suited to poisons than to foods or herbs. Some nontoxic herbs have produced a lot of symptoms in provings, while others have not. Poisons, on the other hand, *always produce symptoms* because that is the nature of toxicity. They contain large amounts of toxins, while nontoxic herbs contain only small amounts of mildly irritating material. These are called "secondary metabolites"; their purpose is to help the plant survive by overcoming environmental stresses. They even include poisons that kill insects and other plants. Secondary metabolites are often bound up in plants with other, antidotal substances that modify and reduce their effect, preventing the living herb from "hurting itself" with its small dose of poison. This "gentle" effect is transferred from the living plant to the medicine.

Opposite Reactions

It was homeopathy that first established the fact that substances could produce opposite effects. Since homeopathic dosages are highly diluted, it was long believed that this was a function of dosage — small amounts produced the opposite effects of large amounts.

In 1876, Hugh Schulz, a pharmacist and phytotherapist in Germany, showed in a series of experiments that small doses of heavy metals had the opposite effects of large doses on yeast colonies. At about the same time, a German psychiatrist named Rudolf Arndt independently observed that "weak stimuli slightly accelerate the vital activity; moderate and strong stimuli raise it; and very strong ones halt it" (Bastide 1998, 3). Schulz realized he had found some evidence for Arndt's assertion, and it became known as the "Arndt-Schulz Law." Both admitted there were exceptions to this "law," so it was sometimes called a "principle."

For over a hundred years, it was supposed that the homeopathic principle was based on Arndt/Schulz. However, decades of research have finally shown that (1) opposite actions are much more complicated than originally believed; (2) Schulz misinterpreted his experiments; and (3) the homeopathic principle is not based on Arndt/Schulz at all.

Extensive modern research by pharmacologists has now shown that there are three kinds of opposite actions (Bastide 1998):

Regulatory. Hormones, minerals, and other physiologically active substances can produce opposite metabolic reactions in large and small doses; this is called the "regulatory effect." In the case of Schulz's experiments, retrospective study showed that the yeast colonies were metabolically stimulated by small doses of heavy metals, while in large doses the metals killed the yeast. However, further research showed that some substances produced opposite results in large and small doses due to toxicology. This was termed the "reverse effect" and was eventually untangled from the regulatory effect.

Reverse. In medical practice it is often observed that two people, given the same dose, experience opposite reactions. It is also found that the same person, given a large and small dose can have opposite reactions. A classic example of the reverse effect in pharmacology is peppermint *(Mentha piperita)*, which produces opposite effects — stimulation and depression — in different people. Research has shown that opposite reactions occur due to shifts in dilution as slight as 1:10. This has been called the reverse effect, or "hormesis." It is not considered a law but a widely observable and often unpredictable phenomenon. It is a very real concern in pharmacological medicine, but so far no way to control or predict this reaction has been found.

The reverse effect is explained as an immunological response; repetition of the small dose stimulates immunity to the large dose. If the exposure is repeated, increasing immune tolerance will often result. This method was used by King Mithridates, who was said to have developed immunity to all the common poisons of his era by building up from small doses to large ones until he no longer reacted to them. (He was eventually killed by a sword.)

Rebound. A third type of oppositional reaction was eventually untangled from the other two. The "rebound effect" occurs due to the passage of time, not to concentration levels.

It has been found that poisonous substances produce an immediate toxicological effect as they impact the system. This is followed by a self-healing response caused by the appropriate reaction of injured bodily systems reacting against the substance. This reaction includes many physiological changes, which are not wholly or even primarily immunological.

The rebound effect is seen in the homeopathic provings, and is the true basis of homeopathy. It accounts for both the primary and secondary symptoms. Because homeopathy also dilutes the substance, the *modus operandi* of the provings became confused with the "reverse effect." It is possible, however, that the dilution of the substance causes a shift so that the primary effect is enhanced by large doses, the secondary by small ones. This would seem to fit with experience—homeopathic and otherwise—but as far as I could tell, this oppositional action is not addressed by the regulatory, reverse, or rebound effect.

The rebound effect has proven to be important in the arena of addiction counseling and medicine because addictive substances cause a "rebound" as the system responds against them and eliminates them. When addiction is maintained, however, there is no rebound effect because of the suppressive effect of the addictive substance. This is undoubtedly how a lot of pharmaceutical drugs (many of which are also physiologically addictive) operate—by suppressing secondary, self-healing effects, interpreted as disease symptoms.

The rebound effect therefore explains a certain amount of drug activity. The reverse effect explains the efficacy of therapeutic applications such as vaccinations, and the regulatory effect explains drugs that are supplementary in action, like thyroxine.

Ironically, it took the reverse effect over fifty years to be taken seriously because of its association with homeopathy—an association that was incorrectly made in the first place. On the other hand, it took almost no time at all for the rebound effect, which does explain homeopathy, to be adopted because of its obvious importance in the assessment and treatment of addiction.

Here is a detailed description of the rebound effect, from M. Bastide (1998, 5):

> Self-recovery is also called the rebound effect and is the consequence of the immunosuppressive effect [of the stressor]. It is a biological phenomenon which exists as a function of time after a strong pharmacological or toxic effect.... The organism presents the opposite manifestations as a dynamic reaction against poisoning. It is not related to a general immunological mechanism (except in an immunosuppressive effect), and has no relationship with the placebo. This self-recovery is the reaction of the living body to aggression, and self-recovery uses the appropriate and specific tools to reach a new equilibrium after the aggression.

The rebound effect is a universal phenomenon that explains sickness and recovery. It has been recognized for some time. The primary and secondary phases of the rebound effect were termed the "disease crisis" and the "healing crisis" by Henry Lindlahr, "the philosopher of naturopathy" (Wood 2000). The disease crisis occurs during the invasion from outside the organism. The "healing crisis" occurs when the organism is recovering. For instance, in an acute fever we often experience a night sweat, after which we feel better and on the road to recovery. In a chronic illness, if we are fortunate enough to recover, we may get a fever or a seemingly acute manifestation of disease, after which we return to health.

The term "healing crisis" goes back to Hippocrates. Both Lindlahr and Hippocrates would induce the healing crisis by a restricted diet (not a full fast) to remove foods difficult for the organism to digest or metabolize. Freed from this burden, the body can rally its resources and more effectively fight the illness. We may say, therefore, that an intuitive understanding of the rebound effect has been a part of medicine since remote periods.

The homeopathic idea is that the remedy reproduces the trauma of the disease as it passed into the organism—the primary effect—and that it unleashes the secondary or healing reaction. Does the rebound effect prove the law of similars? In a strict sense, the answer is yes, because the remedy causes what it cures. However, the rebound effect causes opposing reactions. One could just as well say that homeopathic agents act by the law of contraries, because the secondary symptoms oppose the primary. In other words, homeopathy works by both laws!

If both foods and poisons (including homeopathic remedies) can induce or influence the rebound effect, then herbs must too. However, compared to poisons, most herbs produce a much less noticeable rebound effect because they are not very toxic.

The medicinally active substances in herbs are labeled "secondary metabolites" because they are made by the plant secondary to its primary purpose — eat, drink, procreate. The "primary metabolites" are carbohydrates, lipids, and proteins that we use for food, which do not produce the rebound effect in either the plant or a person. The purpose of the secondary metabolite is to help the herb survive in some way. For instance, cyanogenic glycosides change to cyanide when a deer or beetle bites into the inner bark of a cherry, peach, or apple. This protects the tree. On the other hand, flavonal glycosides give the fruit of these trees strong coloring so that the deer or human will see and eat the fruit and spread the seed.

Secondary metabolites are not only diluted but are usually combined with other substances so that they do not cause the living plant to suffer from their effects. For instance, cyanide is not actually present in the peach bark; it is manufactured only when the bark is injured. If a secondary metabolite were concentrated, it would cause a toxic effect. Apple seeds, for instance, high in cyanide, are eaten by everyone in small amounts. However, if collected and eaten a cup at a time they would kill a person — as happened in one case (Kingsbury 1969).

While herbs usually need to be concentrated to become toxic, toxins have to be diluted in order to make them safe for use as homeopathic remedies. This suggests that while both herbs and homeopathic remedies produce the rebound effect, they act in opposite ways. The herb only gently provokes the primary and secondary responses. Furthermore, because it contains secondary metabolites mixed with naturally occurring dilutants and antidotes, the nontoxic herbal remedy probably provokes elements of the primary and secondary response simultaneously. This explains why some herbs "normalize" or find the middle ground between two opposite activities.

A good example of the opposite actions of an herb are given in the discussion of rhubarb (*Rheum* spp.) in Part II. Here we see the plant recommended for two very opposite constitutions, which we might call the "glutton" and "starvation" types. Rhubarb normalizes between these two opposite poles.

One of the hallmarks of a nontoxic herb is that it operates without producing a strong toxic or rebound effect, yet it eliminates or reduces primary and secondary extremes. A poison, on the other hand, produces a powerful rebound effect. Harnessed as a biomedical drug and given repeatedly, it controls the body and suppresses the symptoms it is directed against. It does not cure or normalize or eliminate primary or secondary symptoms, but forces a continuous response. It is, in fact, just like an addictive drug. It produces effects until it is stopped.

The homeopathic remedy is obviously not able to suppress symptoms—even when a recognized allopathic drug is being used. Pharmaceutical *Atropa belladonna* causes dilation of the sphincter in the eye, while homeopathic *Belladonna* is used to overcome excess dilation. It does not force the organism to respond but sends it through the primary and secondary reactions and back to balanced self-governance. It may normalize between extremes like a nontoxic herb.

Although the reverse effect is no longer associated with homeopathy, it appears to me that the diminution of the dose prevents the homeopathic remedy from forcing the organism. This reduces the primary action, in which the organism can get stuck or addicted, so that it can more easily go through both primary and secondary reactions and back to original balance or homeostasis. It therefore appears that homeopathy is working according to the rebound effect modified by the reverse effect. By comparison, herbs don't need to be reduced in concentration to produce the rebound effect because they are not very toxic and are therefore naturally normalizing between two poles of expression.

Herbs are natural, low-toxicity medicines that act according to what appears to be a universal law of healing—the rebound effect. In addition, they sometimes act through the regulatory effect because they contain small amounts of regulatory substances. They may also act through the vaccination-like reverse effect as demonstrated by the example of Mithridates.

Medical drugs, like addictive substances, force the body into the primary state and keep it there as long as the drug is taken. The symptoms produced in this way suppress some other undesirable symptom. This is a powerful way to influence the organism, almost as ingenious as it is crude. Hahnemann recognized that this approach is different from the principle of contraries (which he named "heter-opathy"); he called it "allopathy," meaning "(the cure) is alien *(allo-)* to the disease *(-pathy)."*

Herbs can also be used in this crude, material fashion to force the body to do something. Herbs, like drugs, can force changes in the body that have nothing to do with the rebound effect. They are, however, seldom strong enough to maintain a primary symptom for a prolonged time. If an herb is used to stimulate some function in the organism that the practitioner deems desirable, this can be an artificial "cure" and not really helpful to the organism (though seldom harmful).

An example of this would be the use of *Echinacea spp.* to boost white blood cell production: is this what the body really needs? An increase in WBC production might be completely unrelated to the processes going on in the body. In acute conditions, the grandmas and physicians of old used diaphoretics (sweat-inducers) to open the pores of the skin, which may have been a better approach to treating acute conditions. Thermoregulatory mechanisms are active all day and night, moderating changes in temperature and humidity through changes in blood flow and perspiration, long before the body initi-ates immune processes such as white-cell production. Influencing the circulation and diaphoresis may therefore be the natural, better way to right the primal wrong. Stimulating white-cell production might be better suited to deeper, more chronic assaults on the body, while unnecessary stimulation might weaken the organism.

This discussion has addressed how herbs do not act in an opposite way from homeopathic remedies and drugs. It appears almost certain, rather, that foods, nontoxic herbs, and poisons all operate on the body via the rebound effect—which is the basis of both sickness and healing.

However, the question of dosage remains. What is the upper limit, above which the herb becomes an overly forceful or toxic substance; and what is the lower limit, below which the herb ceases to produce any reaction in the body? The answer to this question I leave with each practitioner.

Other Differences Between the Sister Arts

Samuel Hahnemann (1755–1843), the founder of homeopathy, taught that it was impossible to know what is going on in the "hidden interior" of the organism. Therefore, he used symptoms as a basis for diagnosis and treatment, without connecting these symptoms to internal processes. Hahnemann's dictum was that the symptoms alone should be used to determine treatment. But it should be evident that knowledge of simple functional pathophysiology helps to interpret and understand the sources of symptoms and how they fit together. Many symptoms, of course, are unexplainable. Symptoms are like the kosher laws—some have obvious significance; others are obvious due to later discoveries; another category may be obvious in the future; and some laws may never be explainable under any rational circumstances.

By comparison, in herbalism one does attempt to understand what is going on in the "hidden interior" of the organism. This is undertaken through the knowledge, as I have shown, of energetics or tissue states, organ affinities, actions, and specific indications. It may be difficult to know what is going on inside the organism, but it is not impossible. Hahnemann is correct in saying that therapeutic accuracy can be derailed by incorrect assumptions about internal processes, and he developed a method that made an end-run around this problem. That, however, does not mean that we need to use it all the time.

The major appeal of homeopathy is that it is based upon a universal law or fixed therapeutic principle, and upon symptoms that are precise and well recorded, having been produced in the healthy and applied to the sick with frequent verification. The disadvantages to homeopathy are (1) the dosages are often so counterintuitively small that it tends to be subjected to feverish opposition from bigots, and (2) the symptoms observed are removed from their physiological context. Homeopaths do not strive to establish the physiological context in which the symptoms were produced, and are therefore less able to interpret disease processes than other medical disciplines.

By comparison, herbs are mostly used empirically, that is to say, on the basis of experience, without reference to a doctrine like similars or contraries. However, herbs are usually prescribed according to the "law of contraries." The stimulant warms the cold tissues, the astringent contracts the relaxed membranes, the laxative promotes peristalsis, etc. This usage is still in accord with the rebound effect, or primary and secondary symptoms, and therefore not in opposition to homeopathic principles.

Herbs are also used according to the "law of similars," but here the reference is to the "doctrine of signatures": the plant may look like a disease or organ, or grow in a place that resembles the disease. For instance, gravel root *(Eupatorium purpureum)*, *Hydrangea* spp., and horsetail *(Equisetum hyemale)* grow by the stream's edge, and are used for the kidneys. Gravel root also has a root system that looks like the capillaries, so it is considered good for stimulating capillary profusion. Herbs have been used empirically, according to the law of similars (especially the doctrine of signatures) and the law of contraries. To discard any one of these tools is to lose out on herbal heritage and power.

Toxic Plants

The area where there is sometimes clear conflict between homeopathy and herbal medicine is in the use of toxic plant medicines. The homeopaths and the eclectics often used remedies such as *Aconitum, Atropa belladonna, Gelsemium,* etc. in opposite fashions. Even here, if we understand the approaches, we see that both methods were skilled and health-promoting, though seemingly in conflict with each other.

Belladonna is used in both homeopathy and eclectic medicine to reduce inflammation accompanied by pounding, pulsating arteries. In biomedicine, it is still used in the form of *atropine* to relax the pupil of the eye. All three schools therefore use the plant to relax the neurovascular system, although the biomedical approach forces the body to react, while homeopathy and eclectic medicine encourage the body to complete its own process through a slight aggravation (displaying primary symptoms) followed by a cure (displaying secondary symptoms). The homeopathic and eclectic uses of *Belladonna* are therefore identical, but opposite to its biomedical use.

Gelsemium causes extreme muscle constriction followed by extreme prostration and relaxation. It is used in eclecticism to relax a tight muscle, while in homeopathy it is used for prostration, exhaustion, and excessive relaxation. Here the use is opposite: The eclectics focus on the primary symptoms, and the homeopaths on the secondary, but both are correct and valuable.

Sometimes the uses are not opposite but virtually unrelated: *Staphysagria* is used in homeopathy for psychological or physical violation, anger, and irritation of extremely sensitive tissues, while in herbalism it is used externally only (due to its toxicity) to kill head lice. That actually is a form of irritation, but is not exactly an opposite!

Bryonia was used by herbalists in Culpeper's day, in small doses, as a purgative. In large doses, it is fearfully cathartic, draining the colon of water and causing a dry, irritable, inflamed state. In homeopathy, *Bryonia* is used for symptoms that are "worse from motion." No explanation of this tissue condition is given, but it is due to the extreme evacuation of fluids and dryness it caused in the provings.

Therefore the original herbal use and the homoeopathic uses are opposites, based on the rebound effect. The eclectics used *Bryonia* for severe heat and dryness, so they used it as the homeopaths did.

In homeopathy, *Aconitum* is used for fever following severe chill, overheating, or animal fear, while in herbalism (both Chinese and older Western traditions) aconite is used externally to deaden pain in cold, arthritic, aging joints, because it numbs the nerves. It is so poisonous that a small dose can kill. The antique medicine bottle I have says to dilute the contents at 1:3,000! In other words, homeopathy uses *Aconitum* to counter the severe chill and fever it would cause as a poison, while herbalism uses it to produce a mild, local inflammation that deadens (but does not kill) the painful nerves. These uses are opposite. How can we say that one is more appropriate than the other?

In order not to cause confusion, *The Earthwise Herbal Repertory* does not include eclectic or other usages based on toxic dosages. This book is intended for use of *relatively nontoxic herbs in safe doses*. I have included a few "active," moderately toxic herbs traditionally used alongside the milder herbs, such as lobelia and kava-kava *(Piper methysticum)*, but not *Aconitum* or other plants poisonous in large doses.

I have also included a few homeopathic remedies in the repertory, simply because they are so useful. Therefore, when the names *Aconitum, Bryonia, Gelsemium, Staphysagria,* etc., appear in the repertory, they refer to the homeopathic dilution. These are prepared on a scale of one to ten, or one to a hundred: 3x refers to a dilution of one part in ten to the third power (1:1,000), 6x to one part in ten to the sixth power (1:1,000,000), 3c to one part in a hundred to the third power (1:1,000,000), 6c to one part in a hundred to the sixth power (1:1,000,000,000,000), etc. The x method is used to make less diluted potencies, the c to make more diluted or "higher" potencies.

Homeopathic Remedies Listed in this Repertory

A small number of homeopathic remedies have been listed in this repertory, for several reasons. First, these are mostly vegetable "polycrests" (remedies with many uses) found in a homeopathic home-remedy kit and commonly used by laypeople as well as professional prescribers. Second, most of these remedies were used by the eclectic medical movement in the nineteenth century and are therefore an important part of our Western herbal heritage. Third, poisons can have virtues, as do nontoxic herbs and foods. Homeopathic remedies that are not toxic are listed as herbs (*Hypericum, Sambucus,* etc.) and can be used in large doses. Fourth, many of these homeopathic agents were listed by Michael Moore in his *Herbal Repertory in Clinical Practice* (1994), and I felt he established a precedent I was happy to follow. Fifth, I use most of these remedies myself in my own herbal practice.

Almost all of the homeopathic remedies are moderate to deadly poisons, and therefore only the homeopathic dosages (which are less than 0.1% of the mother tincture) are recommended, except in certain circumstances. The eclectic use of *Gelsemium* as an antispasmodic is too useful to discard, and therefore it has been preserved, but for *external use only. Staphysagria* is used as the mother tincture, but only on the hair, against lice. Here are the major homeopathic remedies I have included:

Aconitum napellus (Aconite)

Atropa belladonna (Belladonna)

Bryonia alba (White Bryony)

Delphinium staphisagria (Staphysagria, Stavesacre)

Gelsemium sempervirens (Gelsemium)

Rhus toxicodendron (Poison Ivy)

Veratrum viride (American hellebore)

A few other homeopathic remedies have also crept into the pages of this tome.

Conclusion

Both homeopathic and herbal remedies primarily act according to the rebound effect, which encompasses both similarity and contrarity. This repertory, therefore, can be used by both homeopaths and herbalists.

The Traditional Homeopathic Repertory

by David Ryan and Matthew Wood

Two-thirds of our *Materia Medica* are plants, so to
really study homeopathy you should become an
herbalist. You'll know plants.

—ROBIN MURPHY, ND, HOMEOPATH

In 1827, a botanist and lawyer named Baron Clemons Maria Franz
von Boenninghausen was dying of "consumption." In a letter of fare-
well to a fellow member of his regional botanical society, he regretfully
predicted the end of their friendship and correspondence. Unknown
to Boenninghausen, his friend, Dr. Carl Weihe, was a dedicated and
skillful practitioner of the "new system," as homeopathy was often
called at that time. The doctor asked Boenninghausen to tell him his
symptoms, then sent back a homeopathic preparation of *Pulsatilla*,
the windflower. The ailing baron was restored to full health in several
months and, not surprisingly, began the earnest study and practice
of the "new system."

Samuel Hahnemann's "new system" was based on the principle
of "like treats like," or the "law of similars." The ancient form of
this "law" was based on the doctrine of signatures—the medicine
looks like the disease. However, Hahnemann's concept was different,
based on the idea that the substance causes the same symptoms in
the healthy that it cures in the sick.

In order to develop homeopathy, Hahnemann invented a method
called "drug proving": a substance is given to a healthy person in
a safe but symptom-provoking series of doses. The symptoms produced in this manner are used to guide the selection of a remedy
for a sick person with the same symptoms. Through experience,
Hahnemann found that diminishing the amount of the dose reduced

the side effects. Eventually he reduced the dosage to "infinitesimal" levels — minute amounts in dilutions well beyond the point where any substance remained. This unlikely-sounding technique led to the primary criticism of homeopathy, then and now.

But practically, how were symptoms produced by provings linked to the sick? Remember that Hahnemann was groping in the dark at the start. He was inventing or discovering a "new system" that had never before been practiced. Both the provers and the sick had many symptoms. Hahnemann realized that some were more "characteristic" than others, and set the emphasis on these. A characteristic symptom is one that is typical of a remedy in many provers, patients, and diseases. The "characteristic" symptom often indicates one or a few remedies. An example would be "worse from motion," the grand indication for *Bryonia*.

The next generation of homeopaths differentiated between a "characteristic" symptom and a "keynote." The former could be composed of as little as one symptom ("worse from motion") while the latter represents a more developed and unique complex of several symptoms. For example, the homeopathic remedy *Belladonna* is indicated for the simultaneous presence of heat and throbbing in the head. This is considered a keynote symptom because there is a complex of three indications: a sensation (throbbing), a second sensation (heat), and a location (head).

Modern research shows that Hahnemann experimented with many different options in his practice before settling on guidelines for his students. Once he had determined what he thought was appropriate, however, his opinion was usually dogmatic. His basic directives, given in his *Organon of the Medical Art* (1996), comprised the three fundamentals of homeopathic practice: (1) the remedy is applied by the law of similars (like treats like), producing the symptoms it has cured; (2) the remedy should match the totality of characteristic symptoms of the patient; and (3) the remedy should be given in the smallest dose capable of producing a curative response.

Over several decades, Hahnemann and his students generated drug provings for nearly a hundred remedies, many of which are still the bedrock of homeopathy today. His initial pharmacopeia was published under the name *Materia Medica Pura*. The symptoms were "pure" in the sense that they were generated by provings alone. They were also unindexed, with only scant notes on the possible uses or general applications of the medicine.

After practicing his system for over two decades, Hahnemann came to the conclusion that there could be hidden, chronic illnesses lurking in the interior of the organism, encumbering the "vital force" of the patient so that they did not respond in a healthy manner to his well-selected remedies. Instead of concluding that he needed more remedies, Hahnemann felt he needed deeper-acting remedies.

At this point Hahnemann divided the *materia medica,* the symptomology, and the disease states into two classes: (1) acute, localized, or simple chronic diseases and their symptoms, generally suited to treatment by the remedies in *Materia Medica Pura;* and (2) chronic and genetic diseases and symptoms requiring deeper, chronically acting remedies that affect the whole complex to eliminate the "miasmatic taint." This led to the publication of his second major homeopathic pharmacopeia, *The Chronic Diseases.* The majority of remedies in the first group were plants, while those in the second group were mostly of mineral and animal origin. It appears from this selection that Hahnemann conceived the plant remedies to have a less far-reaching action than the second group. This matter of the "difference between the kingdoms," plant, mineral and animal, will be taken up below.

The release of *Chronic Diseases* caused a firestorm of controversy among Hahnemann's followers. It was rightly pointed out that it completely contradicted his previous directives, which dogmatically emphasized prescription based on symptoms alone.

The fact that Hahnemann radically changed his directions for homeopathic practice in mid-career might warn us that we should not consider his dogmatic instructions to be the "only" or "true" basis of homeopathic practice. Furthermore, modern research shows that Hahnemann did not entirely adhere to his own guidelines. Rima Handley (1990) and David Little (2015) trace out the contours of Hahnemann's actual practice late in life. Usually he would give a dose of *Sulphur* to ignite a cleansing metabolic fire and open the channels of elimination. He followed this with a course of remedies suited to the presenting symptoms. After decades of bedside experience, he had memorized two or three basic remedies for each common presentation.

Other modern research, found in *Vitalism* (Wood 2000), shows that Hahnemann used the medical pathology of his era in the analysis of patients, even though he claimed that the prescription should be based upon the symptoms. In two cases, Hahnemann diagnosed an abscess on the liver perforating through the pleura and emptying out through the lungs. This was a rare condition in the nineteenth century; today it is virtually unknown, thanks to antibiotics. In a case witnessed by Dr. Dunscomb, six doctors had made the mistaken diagnosis of tuberculosis before the patient was brought to Hahnemann. He changed the diagnosis to liver abscess and quickly and successfully treated the case. Dunscomb attributed the success of Hahnemann's prescription to the correct pathological diagnosis.

The next several generations of homeopaths were mostly educated doctors already trained to make these kinds of diagnoses themselves, so it should be granted that medical physiology and pathology played a larger role in homeopathy than is generally admitted. Modern homeopaths, by comparison, usually have very little medical training.

Boenninghausen's initial repertories (very different from his final arrangement) appeared late in Hahnemann's career. Until then, the founder's actual practice was based on the pathological presentation, the characteristic symptoms, and the "cheat sheet" of remedies he associated with each common presentation. ("I know many herbalists who practice exactly like this," remarks Matthew.) Some herbalists also use an "opening formula," like Hahnemann's use of *Sulphur.* One thinks immediately of Samuel Thomson's lobelia, cayenne, and bayberry formula.

We assert that the real difference between homeopathy and herbalism is not the law of similars. As we have seen in the last chapter, similars and contraries are both present in the homeopathic provings and remedies because of the rebound effect. The differences in therapeutic approach between Hahnemann and herbalism, as just shown, is less dramatic than is commonly thought. The major innovation introduced by Hahnemann is the prescriptive accuracy that arises from careful cross-referencing of remedy symptoms with the client's symptoms. He originally called his remedies "specifics" rather than "similars," showing that he thought in these terms for a while, before adopting the law of similars as the basis of his new system.

This prescriptive accuracy and symptom detail probably stimulated the eclectic thinking of John Scudder, and led to his development of specific indications. While the idea is similar, the execution is different, because Scudder's specific indications are based on bedside experience and are almost never identical to homeopathic symptoms. Blending of homeopathy and Scudder's specific medicine occurred in the next several generations, on both sides.

The First Homeopathic Repertories

When Boenninghausen began his studies and practice, keynote symptoms were poorly developed, and there were few shortcuts to prescribing homeopathic remedies. Taking a chronic case could easily overrun an hour, with many more hours needed to search for the right remedy in the *Materia Medica Pura* and journals containing new provings. Homeopaths desperately needed a way to arrive at the appropriate prescription quickly and reliably. A major weakness of the "new system" was the lack of a symptom index. Hahnemann realized this, and began a small "lexicon" of symptoms, but it was never completed. In his seventies, he knew he was not up to finishing the task, so he delegated the job to two of his top students, Boenninghausen and G.H.G. Jahr. The latter moved on to other projects.

Boenninghausen's first repertory (1832) covered only the agents in Hahnemann's *Chronic Diseases*. He created a separate repertory (1835) for acute remedies and conditions. He then began to merge the acute and chronic repertories. However, halfway through the revision "it had increased in size beyond all expectation" (Boenninghausen 2007, *vi*). "I gave it up," he explained, "as I saw it was extremely probable that a similar object might be attained in a more simple and satisfactory manner." His grand insight is described in Roberts' introduction to the *Pocket Book:*

> He conceived the figure of a great all-inclusive Symptom Totality, made up of the cardinal points of location, sensation, conditions of aggravation and ameliorations [modalities], and concomitance, under which all symptoms of the *materia medica* and all the symptoms of the disease as well should be covered (Roberts 2007, 26).

Using this model, Boenninghausen found he could simplify symptoms into their four elemental components. This established not only the basis for an easy-to-use repertory but a model for case-taking and study of *materia medica*. It also allows hitherto unknown symptom combinations to be discovered, which led to previously unknown uses of remedies. It is therefore a dynamic, holographic, archetypal approach to symptoms. It is remarkable that Boenninghausen both divided symptoms into their components and also succeeded in bringing them back together into organic patterns. This is the basis of *The Therapeutic Pocket Book,* which first appeared in 1846. For practicality, he includes sections on mind or soul (German *seele*), sleep and dream, and fever, in addition to the basic sections on location, sensation, modality, and concomitant.

Here is a rendering of the "Symptom Totality" into its four major corners, or parts, as conceived by Boenninghausen.

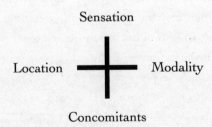

Sensation

Location   Modality

Concomitants

Hahnemann tested and approved this method in his final years. Boenninghausen noted that "the late honored Founder pronounced my idea 'excellent and eminently desirable,' so I had no more misgivings about finishing the work" (Boenninghausen 2007, *vi*).

At the time of his death, Hahnemann's *Organon* and *Chronic Diseases* provided the theory; the ever-expanding homeopathic *materia medica* provided the remedies, and the *Repertory* provided the practical means for choosing remedies. These became the threefold foundation of the new system.

The Complete Symptom

Boenninghausen's approach to the symptom was based on teachings that go all the way back to the ancient Hippocratic physicians. They determined that there were seven basic questions that needed to be asked and answered in order to arrive at a complete understanding of a case. In the twelfth century, the Latin churchmen reduced these to a simple verse that Boenninghausen adopted: *Quis, quid, ubi, quibus auxiliis, cur, quomodo, quando*. This formed the basis of his mature vision of the repertorial template. Here is an expansion and explanation, based on John Henry Clarke's *Clinical Repertory* (1904) and the work of David Little (2015):

I. *Quis* (Who): Who is the patient (constitution, temperament, mind)?

II. *Quid* (What): What is wrong (sensations, complaints, clinical conditions)?

III. *Ubi* (Where): Where is the problem (location)?

IV. *Quibus auxiliis* (With what): What accompanies the problem (concomitants)?

V. *Cur* (Why): How did it start (etiology, causation)?

VI. *Quomodo* (In what way): What makes the complaints better or worse? (This was the origin of the term "modality" as used in homeopathy.)

VII. *Quando* (When): What is the pathological timeline, including changes that occurred?

Robin Murphy stresses that the entry complaint—what the person wants taken care of *(quid)*—should come first. Clarke makes the same adjustment in his *Clinical Repertory*. Without question, the first fact to be established in a case is the goal of the client. What is it we are doing? If, during the course of the case, the practitioner feels a different goal is preferable or attainable, he or she must inform the client and change the goal.

This list is a good guide for any type of holistic case-taking. It reminds us of the "ten questions" or "ten-asking song" in Traditional Chinese Medicine.

Boenninghausen's Advice on Using the Repertory

The baron's advice on using his repertory holds true for other repertories as well, including this one. Boenninghausen wrote:

> Much depends upon whether one is entirely a beginner, or is already somewhat skilled…. But he who knows nothing whatever must, indeed, make a most careful search for everything without exception. The more he knows, the less he has to look for and, finally, only to use it here and there to help his memory (Boenninghausen 2007, *x*).

The "prince of repertory-makers" then gives a case example to illustrate the difference between how a beginner and an experienced homeopath might take a case. It happens that the example fits our purposes, because the remedy is commonly used by herbalists and can also be found by searching the current repertory.

> E.N. of L., a man of about 50 years, of a blooming, almost florid complexion, usually cheerful but during his more violent paroxysms inclined to outbreaks of anger with decided nervous excitement, had suffered for a few months with a peculiar kind of violent pain in the right leg after the previous dispersion allopathically of a so-called rheumatic pain in the right orbit by external remedies, which could not be found out; this last pain

attacked the muscles of the posterior part of the leg, especially from the calf down to the heel, but did not involve the knee or ankle-joint. The pain itself he described as extremely acute, cramping, jerking, tearing, frequently interrupted by stitches extending from within outward; but in the morning hours, when the pain was generally more endurable, it was a dull burrowing with a bruised feeling.

The pain became worse towards evening and during rest, especially after previous motion, while sitting or standing, particularly if he did it during a walk in the open air. While walking the pain jumped suddenly from the right calf into the left upper arm, if he put his hand into his coat pocket or his breast and kept the arm quiet, which was relieved by moving the arm, and then the pain suddenly jumped back into the right calf. The greatest relief was experienced while walking up and down the room and rubbing the affected part.

The concomitant symptoms were sleeplessness before midnight, frequently recurring attacks in the evening of sudden flushes of heat with thirst without previous chill, a disagreeable fatty taste in the mouth, with nausea in the throat, and an almost constant pressing pain in the lower part of the chest and pit of the stomach, as if something there were forcing itself outward (Boenninghausen 2007, *xi*).

Boenninghausen gives examples of how several homeopaths might analyze the case. The wandering pains, fatty taste in the mouth, and sleeplessness before midnight, suggest a condition calling for *Pulsatilla*, but this remedy is not prescribed for anger or the florid, blooming complexion. "Another person who has studied more [thoroughly] the peculiarities of the pains," continues Boenninghausen, "distinctly remembers that *China* [quinine] corresponds to the paralytic and bruised pains as well as to the jerking tearing [pains], and stitches from within outward, and to the pains jumping from place to place."

Looking further, "sleeplessness before midnight, the aggravation during rest, as well as the relief from motion and rubbing, together with the flushes of heat with thirst, correspond to this drug." However, further research would find contradictions; *China* is not recommended for persons of florid, blooming health. The more experienced physician, says the baron, recognizes the symptoms of an "infrequently used remedy," looks up the "few doubtful symptoms," and concludes that the indicated remedy is *Valeriana*. And, indeed, a single dose of "high potency" (30c or 200c) in water, removed "the whole trouble, with all the concomitant symptoms," in three days (Boenninghausen 2007, *xi, xii*).

Matthew's experience illustrates how an herbalist might take this case: The man appears florid and blooming, so he has a "full" or "excess" physique, indicating some degree of heat/excitation. This is his constitution. However, the disease is seen in the cramping, changeable symptoms, indicating predominance of the wind/tension tissue state. The mind displays anger and nervousness, a combination of tension and excitation. Tension frequently relates to gall bladder symptoms (in both Greek and Chinese medicine). Gall bladder symptoms appear in this case—the fatty taste in the mouth, nausea in the throat, and pain in the stomach. However, this conclusion might be too simplistic: the symptoms also look like tension stretching throughout the autonomic nervous system (ANS). That puts the emphasis more on the stomach than the gall bladder.

At this point the experienced herbalist would probably be thinking of a predominately acrid (relaxing), somewhat cooling remedy with an affinity to the gall bladder or stomach and wind conditions. The major remedies that would probably come to mind are *Valeriana, Lobelia,* and *Nepeta* (catnip). The repertory would also lead in this direction.

Lobelia and *Valeriana* are both found in the repertory as acrid, cooling remedies with affinities to the ANS. They are often recommended for full-bodied, muscular people. Neither is specifically a gall bladder remedy, and there is no specific information available for the ANS (perhaps in the next edition of this repertory?) Both act very strongly on the stomach, so the guess about the ANS may be right. The sleeplessness suggests *Valeriana*. Not many people recognize the mental state for this remedy, but it is given in the *Herbal*

Repertory and it cinches the case. In the "Emotions" section, under Concentration, we find "anxiety producing upset stomach in children; aggressive behavior"; under Nervousness, "anger and nervousness"; under Anger, "acute, chronic; holds anger inside, causing knots in stomach, lower back." (Also see "Stomach Problems from Stress.") The notation "in children" shows that sometimes the repertory can be too exact. In repertorizing it is better to include a close or doubtful symptom, rather than to ignore it.

Through this process we arrive at *Valeriana* as the most likely candidate for this case, with *Lobelia* as another possibility. Anyone who also suggested *Nepeta* should be considered a winner; *Nepeta* is an acrid relaxant that contains valerianic compounds and has affinities to the stomach, spasms, anger, and nervousness. Since *Lobelia* enhances the action of other remedies, especially ones to which it is similar, an elegant approach (for an herbalist) would be to combine a small amount of *Lobelia* with the *Valeriana* — see the section on "Adjuvants, Accelerators, and Synergists." Adding *Nepeta* to *Valeriana* would have produced an awkward, redundant formula.

What if the practitioner had given *Lobelia* or *Nepeta* rather than the *Valeriana*? Palliation or cure may have occurred using these remedies. Clarke addresses such a near-hit:

> In most cases there are more remedies than one that will benefit; and if the exact simillimum [related remedy] is not found, the next or the next to that will give a measure of help; so the beginner need not abandon the ideal as too difficult of attainment. Then there are many different kinds of similarity, as well as of degrees, and every kind is available for the prescriber's use. There is similarity between drug and disease in organ affinity; in tissue-affinity; there is similarity of diathesis [constitutional imbalance]; similarity of sensations and conditions — all these and other kinds of like-ness are available for the prescriber (Clarke, 1886).

This "non-perfectionist" advice is much more helpful than idealism.

The Repertory Matures

Boenninghausen's *Therapeutic Pocket Book* soon became a necessary companion for the practicing homeopath. Contributors in succeeding generations wrote additional material to accompany and update it. These included Clarke's *The Prescriber* (1886) and *Clinical Repertory* (1904), and Cyril M. Boger's *Characteristics and Repertory* (1905) and *Synoptic Key* (1931).

All these books are useful for an herbalist wanting to use homeopathic repertories and prescribers; but if only one were chosen, I direct herbalists and budding homeopaths to Boger's *Synoptic Key*. The author omitted a lot of useless symptoms by only including those that were clinically verified. The core is a mere two hundred pages long, compared to five hundred in Boenninghausen's full *Pocket Book*. Boger also focuses on the most important physical symptoms, specifically called the "physical generals," which relate to the whole physical being rather than only the mind or local physical symptoms. Once one understands the *Synoptic Key*, an almost indispensable addition would be S.R. Phatak's *Concise Repertory*, which adds many new remedies and indications.

Laypeople, herbalists, and some neophyte homeopaths are confused by the almost comical detail in traditional descriptions of homeopathic symptoms. To combat this tendency, Boger introduced "physical generals," a category emphasizing broad, systemic symptoms, easy to observe, allowing us to now look up a general condition such as the color and nature of the skin, modalities, temperature, excess or deficiency, etc. This quickly leads to a few remedies, or just one. This is very compatible with the approach taken in this book.

Boger gives a description of his approach to case-taking:

> The spirit of the clinical symptom picture is best obtained by asking the patient to tell his own story, whenever this is possible. This account is then amplified and more accurately defined by the questioner, who should first try and elicit the evident cause and course of the sickness, to which he will add all the things

which now seem to interfere with the sufferer's comfort. Especially should the natural modifiers of sickness — the modalities — be very definitely ascertained. The following are the most vitally important of such influences: Time, Temperature, Open Air, Posture, Being Alone, Motion, Sleep, Eating and Drinking, Touch, Pressure, Discharges, etc.

A consideration of the mental state comes next in order of importance. Here the presence of Irritability, Sadness, or Fear is the ruling factor.

The third step concerns the estimate to be put upon the patient's own description of his sensations. This is a very vital point, and in order not to be misled it is always well to ascertain if any of the following primary sensations are present: Burning, Cramping, Cutting, Bursting, Soreness, Throbbing, and Thirst.

… Next in order of importance comes the entire objective aspect or expression of the sickness: This should especially include Facial Expression, Demeanor, Nervous Excitability, Sensibility, restlessness or Torpor, State of the Secretions, and any abnormal coloring that may be present.

Lastly, the part affected must be determined; this also brings the investigation in touch with diagnosis (Boger 1931, from unpaginated introduction).

The qualities capitalized are rubrics or headings in Boger's *Key*. Notice that Boger, like Boenninghausen, does not go into great detail under emotions and psychology, but only mentions major types of emotion (Sadness, Fear, etc.). This is the approach taken in Traditional Chinese Medicine and in *The Earthwise Herbal Repertory*. The bare essentials of the psychological presentation are often all that is needed; modern homeopaths and herbalists, by comparison, often take extensive psychological profiles but do not understand pathological symptoms. The practitioner can develop his or her own approach to psychological issues.

Not having been trained in psychoanalysis, I prefer to let the physical body guide me to the constitutional remedy whenever I am at

all doubtful of the psychological component, which is fairly often....
The main advantage of this method is that far less psychological
interpretation is required on the part of the practitioner in order to
arrive at the indicated remedy. Interestingly, I have often found that
a remedy selected this way is later discovered to cover very fundamental psychological symptoms in the case that were either missed
or misinterpreted by the practitioner or withheld by the patient (Ian
Watson 2004, 68).

The first major additions to Boenninghausen's work were made by
the English homeopath John Henry Clarke. The first edition of his
Prescriber came out in 1886 and has been in print (with updates) ever
since. In *The Prescriber* he explains, "My work has been to approach
practice from the clinical side. Boenninghausen's work approaches
it from the symptomatic side." Clarke's *Clinical Repertory* (1904) is an
addendum to Boenninghausen's *Pocket Book*.

What is the difference between a repertory and a prescriber? A
repertory is based on cross-referencing symptoms, without including
clinical details, while a prescriber is based on disease names, pathological conditions, and keynote symptoms frequently encountered in
practice. The prescriber is therefore a practical clinical guide, not a
comprehensive index for arriving at a remedy through the analysis
of symptoms.

Because *The Earthwise Herbal Repertory* is based on a system for
cross-referencing symptoms (tissue state, organ, specific indication), it is a repertory. However, it often lapses into the model of
a prescriber since herbalism does not have the rich knowledge of
symptoms that homeopathy possesses. Most of the so-called herbal
"repertories" up to this point have been prescribers. If herbalists are
to incorporate this method from homeopathy, they should understand
such distinctions. This is part of the reason for our extensive treatment of reportorial history and layout in this part of the book.

The Earthwise Herbal Repertory resembles the baron's approach since
it is based on tissue states and organ affinities, which are similar
to sensations and locations. Herbalists have not accumulated much
knowledge of modalities, but to the extent these are known, they

would largely identify tissue states. The practitioner arrives at the remedy (or several remedies) through cross-referencing symptoms, not necessarily by looking up the name of the disease.

A repertory following Boenninghausen and Clarke was compiled by Oscar Boericke and included in the back of the ninth edition of his brother William Boericke's *Pocket Manual of Homoeopathic Materia Medica* (1927). This repertory included many plant remedies, and was used by both Michael Moore and myself (Matthew) in the construction of our repertories. In print to the present, Boericke's is the last of the traditional repertories descended from Boenninghausen until Indian homeopaths began to make new contributions in the 1960s.

A completely different approach to repertory construction was pioneered by James Tyler Kent (1849–1916), the still-controversial revisionist of Hahnemannian homeopathy. Quite remarkably, Kent is the only major homeopath we know of who was educated inside the idiosyncratic walls of the Eclectic Medical Institute during the tenure of Dr. Scudder. We see in him the ruthless independent medical thinking of Scudder and the eclectics, who took "whatever worked" from wherever they wanted. Kent embraced this spirit, but came to despise the "mongrelism" of the eclectics and any homeopaths "tainted" by open-mindedness to other medical systems. Living in St. Louis, isolated from the homeopathic educational lineages established by Hahnemann's followers in Boston, New York, and Philadelphia, Kent's approach was a departure from the past. He developed a completely new interpretation of homeopathy—which, however, he represented as the true, more profound teachings of Hahnemann.

Kent was highly influential, and the split he caused in homeopathic circles has not ended to this day. The homeopathy he formed and shaped is called "classical" or "Kentian" homeopathy, while that which adheres to the teachings of Hahnemann and Boenninghausen we call "traditional."

"Kent, in his writings, admits that he could not use the Boenninghausen method, and it made no sense to him," wrote Julian Winston (2001). He did not think like the baron. Like many nineteenth-century American homeopaths, Kent was a follower of Emanuel

Swedenborg, a visionary who taught that the universe is laid out from an internal essence to the outward physical expression; though the outer person does not necessarily notice it, over the long run the inner self dominates the outer personality. This agreed with an additional law of homeopathy introduced by Constantine Hering, a student of Hahnemann, which is usually called the "law of direction of cure" or "Hering's law." As a cure takes place, writes Hering, the symptoms move from vital to less vital, from inner to outer, top to bottom, and in the reverse order in which they arrived.

Kent called this principle "government from center to circumference." He looked upon it as a universal law, and applied it to every aspect of homeopathy. His repertory is therefore organized to cause the practitioner to analyze the case from the psychological and constitutional indications outwards towards the peripheral, purely physical expression of the disease. This encouraged a tendency in homeopathy to focus more on the psychological and constitutional, and to overlook "mere" physical disease. This tendency increased in the last half of the twentieth century, when most homeopaths no longer had any training in physical medicine.

Using Aristotelian language, already long out of date, Kent organized his information "from generals to particulars," or from the unified theme of a remedy to its particular or local expressions. Combined with his Swedenborgian tendencies, Kent managed to anchor homeopathy into a metaphysical backwater that the rest of the world soon passed by.

Kent lectured on Hahnemann's *Organon* as if the founder's ideas were in concert with his own. He was a persuasive orator, intolerant of other views, and he bent the homeopathic stream towards his own theory and practice. While his contributions are undeniably substantial, he introduced a note of intolerance and a "one-size-fits-all" attitude that has not been healthy for homeopathy. It had already suffered a certain amount of this due to Hahnemann's own penchant for dogmatism and intolerance—though that lessened in his later years as his loving wife apparently smoothed out his sharp edges.

One innovation introduced by Kent, which influenced nearly all homeopathic schools, as well as the development of Dr. Edward Bach's flower essences, and eventually the herbal world as well, was his emphasis on the "essence" or primal unity holding all the properties, uses, pharmacology, and symptoms of a remedy together into a whole. This eventually found its way into herbalism; we see the influence particularly in the approach of Dorothy Hall, Matthew Wood, Eliot Cowan, and Stephen Harrod Buhner. For further studies on Thomson, Hahnemann, Scudder, Kent, and Bach, see *Vitalism* by Matthew Wood (2000).

Robin Murphy suggests that the complex format of Kent's repertory, used in many homeopathic schools, is partly responsible for a high rate of attrition among homeopathic students. Boenninghausen's approach, by contrast, is much gentler on the mind. The simplicity of his *Pocket Book*, and later the condensed clinical repertories based on it, are the remedy for everyone who has ever looked to homeopathy with hope, only to encounter a byzantine maze of shotgun remedies in old books with more Latin abbreviations than a legal document, couched in either overly simplified or agonizingly complex, woefully out-of-date descriptions. Also, Kent did not break the symptoms down, as Boenninghausen did, but used them whole. This made his repertory longer than the Bible!

As homeopathy began to decline in North America in the twentieth century, it began to flourish in India. Before Boger died, he corresponded with homeopaths living on the subcontinent and handed on to them the lineage from Hahnemann, Boenninghausen, and himself. This included S.R. Phatak and the elder Sankaran. Together they reestablished the "traditional" method of prescribing by keynotes, locations, sensations, modalities, and concomitants. Contemporary advocates of this system include David Little, Ian Watson, Helmut Sydow, and Robin Murphy.

The introduction of the personal computer has, in the last twenty-five years, completely revolutionized the homeopathic repertory, many versions of which are available online and as software.

Cross-referencing symptoms is *perfectly* suited to the computer age. Both the Boenninghausen and the Kentian lineages are represented in this renaissance. Roger van Zandvoort is the representative of the traditional, non-Kentian approach. His *Complete Repertory* gives access to the whole plant database of homeopathy (www.completedynamics.com).

The Kingdom Issue

The mineral and animal kingdoms have always shared medical cauldrons with herbs. The old Greek pharmacopeia, like that of the Chinese, is full of all manner of "stuff." Paracelsus vastly expanded the role of minerals when he introduced alchemy into medicine. Culpeper closed his fantastical career focusing on a universal alchemical gold remedy. Mineral and animal remedies rub shoulders with plants in TCM. Homeopathy is preponderantly plant-based, but incorporates nearly everything under the sun—including sunlight itself! Herbalism can be practiced as a primary general medicine, but history suggests that herbalists should know about mineral and animal remedies as well, and homeopathy provides a safe, inoffensive way to use them.

Homeopathic clinician and historian David Little (2015) points out that the superficially acting acute-ailment remedies in Hahnemann's *Materia Medica Pura* tended to be plants, while the deep-acting chronic-ailment remedies in *Chronic Diseases* tend to be mineral and animal in origin. Does this suggest that there is a medicinal difference between kingdoms?

Many of the plant remedies are well known for their role in cases where the organic pathology becomes the active layer and appears as a regional affection. The biochemical qualities of plants differ from the inorganic minerals in that the botanical world represents carbon-based organisms. This structure is founded on protoplasm (CHON) *[carbon/hydrogen/oxygen/nitrogen]*, which reflects the cellular organization as witnessed in the human organism. This is why the plant remedies have special affinities with specific systems, regions, organs, and tissue (Little 2015).

Continuing with this analogy, minerals would be best suited to deep changes on the mineral level of the body—involving primal activities regulated by mineral-dependent electrolytes and enzymes. Animal-based medicines, on the other hand, are associated with the nervous system, as are plant alkaloids, and as such have deep actions in this sphere. Plants act on the cellular level that underlies so much of organic function.

The same distinction between vegetable and non-vegetable medicinal sources seems to appear in biomedicine as well. The innocent, nontoxic herbs of grandma's cupboard are laughed at, while toxic jungle plants containing powerful alkaloids, along with minerals and some animal substances, are the source of much of the pharmacy of modern medicine.

The rebound effect may provide a reason for this difference among kingdoms. Nontoxic herbs, with their secondary metabolites and low-level toxicity, do not easily lock the organism into a primary response, as does a drug or poison. Therefore, they are better suited to diseases where the rebound mechanism is not overwhelmed. Poisons, found in the mineral and animal kingdoms (from snakes, insects, etc.), can force a primary reaction more powerfully and perhaps traumatize the self-healing mechanism more deeply, trapping the body in the primary response. This will suppress the self-healing ability, while plant medicine will support it by normalizing between primary and secondary reactions.

Energetic Expense

Many years ago Matthew noticed a statement by Dr. Edward Bach that herbs have a "positive" healing action, in contrast to the "negative" effect of homeopathic remedies. A letter to the Bach Centre in the UK at that time, asking what this meant, elicited only a kindly response saying that it didn't mean homeopathic remedies are unsafe.

Matthew reported this to me (David), and I contemplated Bach's statement for many years. Without a literary record, which seems to have been lost, we cannot know exactly what the good doctor was thinking. However, his idea stimulated both of us.

Our first consideration is that nontoxic plants may be considered "positive" simply because they are less toxic and more natural and innocuous in their healing effects. Second, the plant organism is analogous to the cellular level of organization that we find in our own bodies. Are they not, therefore, well suited to the treatment of the ills of humanity? The same idea has occurred to other homeopathic practitioners. After spending lifetimes in homeopathy, David Little and Robin Murphy came to the same conclusion: plants are our natural medicine chest. Hahnemann himself never completely abandoned plant remedies; his remedy box at the time of his death still included a handful of herbal tinctures.

Then what would make a homeopathic remedy "negative" in comparison? The potentized homeopathic remedy acts by *forcing* the vital force or immune system to react against it (in the secondary effect following the primary). Robin Murphy notes that this may be an energetically expensive process, and may have a wear-and-tear effect on the vital force or immune system of the patient. The nontoxic herb doesn't force the body like this, unless it is a large dose intended to do so. Several observers note that excessive use of the high potencies (as is common in classical/Kentian homeopathy) can exhaust a person. On the other hand, well-selected lower potencies (more common to traditional homeopathy in chronic disease) seem to wake up the vital force.

Also, as we become more toxic, stressed, and poisoned as a society, the constitutional and chronic disease remedies used by homeopaths—often in broad-spectrum therapy to elicit a response in the organism (*Sulphur* and *Nux Vomica* come to mind)—may be quite stressful to the organism. These are reminiscent of the "heroic" medicine of the old allopaths, or of Samuel Thomson and the "puking doctors" who favored emetic treatments.

Homeopathic remedies—especially the high potencies—do not just cure but more or less command. The vital force is forced to act—and *now!* In this way it is somewhat like allopathy. The rebound effect is especially pronounced in addiction recovery; this warns us not to stimulate the rebound effect in a wanton or careless manner.

Can the Two Sisters Get Along?

Clarke reckoned that thirteen homeopathic remedies were enough to cover half of his cases: *Sulphur, Lycopodium, Calcarea, Arsenicum, Thuja, Aconitum, Nux, Pulsatilla, Silicea, Hepar Sulphuris, China, Belladona, and Bryonia.* Would it not also behoove the herbalist to become familiar with these remedies and their indications?

There are other considerations as well that recommend homeopathy to the herbalist. Where herbs need harvesting, processing, storing, decanting, bottling, labeling, etc., a homeopathic pharmacy can be a thing of compact beauty and versatility. Many herbs are easily available in low-potency homeopathic form. Homeopathic remedies have a shelf life of decades, possibly even centuries, for all practical purposes, despite expiration dates mandated by the FDA. An herbal remedy may also be unavailable in a pinch. With budgets increasingly tight, the low-potency homeopathic remedies made in India are almost free. And it is possible that in the future we may be dealing with remedies becoming unavailable due to excessive government regulation. Even more significantly, homeopathy may provide the only source for botanicals that are becoming unavailable due to environmental stress. Examples here include *Cypripedium pubescens* (lady's slipper) and *Aletris farinosa* (true unicorn root).

Homeopathy can fill gaps in an herbal and/or bodywork practice; it can provide, perhaps most importantly, a whole new way of looking at symptoms, health, and disease.

Homeopathy is a truly practical form of medical alchemy. As a medical system it is portable, life-saving, scientific in its own sphere, and clinically adaptable and flexible beyond virtually all other healing arts in the hands of a competent master prescriber. Yet it has its cost: it requires vital force to digest and assimilate the remedies, and our bodies have a limited amount of this. And the increasing hypersensitivities in increasing numbers of people make it inadvisable to use the high homeopathic potencies.

What do homeopaths need to learn from herbalists? Homeopaths need to recognize that the law of contraries is built into the proving of remedies, and is in fact a basis for prescription as much as similarity. The rebound effect explains both the law of similars and the law of contraries.

What else? Homeopaths tend to be far too wary of the innocent, nontoxic little herb. Herbs in fact have already enriched the homeopathic apothecary. Much of this inclusion resulted from experimentation by doctors who were, in their time, criticized by other homeopaths for being too open-minded. One thinks here of Edwin Hale, William Burt, James Compton Burnett, and William Boericke—who surreptitiously introduced many of John Scudder's specific remedies into homeopathy. Schools are often by their nature creatures of habit, but experimentation should always be allowed.

Bibliography

This section usually goes at the back of a book, but as I learned from David Ryan, it is best to put it at the front when constructing a repertory because there is less interference with the body of the text in which we want to look up medicines.

Azar, Henry. *The Sage of Seville.* Cairo: The American University in Cairo Press, 2008.

Barnes, Broda. *Hypothyroidism.* New York: Harper, 1976.

Bartram, Thomas. *The Encyclopedia of Herbal Medicine.* Christchurch, UK: Grace Publishing, 1995.

Bastide, M. "Basic Research on High Dilution Effects." In *High Dilution Effects on Cells and Integrated Systems.* Edited by Paolo Marotta and Cloe Taddei-Ferretti. River Edge, NJ and London: World Scientific Publishing Co. Pte. Ltd., 1998.

Bhattacharya, A. K. *Eclectic Medicine, or Simple Healing Methods.* New Delhi: Firma KLM Limited Private, 1985.

Bigfoot, Peter and Angelique Zelle. *Venomous Bites and Stings: Natural Remedies.* Roosevelt, AZ: Reevis Mountain School, 1993.

Boenninghausen, C.M. *Boenninghausen's Therapeutic Pocket Book: The Principles and Practicability.* Edited by T.F. Allen. New Delhi: B. Jain, 2007.

Boericke, William. *Pocket Manual of Homoeopathic Materia Medica.* Philadelphia: F. E. Boericke, 1927.

Boger, Cyril. *A Synoptic-Key to Materia Medica.* Parkersburg, WV: Privately published, 1931.

British Herbal Medicine Association. *A Guide to Traditional Herbal Medicines.* Bournemouth, Dorset: BHMA Publishing, Ltd., 2003.

_____. *British Herbal Pharmacopoeia 1983.* Bournemouth: BHMA Publishing, Ltd., 1999.

Bruton-Seal, Julie and Matthew Seal. *The Herbalist's Bible: John Parkinson's Lost Class Rediscovered.* Ludlow: Merlin Unwin, 2014.

Buhner, Stephen Harrod. *The Secret Teachings of Plants.* Rochester, VT: Bear & Company, 2004.

Bunce, Larkin, Caroline Gagnon, Michael Tierra, Matthew Wood, Cathy Skipper, Robin Rose Bennett, Michael Vertolli, and Jessica Aveni. "Herbs For Depression: Eight Herbalists Share Strategies," posted December 2, 2013 by Melanie Pulla, www.herbgeek.com/herbs-for-depression-eight-herbalists-share-strategies/

Burnett, J. Compton. *The Diseases of the Liver.* Philadelphia: Boericke & Tafel, 1895.

Chevallier, Andrew. *Herbal Medicine for the Menopause.* Rochester, UK: Amberwood Publishing Ltd., 2001.

Christopher, John R. *School of Natural Healing.* 25th anniversary edition. London: Atlantic Books, 1991.

Clarke, John Henry. *A Clinical Repertory to the Dictionary of Materia Medica: Together with Repertories of Causation, Temperaments, Clinical Relationships, Natural Relationships.* London: Homoeopathic Publishing Company, 1904.

_____. *The Prescriber: a Dictionary of the New Therapeutics.* 9th ed. (1st ed. 1886.) Saffron Walden, UK: The C.W. Daniel Company, Ltd., 1992.

Cook, William. *The Physiomedical Dispensatory.* Cincinnati: Privately published, 1869.

Crellin, John K. and Jane Philpott. *Trying to Give Ease: Tommie Bass and the Story of Herbal Medicine.* Chapel Hill: Duke University Press, 1990.

Cowan, Eliot. *Plant Spirit Medicine.* Columbus, NC: Granite Publishing LLC, 1995.

Culpeper, Nicholas. *The Complete Herbal and English Physician.* 300-year anniversary edition. Birmingham: The Kynoch Press, 1953.

Dash, George E. "How Remedies Act on the Skin." *The Eclectic Medical Gleaner* 4, no. 1 (1908).

D'Castro, J. Benedict. *Logic of Repertories.* Delhi: B. Jain Publishers, Pvt., Ltd., 2004.

Ellingwood, Finley. *The American Materia Medica: Therapeutics and Pharmacognosy,* Reprint. (1st ed. 1919.) Sandy, OR: Eclectic Publications, 1995.

Fernie, William. *Herbal Simples Approved for Modern Uses of Cure.* 2nd edition. Philadelphia: Boericke and Tafel, 1897.

Foreman, Richard and James W. Mahoney. *The Cherokee Physician.* Asheville, NC: Edney & Dedman, 1849. http://docsouth.unc.edu/nc/foreman/menu.html

French, J.M. "Chelidonium Majus." *The Eclectic Medical Gleaner* 4, no. 1 (1908).

Green, James. *The Male Herbal: The Definitive Health Care Book for Men and Boys.* Berkeley, CA: Crossing Press, 2007.

Grieve, Maude. *A Modern Herbal.* Online edition. (1st ed. 1931.) Available at http://www.botanical.com/botanical/mgmh/mgmh.html.

Griggs, Barbara. *Green Pharmacy.* Rochester, VT: Healing Arts Press, 1997.

Gümbel, Dietrich. *Principles of Holistic Therapy with Herbal Essences.* Heidelberg: Haag, 1986.

Hahnemann, Samuel. *Organon of the Medical Art.* 6th edition. Edited by Wenda Brewster O'Reilly. Redmond, WA: Birdcage Books, 1996.

Hale, Edwin M. *Materia Medica and Special Therapeutics of the New Remedies.* Philadelphia: F.E. Boericke, 1885. Available at http://onlinebooks.library.upenn.edu/webbin/book/lookupname?key=Hale%2C%20Edwin%20M.%20(Edwin%20Moses)%2C%201829-1899

Hall, Dorothy. *Dorothy Hall's Herbal Medicine.* Melbourne: Lothian, 1998.

Handley, Rima. *A Homeopathic Love Story: The Story of Samuel and Mélanie Hahnemann.* Berkeley, CA: North Atlantic Books, 1990.

Harper-Shove, F. *Prescriber and Clinical Repertory of Medicinal Herbs.* Bradford: Health Science Press, 1938.

Hershoff, Asa and Andrea Rotelli. *Herbal Remedies: A Quick and Easy Guide to Common Disorders and Their Herbal Treatments.* New York: Avery, 2001.

Hoffman, David. *The New Holistic Herbal.* New York: HarperCollins Publishers Limited, 1991.

Hool, Richard Lawrence. *Common Plants and Their Uses in Medicine.* Lancashire, UK: Lancashire Branch of the NAMH, 1922.

Howard, Horton. *An Improved System of Medicine.* Columbus, OH: Privately published, 1832.

Huang Huang. *Ten Key Formula Families in Chinese Medicine.* Translated by Michael Max. Seattle: Eastland Press, 1994.

Hueneke, Pati Solva. *Living in the Golden Light: Healing with the Golden Angels of the Five Elements and the Gold Light Plant Essences.* Bloomington, IN: Balboa Press, 2010.

Jones, Eli G. *Cancer: Its Causes, Symptoms, and Treatment.* New Delhi: B. Jain Publishers Ltd., 2004.

Jones, Stacy. *The Medical Genius: A Guide to the Cure.* Philadelphia: John C. Winston & Co., 1894. Available at https://archive.org /details/medicalgeniusag01jonegoog

Kenner, Dan and Yves Requena. *Botanical Medicine: A European Professional Perspective.* Brookline, MA: Paradigm Publications, 2001.

Kent, Janet. *Ease Your Mind: Herbs for Mental Health.* Asheville, NC: Medicine County Herbs, 2014.

Kingsbury, John M. *Deadly Harvest: A Guide to Common Poisonous Plants.* New York: Holt, Rinehart and Winston, 1969.

Kress, Henrietta. *Practical Herbs.* Helsinki: Privately published, 2011.

Kuhn, Merrily A. and David Winston. *Herbal Therapy and Supplements: A Scientific and Traditional Approach.* 2nd edition.

Philadelphia, etc.: Wolters/Kluwer, Lippincott Williams and Wilkins, 2008.

Light, Phyllis. *Dysfunctions of the Endocrine System: Causes, Symptoms, and Remedies: A Practical Guide.* Arab, AL: Self-published, 2001.

Little, David. *The Homoeopathic Compendium.* 6 vols. Privately published, 2015. www.similimum.com

Marinelli, Ralph *et al.* "The Heart is not a Pump: A Refutation of the Pressure Propulsion Premise of Heart Function." *Frontier Perspectives* 5, no. 1 (1995). Accessed April 3, 2016. www.rsarchive.org /RelArtic/Marinelli/

Massinger, O. L. "Echinacea Angustifolium." *The Eclectic Medical Gleaner* 4, no. 1 (1908).

Mills, Simon. *Out of the Earth: The Essential Book of Herbal Medicine.* London, New York, Toronto, Sidney, Auckland: Penguin Books, Viking Arkana, 1991.

Moore, Les. Classical Formulas in the Western Herbal Tradition. Shortsville, NY: Self-published, 2002.

Moore, Michael. *Herbal Repertory in Clinical Practice: A Manual of Differential Therapeutics for the Health Care Professional.* 3rd ed. Albuquerque, AZ: Southwest School of Botanical Medicine, 1994.

Murphy, Robin. *Case Analysis and Prescribing Techniques.* New Delhi: B. Jain, 2006.

Occom, Samson. "Herbal remedies and letter fragment." https://collections.dartmouth.edu/occom/html/diplomatic /754900-2-diplomatic.html

Orr, Althea Northage. "The Use of Nervines and Other Herbs in the Treatment of Mental and Nervous Disorders." http://www .transformationaltechniques.com/wp-content/uploads/2012/03 /Use-of-Nervines-and-Other-Herbs-in-the-Treatment-of-Mental-and-Nervous-Disorders.pdf)

Parton, Frank. *Herbal.* London: Self-published, 1931.

_____. *Miracle Workers From the Fields and Hedgerows, A New Herbal with Remedial Diet.* London: The C. W. Daniel Company, 1935.

Phatak, S.R. *A Concise Repertory of Homeopathic Medicines*. New Delhi: B. Jain, 2004.

Pischinger, Alfred. *The Extracellular Matrix and Ground Regulation: Basis for a Holistic Biological Medicine*. Berkeley, CA: North Atlantic Books, 2007.

Pollack, Gerald H. "The Fourth Phase of Water: Implications for Energy and Health." *Wise Traditions in Food, Farming and the Healing Arts* 16, no. 4 (2015).

Porcher, Francis Peyre. *Resources of the southern fields and forests, medical, economical, and agricultural, being also a medical botany of the Confederate States, with practical information on the properties of the trees, plants, and shrubs*. Originally published 1863. Delhi: Gyan Books Pvt. Ltd., 2013.

Powell, Eric. *The Natural Home Physician*. Bradford: Health Science Press, 1962.

Priest, A.W. and L.R. Priest. *Herbal Medication: A Clinical and Dispensary Handbook*. London: L. M. Fowler and Co., Ltd., 1983, reprinted 2001.

Rafinesque, Constantine. *Manual of the medical botany of the United States, containing description of fifty-two medicinal plants, with their names, qualities, properties, history, &c*. Reprinted from 1828–1830 edition. Delhi: ReInk Books, 2014.

Rippe, Olaf and Margret Madejsky. *Die Kräuterkunde des Paracelsus*. 2nd ed. Baden and Munich: AT Verlag, 2013.

Salmon, William. *Botanologia, or The English Herbal*. London, Printed by I. Dawks for H. Rhodes and J. Taylor, 1710.

Schulze, Richard. *Dr. Schulze's 2011 Herbal Product Catalog*. Marina del Rey, CA: American Botanical Pharmacy, 2011.

Scudder, John M. *Materia Medica and Therapeutics*. 12th ed. Cincinnati: The Scudder Brothers Company, Publishers, 1898.

Sedlacek, Trilby. *Materia Medica for Women's Active Sex Life*. Handout. Cedar Rapids: GreenAngelsHerbs.com, 2015.

Selye, Hans. *The Stress of Life*. Revised edition. New York, etc.: The MacGraw-Hill Companies, Inc., 1976.

Sherman, John. *The Complete Botanical Prescriber.* 3rd ed. Privately published, 1993.

Simeon, Albert T. *Man's Presumptuous Brain: An Evolutionary Interpretation of Psychosomatic Diseases.* New York: Penguin Group (USA) Incorporated, 1962.

Thomson, Samuel. *New Guide to Health: or Botanic Family Physician ... To Which is Prefaced, A Narrative of the Life and Medical Discoveries of the Author.* Boston: Privately published, 1835.

Thurston, Dr. Joseph M. *The Philosophy of Physiomedicalism.* Richmond, IN: Nicholson Printing and Mfg. Co., 1900.

Tierra, Michael. *Planetary Herbology.* Twin Lakes, WI: Lotus Press, 1992.

————. *The Way of Herbs.* New York: Pocket Books, 1998.

Tilke, Samuel Westcott. *Practical reflections on the nature and treatment of disease: Founded upon sixteen years' experience in the cure of gout, rheumatism, scrofula, fever,... with suggestions for its improvement.* 5th edition. London: Self-published, 1844.

Treben, Maria. *Health From God's Garden.* Wellingborough, UK and Rochester, VT: Thorson's, 1987.

————. *Health Through God's Pharmacy: Advice and Proven Cures with Medicinal Herbs.* 29th edition. Steyr, Austria: Ennsthaler Publishing, 2003.

Turner, William. *A New Herball.* Facsimile of the first editions of 1551, 1562, and 1568. Edited by George T.L. Chapman

Vogel, Virgil. *American Indian Medicine.* Norman, OK: University of Oklahoma Press, 1970.

Waterhouse, E. R. "Tongue Diagnosis." *The Eclectic Medical Gleaner* 4, no. 1 (1908).

Watson, Ian. *A Guide to the Methodologies of Homeopathy.* Cornwall, UK: Cutting Edge Publications, 2004.

Weed, Susun. *Breast Cancer? Breast Health! The Wise Woman Way.* Woodstock, NY: Self-published, 1996.

————. *Down There: Sexual and Reproductive Health the Wise Woman Way.* Woodstock, NY: Self-published, 2011.

_____. *New Menopausal Years: The Wise Woman Way—Alternative Approaches for Women 30–90*. Woodstock, NY: Self-published, 2002.

_____. *Wise Woman Herbal for the Childbearing Year*. Woodstock, NY: Self-published, 1996.

Weiss, Rudolf Fritz. *Weiss's Herbal Medicine*. New York: Thieme, 1994.

Winston, David. *The Energetics of Herbs: "The 10 Tastes."* American Herbalists Guild Conference Proceedings, 2006.

_____. *Herbal Therapeutics: Specific Indications for Herbs and Herbal Formulas*. 10th ed. Broadway, NJ: Herbal Therapeutics Research Library, 2013.

_____. *The 10 Tastes Pamphlet: The Energetics of Herbs*. Broadway, NJ: Self-published, 1999.

Winston, David and Steven Maimes. *Adaptogens: Herbs for Strength, Stamina, and Stress Relief*. Rochester, VT: Healing Arts Press, 2007.

Winston, Julian. "The Boenninghausen Repertory: Therapeutic Pocket Book Method." In *The American Homeopath* 7 (2001). http:/minimum.com, accessed January 17, 2016.

Wood, Matthew. *The Earthwise Herbal: A Complete Guide to Old World Medicinal Plants*. Berkeley: North Atlantic Books, 2008.

_____. *The Earthwise Herbal: A Complete Guide to the New World Medicinal Plants*. Berkeley: North Atlantic Books, 2010.

_____. *The Practice of Traditional Western Herbalism*. Berkeley: North Atlantic Books, 2004.

_____. *Vitalism: The History of Homeopathy, Herbalism, and Flower Essences*. Berkeley: North Atlantic Books, 2000.

Wood, Matthew, Francis Benaldo Begnoche, and Phyllis Light. *Traditional Western Herbalism, Pulse Evaluation: A Conversation*. N.p.: Lulu Publishing Services, 2015.

Indications from Oral Sources

When a name is not listed in the bibliography, the reader may presume that I am quoting (or closely paraphrasing from) a conversation I had with an herbalist or information from a class I attended. Direct quotations from books, printed matter, or the Internet are sourced, while oral sources are not.

In this regard, I would like to thank and acknowledge the following herbal practitioners for their verbal contributions to this repertory: 7Song, Tim Bernard, Rachel Bowen, Sondra Boyd, Rico Cech, Glenda Croft, Tis Mal Crow, Brent Davis, Christine Dennis, Sean Donahue, Bernadette Dowling, Jane Doyle, Kim Dudley, Tim Dymond, Jolie Elan, Erica Fargione, Libby Fenton, Pam Fischer, Margi Flint, Wendy Fogg, Kate Gilday, Christopher Hobbs, Mark Jensen, Paula Jensen, Keewaydinoquay, Bonnie Krekow, Judy Leiblen, William LeSassier, Phyllis Light, Jim MacDonald, Darrel Martin, Mary Pat Palmer, Bianca Patel, Erin Piorier, Sajah Popham, Paul Red Elk, John Redden, Robert Rogers, Keva Rose, Tony Seifert, Nicholas Schnell, Jill Stansbury, Brandt Stickley, Jennifer Tucker, Nancy Welliver, Lise Wolff, Susan Yerigan, and others. If I have forgotten someone, I apologize—and please let me know.

I am also indebted to David Ryan for helping me understand the definition and logic of a homeopathic repertory, and for helping me design the present herbal repertory for the ease of use by the reader. We thank Roger Van Zant for checking over our ideas on the homeopathic repertory.

PART II: THE REPERTORY

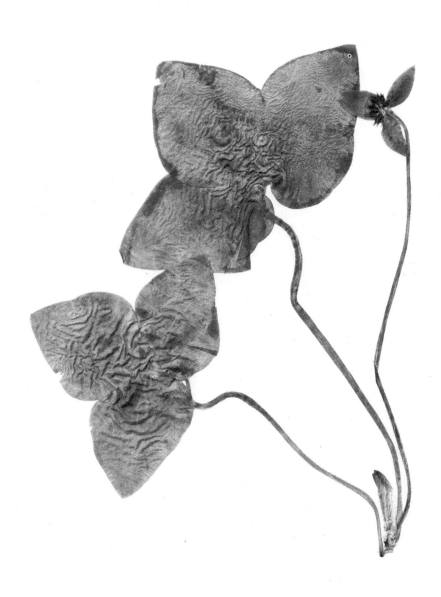

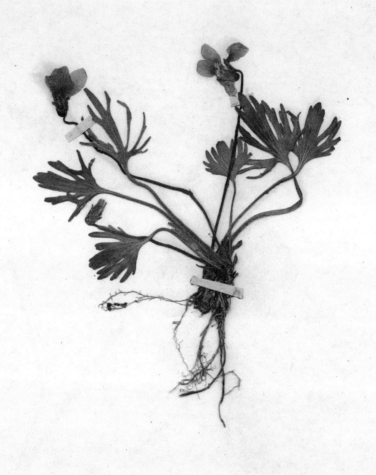

1. List of Herbs

Variations in scientific names of plants have always occurred but are especially frequent today, when research on plant genomes are leading to new discoveries about the true relationships between plants. This can be expected to continue after the publication of this book. I was educated in botany forty-five years ago and in herbalism over the succeeding decades, and like many older herbalists I am used to "the old names" and not always current on new names. So, I have kept a considerable number of the old names that I am familiar with in place. This will be inconvenient to manufacturers of plant products, who now have to have the most recent name on their labels, according to regulations set in place by the FDA in the last several years. Unfortunately, homeopathy, which is also regulated by the FDA, and also uses many of the old names that herbalists always used, is allowed to use these names because they are established in the U.S. Homeopathic Pharmacopeia, which is official with the FDA. Therefore, the relationships between herbs and homeopathic remedies, and between modern herbs and herbs as named in the old books will be somewhat confusing. New names will undoubtedly appear after the publication of this book and this is not something I am going to try to correct, if there should be a future edition. Indeed, I have used some names that have already been changed in the last decade because I am so familiar with them. Others are subject to dispute and it is not always clear to an outsider what is the accepted botanical name — it may not yet be agreed upon. I have attempted to include all the major new and old names in the following list, but some are probably missing.

Common names are also often peculiar to herbalists, as they are to farmers, florists, grocers, horticulturalists, and the writers of plant guides on the internet or on paper. The shopper says "celery," while the herbalist says "celery seed" because we are not thinking of the vegetable. We don't want the listener to think we are referring to the vegetable. History also enters into nomenclature. The horticulturist may say "queen of the meadow" while we say "gravel root," because of the way gravel sticks between the roots and also because it treats gravel. We might also say "Joe Pye weed" in remembrance of the Indian medicine man who first introduced this herb into the consciousness of white and black American herbalists. Southern herbalists might use "queen of the meadow" as the common expression in their area, while Northern herbalists avoid the term since for them it refers to two completely different medicinal plants, *Eupatorium purpureum* and *Filipendula ulmaria*. Common names are legion; I have kept to the ones I would use in conversation with herbalists—but correct form is what you use, as long as others understand you.

Abies balsamea	Balsam Fir
Abies canadensis (see *Tsuga canadensis*)	
Acacia catechu	Black Catechu
Aceticum acidum	Cider Vinegar
Achillea millefolium, A. lanulosa	Yarrow
Aconitum napellus	Aconite (extremely toxic; homeopathic only)
Acorus calamus	Sweet Flag (not approved by FDA for internal consumption)
Actaea racemosa (see *Cimicifuga racemosa*)	
Adiantum spp.	Maidenhair Fern
Aesculus glabra	Ohio Buckeye
Aesculus hippocastanum	Horse Chestnut
Agastache foeniculum	Anise Hyssop
Agrimonia eupatoria, A. spp.	Agrimony
Agropyron repens	Couch Grass
Ajuga reptans	Bugle

| *Albizia julibrissin* | Albizia |
| *Alcea rosea* | Hollyhock |

(Note: *Alcea* can be used as a substitute for *Althaea*.)

Alchemilla officinalis, *A. mollis,* etc.	Lady's Mantle
Aletris farinosa	True Unicorn Root (environmentally endangered; homeopathic)
Allium cepa	Red Onion
Allium sativa	Garlic
Allium ursinum	Ransoms
Alnus rubra	Red Alder
Alnus serrulata	Tag Alder
Aloe barbadensis	Purging Aloe (purgative; small dose or homeopathic)
Aloe vera	Aloe Vera
Alpinia officinarum	Galangal (toxicity disputed)
Althaea officinalis	Marshmallow
Althea rosea	Hollyhock
Amanita muscaria	Fly Agaric Mushroom
Ambrosia artemisiifolia	Ragweed
Ammi visnaga	Khella
Ampelopsis hederacea	Virginia Creeper (see *Parthenocissus quinquefolia*)
Amygdalus persica	Peach
Anagallis arvensis	Scarlet Pimpernel
Ananas comosus	Pineapple
Andrographis paniculata	Kalmegh
Anemone pulsatilla, A. wolfgangia	Pulsatilla (mildly toxic; small dose or homeopathic)
Anemopsis californica	Yerba Mansa
Anethum graveolens	Dill

Angelica archangelica	Angelica (European)
Angelica sinensis	Chinese Angelica
Anthemis cotula	Mayflower
Anthemis nobilis (Chamaemelum nobile)	Roman Camomile
Anthriscus cerefolium	Chervil
Aphanes arvensis	Parsley Piert
Apium graveolens	Celery Seed
Apocynum androsaemifolium	Werewolf Root (small dose)
Apocynum cannabinum	Indian Hemp (small dose)
Aquilegia canadensis, A. vulgaris	Columbine
Aralia californica (cognate with A. racemosa)	California Spikenard
Aralia hispida	Bristly Sarsaparilla
Aralia nudicaulis	Wild Sarsaparilla
Aralia racemosa	American Spikenard
Arctium lappa, A. minus	Burdock
Arctostaphylos uva-ursi	Bearberry
Argemone mexicana	Prickly Poppy
Aristolochia serpentaria	Virginia Snakeroot (toxic; small or homeopathic dose)
Armoracia rusticana	Horseradish
Arnica montana	Arnica (toxic; external or homeopathic only)
Artemisia abrotanum	Southernwood
Artemisia absinthium	Wormwood (not for persistent, large-dose usage)
Artemisia annua	Sweet Annie
Artemisia ludoviciana	Wood Sage
Artemisia vulgaris	Mugwort
Arundo spp.	Reedgrass (nontoxic homeopathic)

Asafoetida ferula	Asafetida
Asarum canadense	Wild Ginger
Asclepias asperula	Antelope Horns ·
Asclepias syriaca	Milkweed
Asclepias tuberosa	Pleurisy Root, Butterflyweed
Asparagus officinalis	Asparagus
Asparagus racemosa	Shatavari
Asperula odorata	Sweet Woodruff
Asplenium scolopendrium	Hart's Horn Fern (formerly *Phyllitis scolopendrium* and *Scolopendrium vulgare*)
Aster novae-angliae	New England Aster
Astragalus membranaceus	Astragalus
Atractylodis macrocephalae	Atractylodis
Atropa belladonna	Belladonna (toxic; homeopathic only)
Avena sativa	Milky Oatseed

(Note: Oatstraw, from *Avena*, has not been given a separate listing in this repertory; it can be used when a mineralizing effect is desired.)

Azadirachta indica	Neem
Bacopa monnieri	Brahmi
Ballota nigra	Black Horehound
Balsamorhiza sagittata	Balsam Root
Baptisia tinctoria	Wild Indigo
Barosma betulina	Buchu
Bellis perennis	Daisy
Berberis aquifolium, B. repens (see *Mahonia*)	
Berberis vulgaris	Barberry Root
Beta vulgaris	Beet
Betonica officinalis (see *Stachys*) ·	

Betula lenta, B. spp.	Birch (inner bark)
Bidens spp.	Spanish Needles
Borago officinalis	Borage (pyrrolizidine toxicity; small dose)
Boswellia serrata	Frankincense
Bryonia alba	White Bryony (toxic; homeopathic)
Bupleurum chinense	Bupleurum
Calendula officinalis	Calendula
Calluna vulgaris	Heather
Camellia sinensis	Green Tea
Capsella bursa-pastoris	Shepherd's Purse
Capsicum annum	Cayenne
Carbo vegetabilis	Charcoal (homeopathic)
Carica papaya	Papaya
Carthamus tinctorius	Safflower
Carum carvi	Caraway
Cascara sagrada	Cascara
Cassia acutifolia	Senna (purgative)
Castanea sativa	European Chestnut
Caulophyllum thalictroides	Blue Cohosh
Ceanothus americanus, C. spp.	Red Root
Celastrus scandens	Bittersweet Vine
Centaurium erythraea	Centaury
Centella asiatica	Gotu Kola
Cephaelis ipecacuanha	Ipecac (emetic; small or homeopathic dose)
Cetraria islandica	Iceland Moss
Chamaelirium luteum (see *Helonias*)	

Chamomilla matricaria	Chamomile (old name for *Matricaria recutita*)
Chelidonium majus	Celandine (mild toxicity; small or homeopathic dose)
Chelone glabra	Turtleshead, Balmony
Chimaphila umbellata	Pipsissewa
Chionanthus virginicus	Fringetree
Chondrus crispus	Irish Moss
Chrysanthemum morifolium	Chrysanthemum
Cichorium intybus	Chicory
Cimicifuga racemosa	Black Cohosh, Black Snakeroot
Cinchona calisaya	Quinine
Cinerarea maritima	Dusty Miller
Cinnamomum cassia	Cinnamon (twig)
Cinnamomum vera	Cinnamon (bark) (formerly *C. zeylanicum*)
Cistis canadensis (see *Helianthemum canadense*)	
Citrus aurantium	Orange Peel
Citrus limonum	Lemon
Clematis virginica	Old Man's Beard (toxic; small or homeopathic dose)
Cnicus benedictus	Blessed Thistle
Codonopsis pilulosa	Tang Shen
Cola acuminata	Kola Nut
Coleus forskohlii	Coleus
Collinsonia canadensis	Stone Root
Commiphora molmol (*C. myrrha*)	Myrrh
Commiphora muki	Guggul
Comptonia asplenifolia	Sweetfern

Conium maculatum	Poison Hemlock (extremely toxic; homeopathic only)
Convallaria majalis	Lily of the Valley (careful dosage)
Coptis trifolia	Goldthread
Cordyceps sinensis	Cordyceps
Coriandrum sativum	Coriander (seed)
Cornus florida	Florida Dogwood
Cornus officinalis	Japanese Dogwood
Corydalis canadensis (see *Dicentra canadensis*)	
Crataegus spp.	Hawthorn
Crocus sativus	Saffron
Cucumis sativus	Cucumber
Cucurbita citrullus	Watermelon Seed
Cucurbita pepo	Pumpkin Seed
Curcuma longa	Turmeric
Cynara scolymus	Artichoke Leaf
Cypripedium pubescens	Lady's Slipper (no longer used due to environmental concerns)
Datura stramonium	Datura (toxic; homeopathic only, or external)
Daucus carota	Wild Carrot, Queen Anne's Lace
Delphinium staphysagria	Staphysagria (homeopathic dose or external)
Dicentra canadensis	Turkey Corn
Dicentra cucullaria	Dutchman's Breeches

(Note: *D. cucullaria* is widely collected in place of *D. canadensis* and is perhaps medicinally interchangeable with it.)

Dioscorea villosa	Wild Yam
Dipsacus fullonum (*D. sylvestris*)	Teasel
Drosera rotundifolia	Sundew

Echinacea angustifolia, E. purpureum	Echinacea
Echium vulgare	Blue Devils
Elletaria cardamomum	Cardamom
Eleutherococcus senticosus	Eleuthero
Epilobium spp.	Willow Herb
Equisetum arvensis, E. hyemale	Horsetail, Shavegrass (infusion, decoction, or tincture; the *marque* or substance is not to be consumed due to sharp silicon fibers)
Erigeron canadensis (Conyza canadensis)	Daisy Fleabane
Eriodictyon glutinosum	Yerba Santa
Eryngium maritimum	Sea Holly
Eryngium yuccifolium	Rattlesnake Master

(Note: These two *Eryngiums* are very similar, but tradition assigns different actions to them.)

Eschscholzia californica	California Poppy (avoid before driving)
Eucalyptus spp.	
Euonymus atropurpureus	Wahoo
Eupatorium cannabinum	Hemp Agrimony
Eupatorium perfoliatum	Boneset
Eupatorium purpureum	Gravel Root
Eupatorium rugosum	White Snake Root
Euphorbia pilulifera	Euphorbia (mild toxicity; small dose)
Euphrasia officinalis	Eyebright
Fagopyrum esculentum	Buckwheat
Ficaria verna	Figwort (see *Ranunculus ficaria*)
Ficus spp.	Fig
Filipendula ulmaria	Meadowsweet

Foeniculum vulgare	Fennel
Fomes officinalis	Quinine Conk
Fouquieria splendens	Ocotillo
Fragaria vesca	Strawberry (leaf)
Frasera canadensis	Colombo
Fraxinus americana	White Ash
Fucus vesiculosus	Bladderwrack
Fumaria officinalis	Fumitory
Galega officinalis	Goat's Rue
Galium aparine	Cleavers
Galium odoratum	Sweet Woodruff (*see Asperula odorata*)
Ganoderma lucidum	Reishi Mushroom
Gaultheria procumbens	Wintergreen
Gecko spp.	Gecko (lizard)
Gelsemium sempervirens	Yellow Jessamine (toxic; homeopathic or external only)
Genista tinctoria	Plantagenet
Gentiana lutea	Gentian
Geranium maculatum	Wild Geranium
Geranium robertianum	Herb-Robert, Storksbill

(Note: *G. robertianum* can be used like *G. maculatum*.)

Geum rivale	Water Avens
Geum urbanum	City Avens
Gillenia trifoliata	Bowman's Root
Gingko biloba	Gingko
Glechoma hederacea	Ground Ivy
Glycyrrhiza glabra	Licorice
Gnaphalium obtusifolium	Rabbit Tobacco
Gnaphalium uliginosum	Marsh Everlasting

(Note: The *Gnaphaliums* above are used interchangeably.)

Goodyeara pubescens	Rattlesnake Plantain
Gossypium herbaceum	Cotton Root (abortive)
Grifola frondosa	Maitake Mushroom
Grindelia spp.	Gumweed, Tarweed
Guaiacum spp.	Guaiac
Gymnema sylvestre	Gymnema
Hamamelis virginiana	Witch Hazel
Handroanthus spp.	Pau d'Arco (usually listed under former name, *Tabebuia*)
Harpagophytum procumbens	Devil's Claw
Hedeoma pulegioides	American Pennyroyal
Helianthemum canadense	Scrophulawort, Rock Rose (also *Cistus canadense*)
Helianthus annuus	Sunflower Seed
Helichrysum italicum	Helichrysum
Helonias luteum	False Unicorn Root
Heracleum lanatum	Cow Parsnip
Hericium spp.	Hericium Mushroom
Hernaria glabra	Herniawort
Hibiscus spp.	Hibiscus
Hieracium pilosella	Mouse Ear
Humulus lupulus	Hops
Hydrangea arborescens	Hydrangea
Hydrastis canadensis	Goldenseal
Hydrocotyle asiatica	Gotu Kola (old name for *Centella*)
Hypericum perforatum	St. John's Wort (can cause sun sensitivity)
Hyoscyamus niger	Witch's Hat (toxic; homeopathic only)
Hyssopus officinalis	Hyssop
Ignatia amara	St. Ignatia's Bean (exotic toxic; homeopathic)

Ilex aquifolium	English Holly
Ilex paraguariensis	Yerba Mate.
Illicum verum	Star Anise (cousins have mild toxicity)
Inonotus obliquus	Chaga Mushroom
Inula helenium	Elecampane
Ipecacuanha (see *Cephaelis ipecacuanha*)	
Iris versicolor	Blue Flag
Isatis tinctoria	Indigo
Jeffersonia diphylla	Twinleaf
Juglans cinerea	Butternut (purgative)
Juglans nigra	Black Walnut (purgative)
Juglans regia	English Walnut (purgative)
Juniperus communis	Juniper
Krameria triandra	Krameria, Ratanhia
Lactuca virosa	Wild Lettuce
Lamium spp.	Dead Nettle
Larix laricina	Larch, Tamarack
Larrea divaricata	Chaparral (not approved by FDA; moderate doses)
Lavandula spica	Lavender
Ledum groenlandica, L. palustris	Labrador Tea

(Note: *Ledums* above were recently renamed *Rhododendrum groenlandicum, R. tomentosum.*)

Lentinula edodes	Shiitake Mushroom
Leonurus cardiaca	Motherwort
Lepidium meyenii	Maca
Levisticum officinale	Lovage
Liatris spicata	Corn Snakeroot
Ligusticum porteri	Osha

Lilium candidum	Madonna Lily (interchangeable with the following)
Lilium longiflorum, L. brownii	Easter Lily
Lilium tigrinum	Tiger Lily
Linum usitatissimum	Flaxseed (the fresh seed is ground to make a poultice or for internal consumption; the refrigerated fresh oil is taken internally; the oxidized or aged oil, called linseed oil in the United States, is toxic; the name linseed can mean flaxseed in other countries)
Liriodendron tulipifera	Tulip Tree
Liriosma ovata	Muira Puama
Lithospermum officinale	Gromwell
Lobelia inflata	Lobelia
Lomatium dissectum	Bear Root
Lonicera spp.	Honeysuckle (flowers; berries are toxic)
Lycium chinensis	Goji, Lycii Berry
Lycopodium clavatum	Wolf's Foot Club Moss (homeopathic, occasionally herbal)
Lycopus virginicus, L. americanus, L. europaeus	Bugleweed
Lysimachia nummularia	Moneywort
Mahonia spp.	Oregon Grape Root
Majorana hortensis	Marjoram (also *Origanum majorana*)
Malus spp.	Crab Apple
Malva neglecta	Low Mallow
Marrubium vulgare	White Horehound
Matricaria recutita, M. chamomilla	German Camomile (see *Chamomilla*)
Medicago sativa	Alfalfa

Melaleuca alternifolia	Tea Tree, Cajeput
Melilotus officinalis	Yellow Clover
Melissa officinalis	Lemon Balm
Menispermum canadense	Moonseed
Mentha arvensis	Wild Mint
Mentha piperita	Peppermint (long-term use not advised)
Mentha pulegium	English Pennyroyal
Mentha spicata	Spearmint
Menyanthes trifoliata	Bogbean, Bog Trefoil
Mitchella repens	Partridge Berry
Momordica charantia	Bitter Melon
Monarda fistulosa	Wild Bergamot
Monarda punctata	Horse Mint

(Note: The two *Monardas* above are not identical in action.)

Monotropa uniflora	Ghost Pipe
Myrica cerifera	Bayberry
Myristica fragrans	Nutmeg
Nepeta cataria	Catnip
Nepeta hederacea (see *Glechoma hederacea*)	
Nigella sativa	Black Cumin
Nuphar lutea	Yellow Water Lily
Nux vomica (exotic toxic; homeopathic)	
Nymphaea odorata	White Water Lily
Ocimum sanctum, O. tenuiflorum	Holy Basil
Oenothera biennis	Evening Primrose
Olea europaea	Olive (leaf and oil)
Ononis spinosa	Restharrow
Onosmodium spp.	False Gromwell

Oplopanax horridus	Devil's Club
Opuntia spp.	Opuntia, Prickly Pear
Origanum majorana (see *Majorana hortensis*)	
Origanum vulgare	Oregano
Osmorhiza longistylis	American Sweet Cicely
Osmunda regalis	Royal Fern
Oxydendrum arboreum	Sourwood
Paeonia lactiflora	White Peony
Panax ginseng	Chinese Ginseng, Red Ginseng
Panax notoginseng	Tienchi Ginseng
Panax quinquefolius	American Ginseng
Papaver somnifera	Opium Poppy (flowers and seeds only; latex is illegal)
Parietaria officinalis	Pellitory-of-the-Wall
Parthenocissus quinquefolia	Virginia Creeper (see *Ampelopsis hederacea*)
Passiflora incarnata	Passionflower
Pedicularis spp.	American Betony
Persicaria maculosa (see *Polygonum persicaria*)	
Petasites officinalis	Butterbur
Petroselinum sativum	Parsley
Peumus boldus	Boldo
Pfaffia paniculata	Suma
Phaseolus spp.	Bean (pod)
Phyllitis scolopendrium (see *Scolopendrium vulgare*)	
Phytolacca decandra	Poke Root (toxic; small or homeopathic dosage)
Picraena excelsa	Quassia
Pilocarpus jaborandi	Jaborandi (toxic; small dose)

Pimpinella anisum	Anise
Pinus strobus	White Pine
Piper cubeba	Cubeb
Piper methysticum	Kava-Kava
Piper nigrum	Black Pepper
Piscidia erythrina, P. piscipula, P. communis	Jamaica Dogwood
Plantago major, P. lanceolata	Plantain
Plantago psyllium, P. ovata	Psyllium (seed, husk)
Platanus occidentalis	Sycamore
Pleurotus ostreatus	Oyster Mushroom
Podophyllum peltatum	Mayapple (toxic; small or homeopathic dose)
Polemonium reptans	Jacob's Ladder
Polygala senega	Seneca Snakeroot
Polygonatum spp.	Solomon's Seal
Polygonum aviculare	Knotgrass
Polygonum bistorta, P. bistortoides	Bistort
Polygonum hydropiperoides, P. punctatum	Knotweed, Smartweed
Polygonum japonica	Japanese Knotweed
Polygonum multiflorum	Ho Shu Wu
Polygonum persicaria	Peach-leaved Knotweed (now *Persicaria maculosa*)
Polymnia uvedalia	Bear's Foot
Populus gileadensis	Balm of Gilead
Populus tremuloides	Trembling Aspen
Potentilla tormentilla, P. erecta	Tormentil
Primula veris	Cowslip
Propolis	Bee Secretion
Prunella vulgaris	Self-Heal, Heal-All

Prunus domestica	Plum, Prune
Prunus persica (see *Amygdalus persica*)	
Prunus pygeum	*Pygeum*
Prunus serotina	Wild Cherry
Prunus spinosa	Blackthorn
Pseudognaphalium (see *Gnaphalium*)	
Psilocybe spp.	Psilocybin Mushroom (illegal)
Ptelea trifoliata	Wafer Ash
Pulmonaria officinalis	Lungwort
Pulsatilla vulgaris	Pulsatilla (old name but official in U.S. Homeopathic Pharmacopeia)
Ranunculus bulbosus	Bulbous Buttercup
Ranunculus ficaria (see *Ficaria verna*)	Figwort
Raphanus sativa	Black Radish (leaf)
Rauwolfia serpentaria	Rauwolfia (prescription only)
Rehmannia glutinosa	Rehmannia
Rhamnus frangula, R. cathartica (purgative; substitutes for the following)	
Rhamnus purshiana	Cascara Sagrada (purgative)
Rheum officinale, *R. palmatum, R. rhaponticum*	Rhubarb (purgative)
Rhodiola spp.	Rose Root
Rhododendrum groenlandicum, *R. tomentosum* (see *Ledum groenlandicum* and *L. palustre*)	
Rhus aromatica	Fragrant Sumach
Rhus coriaria	Kurdish Sumach
Rhus glabra	Smooth Sumach

Rhus typhina	Staghorn Sumach

(Note: All above are fairly interchangeable, and are identified as *Rhus* spp. They are not to be mistaken with *R. toxicodendrum*, poison ivy, which is only used in homeopathic form.)

Rhus toxicodendron	Poison Ivy (homeopathic only)
Ribes nigrum	Black Currant
Ricinus communis	Castor Oil
Rosa spp.	Rose, Wild Rose (hips, petals, seeds)
Rosmarinus officinalis	Rosemary
Rubia tinctoria	Dyer's Madder
Rubus canadensis, R. idaeus, R. strigosus	Raspberry
Rubus fruticosus, R. villosa	Blackberry (root bark, leaf)
Rumex acetosella	Sheep Sorrel
Rumex crispus	Yellow Dock, Curly Dock
Ruscus aculeatus	Butcher's Broom
Ruta graveolens	Rue
Quercus alba	White Oak
Sabal serrulatum	Saw Palmetto (*Serenoa repens*)
Saccharum officinarum	Refined White Sugar
Salix alba	White Willow
Salix nigra	Black Willow
Salvia apiana	White Sage
Salvia miltorrhiza	Chinese or Red Root Sage
Salvia officinalis	Sage
Salvia sclarea	Clary Sage
Sambucus ebulus	Dwarf Elder
Sambucus nigra, S. canadensis	Elder

Sanguinaria canadensis	Bloodroot (excoriative, extremely active; small or homeopathic dose only)
Sanguisorba officinalis, S. minor	Salad Burnet
Sanicula europaea	Sanicle
Saponaria officinalis	Soapwort
Sarothamnus scoparius (see *Scoparium cytisus, Cytisus scoparius*)	
Sassafras albidum	Sassafras
Satureja hortensis	Summer Savory
Satureja montana	Winter Savory

(Note: *S. hortensis* and *S. montana* are interchangeable)

Saxifraga pensylvanica	Saxifrage
Schisandra chinensis	Schizandra
Scolopendrium vulgare	Hart's Horn Fern (see *Asplenium scolopendrium*)
Scoparium cytisus	Broom Tops (active) (see *Sarothamnus*)
Scrophularia nodosa,	Figwort, Pilewort (*S. marilandica,* other *S.* spp.)
Scutellaria laterifolia	Skullcap
Selenicereus grandiflorus	Queen of the Night Cactus
Senecio aureus	Life Root (pyrrolizidine alkaloids; small or homeopathic dose)
Senecio jacobaea	Common Ragwort (pyrrolizidine alkaloids; small or homeopathic dose)
Senega (see *Polygala senega*)	
Sepia officinalis	Squid ink (homeopathic)
Serenoa (see *Sabal*)	
Sesamum indicum	Sesame Seed

Sida acuta	Wiregrass
Silphium integrifolium	Compass Plant
Silybum marianum	Milk Thistle
Sinapis alba	White Mustard
Sinapis nigra	Black Mustard
Smilacina racemosa	False Solomon's Seal (recently *Maianthemum racemosum*)
Smilax spp.	Sarsaparilla
Solanum dulcamara	Bittersweet Nightshade (toxic; small or homeopathic dose)
Solidago virga-aurea S. *canadensis, S.* spp.	Goldenrod
Spongia tosta (homeopathic)	Toasted Sponge
Squilla maritima	Siberian Squills (small dose only)
Stachys officinalis	Wood Betony (formerly *Betonica officinalis*)
Stachys palustris	Woundwort
Stellaria media	Chickweed
Stillingia sylvatica	Queen's Delight
Stramonium	Datura (see *Datura stramonium;* toxic, homeopathic only)
Styrax spp.	Gum Benzoin
Symplocarpus foetidus	Skunk Cabbage
Syzygium cumini	Jambul
Tabebuia	Pau d'Arco (see *Handroanthus*)
Tanacetum balsamita	Costmary
Tanacetum parthenium	Feverfew
Taraxacum officinalis	Dandelion
Teucrium chamaedrys	Germander
Thuja occidentalis	Northern White Cedar (homeopathic and herbal)

Thymus serpyllum	Mother of Thyme
Thymus vulgaris	Thyme
Tilia spp.	Linden, Lime Tree
Trametes versicolor	Turkey Tail Mushroom
Tribulus terrestris	Goat's Head Sticker
Trifolium pratense	Red Clover
Trifolium repens	White Clover
Trigonella foenum-graecum	Fenugreek
Trillium spp.	Trillium, Birth Root
Triticum repens (see *Agropyron repens*)	
Tsuga canadensis	Canada Hemlock

(Note: Not to be confused with *Conium maculatum,* Poison Hemlock.)

Turnera diffusa	Damiana
Tussilago farfara	Coltsfoot
Ulmus fulva (U. rubra)	Slippery Elm
Umbellularia californica	California Bay Laurel
Uncaria tomentosa	Cat's Claw
Urtica dioica, Urtica spp.	Nettles, Nettle
Usnea barbata	Usnea
Ustilago maydis	Corn Smut
Vaccinium macrocarpon	Cranberry
Vaccinium myrtillus	Bilberry

(Note: Other *Vaccinium* species can substitute for *V. myrtillus.*)

Vaccinium spp.	Blueberry, Huckleberry
Valeriana officinalis	Valerian
Veratrum viride	American Hellebore (toxic; homeopathic dose only)
Verbascum thapsus	Mullein (leaf, root)
Verbena hastata	Blue Vervain

Verbena officinalis	Vervain

(Note: These two verbenas can be used interchangeably.)

Veronica officinalis	Speedwell and other *V.* spp.
Veronicastrum virginicum	Culver's Root (purgative)
Viburnum opulus	Crampbark
Viburnum trilobum	American Cranberrybush

(Note: These are referred to in the repertory as *Viburnum* spp.)

Viburnum prunifolium	Black Haw
Vinca major	Greater Periwinkle
Vinca minor	Lesser Periwinkle
Viola odorata, V. spp.	Blue Violet
Viola tricolor	Pansy
Viscum album	Mistletoe (moderate dosage)
Vitex agnus castus	Chaste Berry
Vitis vinifera	Grape
Withania somnifera	Ashwaganda
Xanthium spp.	Cocklebur
Xanthorrhiza apiifolia	Yellowroot
Yucca filamentosa	Yucca
Zanthoxylum americanum	Prickly Ash (large dose painful to consume)
Zea mays	Corn Silk
Zingiberis officinale	Ginger

2. Energetics:
Constitutions and Tissue States

The most effective constitutional system for medical use is based on physical build (thin/medium/thick), because build is closely related to long-term health developments. Thin people tend to get the same diseases, based on undernourishment and nervousness; medium-built people fall prey to accidents and heat-related problems; and thick people tend to suffer from lack of exercise and overeating. There are several alternative medical systems that divide people into three such groups. The oldest is the system of *tridosha* in Ayurvedic medicine, which is thousands of years old. This correlates neatly with systems that were independently developed in the nineteenth- and twentieth-century in conventional and alternative Western medicine. Like most American herbalists, we use the Ayurvedic terms *vata, pitta*, and *kapha*, which correlate with thin, medium, and thick.

The energetic system used here is the "tissue state" model of the physiomedicalists, because it is best suited to the Western herbal model (out of which it evolved). However, all energetic systems have characteristics in common. The most effective way to describe energetics in a holistic framework is binary—yin and yang, excess and deficient, hot and cold, tense and relaxed, damp and dry, etc. The tissue state model uses three binary sets (excitation/depression, atrophy/stagnation, tension/relaxation, or heat/cold, dry/damp, tense/relaxed).

The Ayurvedic or Tridoshic Constitutions

The trifold system of analysis in Ayurvedic medicine is thousands of years old. It is based on the idea of three different "tints" or "tinctures" *(doshas)* entering into the composition of each person. The doshas are derived from the five elements of India. Air and Ether (dryness and wind) produce the thin, dry, nervous type *(vata)*. Fire and the oil aspect of Water or liquid create the strong, medium-built, ardent type *(pitta)*. Earth and the watery aspect of Water create the thick, damp, well-nourished, purposeful type *(kapha)*. These correspond almost exactly with a system developed independently in the West in the nineteenth century in which constitutions were described as *nervous* (thin), *motive* (robust), and *vital* (visceral, thick).

In the twentieth century, psychologist William Sheldon determined through extensive population studies that there are three basic somatotypes, with corresponding psychic tendencies: *ectomorph* (thin), *mesomorph* (medium), and *endomorph* (thick). His theory is that, in the ectomorph, the organs of the fetal ectoderm (nervous system and skin) predominate, while in the mesomorph the fetal mesoderm (muscles and bones) dominates, and in the endomorph it is the vital organs (gastrointestinal, lymph, and endocrine systems, etc.). This is an extremely useful categorization from a therapeutic standpoint; we often find stress (excess or deficiency) in the organs emphasized in the three types.

Dosha can refer either to the congenital constitution or to disorders created by what biomedicine calls "stress." Sometimes the constitution is the source of the problem, while at other times the disease pattern has been superimposed on the constitution. Thus, we might treat either the innate constitution or the imposed pathology.

Some remedies act more on the constitution, while others act more on the pathological imbalance. For instance, *Lycopodium* is an excellent remedy for the vata constitution, while *Althaea officinalis* (marshmallow) is an excellent remedy for a person who is suffering from dryness, no matter what their constitution. On the other hand, *Lycopodium* is sometimes indicated for a superimposed condition, while *Althaea* fits a congenital constitution. For this reason, descriptive keywords in the repertory such as damp, dry, thin, medium, or nervous are not usually designated as constitutional; they often only refer to temporary pathology. Only when the remedy has traditionally been associated with the congenital constitution, gender or age will that be designated.

The Three Doshas

The *vata* dosha is composed of the elements of air and ether, which translate to dry and tension (lack of space causes tension), so the vata person has less digestive juices, causing a thin, dry constitution. He or she is more nervous from tension and thin physique—lack of "insulation" around the nerves makes them more sensitive. In Western constitutional terms this type would be described as an "ectomorph," "asthenic," or "nervous constitution." The ectomorphic constitution is associated with the ectodermic layer of the fetus that develops into the nerves, senses, and skin. Vata conditions are drying, nervous, tense, and wasting.

Pitta is framed from the elements of fire and water. However, in Ayurveda "water" is broken into the two liquids: water and oil. Fire is composed of oil, not water per se. This makes much more sense. The pitta person is active, ardent, a "doer," and is warm or hot and combustive. The oil is like a fuel that burns up. The build in medium, with red or sallow, dark complexion, and firm, active muscles. Some pitta people are blond, red haired, red-blond, or fiery in complexion, while another kind is a dark, lean, and sallow—what the Greeks would have called the "choleric type." In Western terms, this constitutional type is the "mesomorph," whose system emphasizes the mesoderm that forms the muscles of the body, including the heart. Pitta conditions are excessively warm, hot, and combustive.

Kapha is composed from the elements of earth and water, so it is slower moving, gentler, and more relaxed as a doshic influence and as a constitutional type. "Water" in this instance contains both water and oil. The former is relaxing and cooling, the latter lubricating and relaxing. Together with the solid earth, this makes the kapha constitution cool, relaxed, slow, and heavy, with tendencies to retention and stagnation. Unlike vata, this type is well-nourished; with age kapha people can become overweight. More than anything, however, kapha is relaxed. In Western terms kapha is analogous to the "endomorph" made from the endomorphic level of the endoderm, which develops into the organs, bowels, viscera, glands, and endocrine system.

Hence, the kapha person has a strong digestion and metabolism—too strong, perhaps. Kapha conditions are damp, cold, stagnant, slow, sluggish, dull, thick, sthenic.

Vata (Ectomorph, Asthenic, Thin)

• Albizia ("lost capacity to feel joy"—Donahue) • Althaea (dry mucosa and skin) • Ballota (nerve debility) • Amygdalus (delicate constitution with pale skin) • ANGELICA (dry, thin, pallid; poor digestion and gas, but tendency to accumulate fluids) • ARALIA RACEMOSA (warming nutritive; weak, enfeebled nervous system; anemia, general debility) • ARCTIUM (worry, dryness, poor lipid digestion) • AVENA (frazzled, oversensitive, hyperreactive; nerve exhaustion) • BETONICA (thin, elderly) • Borago ("nervous wreck") • Capsella (muscle atrophy; fibroids, weak uterine muscles) • Celastrus (thin, withered, dry and delicate state with poor nutrition and low anabolism) • Cetraria (weakness in children and elderly; chronic, congenital) • Chondrus (similar to Cetraria) • CINNAMOMUM CASSIA (thin, fair; moist skin, sweats easily—Huang) • Codonopsis (sweet and moist nutritive; weak, thin, nervous, dried out, tired, bloated, shallow respiration) • Dioscorea (thin and undernourished; intestinal and other spasms; poor assimilation by small intestine; decalcification, especially in the hip joints) • ELEUTHEROCOCCUS (nervous; dark circles under the eyes) • Galium (nerve disease) • Gnaphalium (thin, nervous) • Hydrangea (thin, dry, nervous, weak) • Inula (thin and pale) • Lavendula (apply oil on side of head; nervousness, exhaustion, tension, extreme mental states; panic, anxiety, irritability; headache) • Leonurus (freaked-out expression; poor bone development) • LYCOPODIUM (homeopathic; thin, withered, dry, and full of gas) • Lycopus (nervous; looks like a hunted animal) • Medicago sativa • MELISSA (nervous) • Mitchella (women; thin, tall, angular, dark-haired, athletic, too much in their minds) • Nuphar (dry vagina; pelvic tension) • Nymphaea (weakness, exhaustion, "pinings, wasting and consumption"—Salmon)

• Origanum (high-strung persons who push themselves to tiredness, but can't relax) • PANAX QUINQUEFOLIUS (neurasthenia, loss of fluids, dry, atrophy, debilitated habits, exhaustion
of brain and nervous system) • POLYGONUM MULTIFLO-
RUM (aging and drying of joints; dry throat, thirst, cough due
to dry lungs; gray hair from kidney-yin deficiency) • Prunus
serotina (thin people that are too hot) • Rhus spp. (nervousness,
weakness; children and the elderly) • Rosa (asthenic and anemic) • Scutellaria ("sedates fire in the small intestine that would
otherwise burn energy too quickly; good for skinny people;
holds energy in the body, good for overthinkers; the perfect
nervine; doesn't drag on the rest of the system"—LeSassier)
• SALVIA (dry, withered; premature menopause, andropause—
Light) • Selenicereus (thin, nervous, neurasthenic; hyperthyroidism, heart palpitations and irregularities) • Stellaria (weedy,
thin, dry, and malnourished) • Tilia (see *Pitta*) • TRIFOLIUM
(insufficient secretions) • Verbascum (general dryness and atrophy) •·Vinca (sclerosis, hardening processes) • Vitex • WITH-
ANIA ("depleted, exhausted, underweight"; "elderly with poor
memory"—Kuhn and Winston).

Pitta (Mesomorph, Medium)

• ACHILLEA (robust, sanguine persons with red, full-blooded
complexion, blue veins) • Amygdalus (fair, thin-to-medium
build, common with histaminic irritation) • Arnica (athletic constitution) • BUPLEURUM ("medium to slightly thin"; dark-
yellow, greenish-yellow, greenish-pale, lusterless complexion;
firm muscles, dry skin; "wiry to thin pulse"—Huang) • Eupatorium perfoliatum • Galium (cooling) • Gnaphalium (allergies)
• Hydrangea (hard, bitter, willful, stubborn, cynical) • Lobelia
(often full-muscled) • MEDICAGO SATIVA • Monarda fistulosa (robust, passionate, creative) • Nuphar • Passiflora (driven,
type-A people; use during the day) • Prunus serotina (specific
for the problems of redheads) • RHEUM (*pitta/kapha*; large,
strong, hot—Huang) • RUMEX CRISPUS (large, strong; red

cheeks, yellow around nose, mouth, eyes; strong digestion; *pitta*, aging into *kapha*) • Scutellaria (reduces heat; see *vata*) • TILIA (*vata/pitta;* "race-horse type, whose energies are squandered in quick speech and a mind that flits from subject to subject"— Parton) • Valeriana (full, excitable) • Zea mays • Zingiberis (muscle relaxant).

Kapha (Endomorph, Plethoric, Thick)

• Acorus (boggy digestion and cloudy thinking, thick white coat on tongue corresponding to "phlegm misting the orifices of the heart"—Donahue) • Angelica (excess mucus, dry) • Arctostaphylos (relaxed, toneless tissues with draggy, weighty feeling; feeble circulation, lack of innervation) • Capsicum • Chimaphila (great *kapha* eliminator; water retention; kidney and spleen yang deficiency) • Commiphora myrrha (relaxation and depression, poor circulation and depressed cell life) • Comptonia (cold center; diarrhea; spleen yang deficiency) • Gnaphalium (middle-aged, adrenocortical-dominant men with big, muscular bellies; to reduce cortisol) • Guaiacum (heavy, damp, cold, depressive; stomach depressed) • Helichrysum (essential oil; same as Gnaphalium) • Myrica (boggy mucosa) • Oplopanax (bogged down, unable to assert self, "water failing to become wood"— Donahue) • Phytolacca (large, bulky persons with large glands, breasts, swellings, and congestions) • RHEUM (robust, strong, firm muscles; reddish, oily, or greasy and dirty skin; thick, darkened, red lips; large appetite—Huang) • RUMEX CRISPUS (similar to Rheum but less intense personality—Wood) • Satureja (endocrine, adrenocortical and sympathetic nervous system deficiencies; stimulates cerebral cortex and sexual glands; weak immune system—Kenner, Requena) • Trigonella (averse to exercise, overweight; slack muscle tone, stagnant lymphatics) • Tsuga canadensis (warms the kidneys and feet) • Zingiberis (large, damp, cold).

Appearance under one dosha does not rule out application in another.

The above designations into the three categories are based on the experience of myself and others. The only source book I have found that uses this system, and from which I have drawn heavily to confirm or add to the above lists, is *The Male Herbal* by James Green (2007). He names three types: the seer *(vata)*, warrior *(pitta)*, and monarch *(kapha)*.

Energetics of Western Herbalism

In order to practice herbalism in a holistic fashion, we need a system for recognizing and describing patterns. Throughout the Old World, we find some form of "humoral" medicine in which the body (and its medicines) are analyzed in terms of hot and cold, damp and dry conditions. Nineteenth-century botanical doctors worked out a model of three, four, or six "tissue states." I have combined the Greek qualities (hot, cold, etc.) with the tissue states of the nineteenth century physiomedicalists (excitation, relaxation, etc.).

Greek, Chinese, and Ayurvedic medicine has been designated as "humoral" by historians of medicine. However, both ancient and modern people also thought in terms of "energy," vital force, qi, or prana, and today the term "energy medicine" or "energetics" is popular while "humoralism" is only used in academia. Of course, "energy" can be considered a "humor" or substance.

The energetic model we use in Western herbal medicine comes from a combination of the Greek system, nineteenth century physiology, and the practices of Native American people. Indian medicine is usually considered "animistic" (spirit-based), but it is also based on the elimination of humors through the use of the sweat lodge, purging, and emesis, so it too should be considered humoral (or energetic) – as well as animist. See Virgil Vogel's *American Indian Medicine* (1970) for extensive accounts of Native American health practices.

Samuel Thomson, the popularizer of herbal medicine in North America, absorbed the teachings of his mentor, Mrs. Benton, the "wise woman" in the neighborhood. Her emphasis was on keeping the perspiration healthy. This is a Native teaching, not Greek or

European. Thomson taught that it was necessary to maintain healthy perspiration by "warming the center" and "keeping open the skin" by expelling cold from inside to outside.

Thomson's model was developed further by Dr. Alva Curtis, who taught that the body reacts to stimulation in a threefold cycle—excitation, contraction, and relaxation. This is based on Albert Haller's observation in the mid-eighteenth century that the motor nerves operate in these three phases. This observation is still a foundation of modern neuroscience; it is called the "E-C-R cycle." Curtis, however, extended the observation to propose that all bodily activity follows this cycle. This idea was taken up by the physiomedicalists (followers of Thomson and Curtis) and enlarged to six imbalances: excitation, depression, atrophy, stagnation, contraction or tension, and relaxation. I have called this "the forgotten energetics of Western herbalism." See my work *Vitalism* (2000) for information on Thomson, Curtis, and physiomedicalism and *The Practice of Traditional Western Herbalism* (2004) for the tissue states in particular. We no longer need to call it "forgotten."

A similar generalization about disease processes following a threefold cycle was made in the twentieth-century by Dr. Hans Selye, discoverer of the function of the adrenal cortex and originator of the medical concept of "stress":

> We have illustrated, with many examples, that the most varied manifestations of disease depend upon a tripartite mechanism consisting of: (1) the direct action of the external agent—the apparent pathogen; (2) factors that inhibit this action; and (3) factors that facilitate this action (Selye 1974, 314).

Selye further notes that "all bodily activities" tend to move through three stages and are therefore "triphasic." As an example, he cites the inflammatory response:

> If virulent microbes get under the skin, they first cause what we call acute inflammation (reddening, swelling, pain); then follows chronic inflammation (ripening of a boil or abscess); and finally an exhaustion of tissue resistance, which permits the inflamed,

purulent fluid to be evacuated (breaking through of an abscess) (Selye 1974, 473).

The rebound effect is an example of a triphasic reaction: pathogenic attack or trauma; primary response (resistance); secondary response (recovery). For centuries we have used the vast majority of herbs, in almost all traditions, to antidote the rebound effect. However, Selye's observations also form the basis of our understanding of how adaptogens work (Winston and Maimes, 2007). The adaptogen gives the organism greater "nonspecific resistance" to all stimulae, so that the extreme reactions to the rebound effect are lessened and it is less likely to be traumatized by the extreme reactions.

The Six Tissue States

The followers of Alva Curtis were called the "physiomedicalists." In the generation following Curtis, Dr. Joseph M. Thurston (1900) identified six different "tissue states." These correspond to the three phases, in excess or deficiency: excitation (overstimulation), depression (understimulation), contraction (tension), relaxation (lack of tension), atrophy (lack of fluid), and torpor (excess of fluid). In a late physiomedical work, A.W. and L.R. Priest (1982, 34) describe only four tissue states: stimulation, sedation, constriction, and relaxation, which can be visualized as follows:

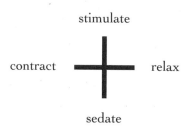

stimulate

contract — relax

sedate

Thurston's sixfold model represents the entire scope of Greek energetics, including the four qualities and the two tissue states (constriction, relaxation) used by various schools of Greek medicine. They align fairly closely (though not perfectly), as follows:

Heat	Excitation, Irritation, Stimulation
Cold	Depression
Dryness	Atrophy
Dampness	Stagnation
Tension	Tension, Constriction, Contraction
Relaxation	Relaxation

In traditional Chinese and Greek medicine, the state called "relaxation" here is often identified with "dampness" because the tissues are damp, with fluid flowing out of open, relaxed pores. This is a "damp flowing" state. This gives us two damp states: stagnation and relaxation. For ease of use I have kept tension and relaxation as a pair and left out the relationship between relaxation and dampness in the repertory.

The original Latin terms for tension and relaxation were *status strictus* and *status laxus*. The TCM term for tension is "wind." The Ayurvedic equivalent is "space" or "ether" – when there is a lack of space there is tension.

The chart on the following page shows the relationship between the three *doshas* (constitutions) and the six tissue states.

Heat/Excitation

This tissue state depends on an *exaggeration* of function. The tissues are overstimulated; circulation and innervation are accelerated. Blood rushes to an area that is over-functioning, resulting in the classical symptoms of inflammation—heat, redness, swelling, and pain. This tissue state, however, is not equivalent to inflammation, which can also result from cold, spasm, dryness, and dampness. Rather, the organism is in a condition where it is too easily pushed into inflammation.

Symptoms of heat: heat, redness, swelling, and tenderness associated with autoimmune excess and exaggeration of function; pink-red (carmine) to dark-red mucosa and skin; dark and concentrated urine;

The Six Tissue States and the Three Doshas of Ayurveda

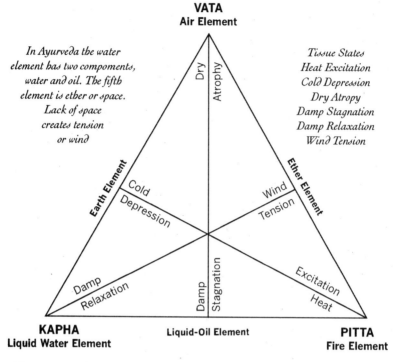

VATA
Air Element

In Ayurveda the water element has two compoments, water and oil. The fifth element is ether or space. Lack of space creates tension or wind

Tissue States
Heat Excitation
Cold Depression
Dry Atropy
Damp Stagnation
Damp Relaxation
Wind Tension

Dry   Atrophy

Earth Element   Cold Depression   Wind Tension   Ether Element

Damp Relaxation   Damp Stagnation   Excitation Heat

KAPHA
Liquid Water Element

Liquid-Oil Element

PITTA
Fire Element

Vata consists of air and ether • Kapha of water and earth • Pitta of fire and oil

pulse is elevated (beats toward the surface, high in the artery), large, rapid, quick; tongue is elongated, pointed, carmine-red, flame-shaped.

Recommended herbs for heat: • Achillea (excitation, depression, relaxation; capillary stasis from venous relaxation) • Amygdalus (excitation, atrophy, immune excess) • Asperula (excitation, depression) • Citrus limonum (excitation, relaxation) • Crataegus (excitation; cardiovascular, mind) • Cucurbita citrullus (excitation, atrophy; kidneys) • Curcuma • Galium (excitation, atrophy; lymph, kidneys, nerves) • Lonicera (excitation) • Lavendula (excitation, tension; circulation, nerves) • Medicago sativa (excitation, torpor, atrophy) • Melilotus (excitation from blood stagnation or tissue depression) • Melissa (excitation; nervous system) • Nigella sativa (both excess and deficiency) • Passiflora incarnata • Prunus serotina (excitation; lungs, heart, small intestine, skin, mind, emotions) • Rheum (excitation, tension; colon; "restless spirit, irritability, easily excited, and fever with sweating"—Huang) • Ribes nigrum (excitation; adrenal cortex) • Rosa (excitation, relaxation; rose hips) • Rumex acetosa (excitation) • Rumex crispus (excitation, relaxation, torpor; colon, liver, skin) • Sambucus spp. (excitation; perspiration; channels of elimination) • Trifolium pratense (excitation; cools through the surface, thins blood) • Vaccinium macrocarpon (excitation, relaxation) • Vaccinium myrtillus (excitation; high blood sugar) • Viburnum trilobum (excitation, tension).

Cold/Depression

This tissue state represents the opposite condition to heat/excitation: tissues fail to respond to stimulation; hence there is a generalized or local depression. The extremities are usually cold; the skin is cold and inactive, failing to perspire and lacking water and oil. The complexion is pale due to lack of blood at the surface, or lack of good blood; or it may be darkish due to lack of oxygen (grey), coagulation (blue), sepsis (purple), or necrosis (black).

Symptoms of cold: deep cold; tissues are pale, white, dark, grey, blue, purple, or black, indicating decreased oxygenation; lessened sensation and function; lack of response to stimulation; cold hands and feet (also see wind/tension); low and slow pulse; pale or dark tongue body.

Recommended herbs for cold: • Achillea (depression, excitation, relaxation; vascular system) • Anethum (diffusive; depression) • Angelica archangelica (warming/stimulating; dries water, generates oil) • Arnica (warming/stimulating; congealed blood) • Artemisia absinthium (warming/stimulating, softening, anthelmintic) • Artemisia annua (warming/stimulating, antiperiodic, antimicrobial) • Artemisia vulgaris (warming/stimulating, softening; uterus) • Baptisia (stimulating, antiseptic, antimicrobial) • Barosma (warming/stimulating, antiseptic; urinary tract) • Calendula (warming/stimulating, antiseptic; lymph/immune) • Capsella bursa-pastoris (stimulating, emollient) • Capsicum (stimulating; heats the interior, cools the exterior) • Carthamus (warming/stimulating; congealed blood) • Curcuma (inflammatory conditions from tissue depression; bacteria living off debris) • Echinacea (stimulating/cooling, antiseptic) • Erigeron (stimulating, astringent) • Foeniculum (mildly warming/stimulating) • Gnaphalium obtusifolium (warming/stimulating, sweet/nourishing, blood-thinning) • Helianthus (warming/stimulating, oily/nourishing) • Helianthemum (stimulating antiseptic) • Helichrysum (warming/stimulating, sweet/nourishing, blood-thinning) • Hyssop (warming/stimulating, opening/moistening) • Inula (warming/stimulating, carminative, thinning/mucolytic) • Isatis (stimulating antiseptic) • Juglans nigra (warming/stimulating, alterative, anthelmintic; hull) • Larrea (warming/stimulating, alterative) • Monarda fistulosa (stimulating, warming/cooling) • Origanum (warming/stimulating, relaxing) • Pinus strobus (stimulating antiseptic, expectorant) • Propolis (warming/stimulating) • Rosmarinus (warming/stimulating, drying; circulation and nerves) • Rubia tinctorum (depression; blood) • Salvia (warming/stimulating, astringent to water, nutritive to oil) • Sassafras (warming/stimulating, blood-thinning) • Sinapis (stimulating carminative) • Solidago spp. (stimulating, carminative) • Thymus (warming/stimulating, antibacterial) • Turnera (stimulating, relaxing) • Tsuga canadensis (warming/stimulating, penetrating topical) • Zingiberis (warming/stimulating, acrid/relaxing, sweet/nourishing).

Tension

This tissue state is called "wind" in Traditional Chinese Medicine. It includes both psychological and physical tension, and corresponds to conditions occurring due to nervous constriction, tension, and spasm.

These range from closure of the sweat pores to torsion, convulsion, and epilepsy, including spasm, chills, chills alternating with fever, sudden onset of symptoms, alternating or periodic symptoms (diarrhea alternating with constipation, chills with fever, or chills at a specific time of day), backward-type movements (hiccough, nausea, esophageal reflux, vomiting), uncontrollable movement, trembling, shaking, etc. All of these are connected to imbalances of the nerves; without nerves, there would be no wind/tension tissue state.

Symptoms of tension: tension of mind, body, or both; symptoms come on suddenly; symptoms repeat or alternate (diarrhea alternates with constipation, or chills alternate with fever); gas and bloating comes and goes suddenly; symptoms reverse direction of normal movement (hiccough, nausea, vomiting); cold hands and feet; cold in the joints; tongue tremors; pulse wiry, tense, resistant, hard.

Recommended herbs for tension: • Agrimonia (relaxing astringent) • Chamomilla (relaxing, stimulant, bitter and sweet digestive tonic) • Cnicus (bitter acrid antiperiodic, alterative) • Cornus florida (bitter acrid antiperiodic) • Dipsacus sylvestris (bitter acrid antiperiodic) • Eupatorium perfoliatum (bitter acrid antiperiodic, diaphoretic) • Lactuca (bitter acrid relaxant, antiperiodic) • Lobelia (acrid diffusive relaxant, antispasmodic, diaphoretic) • Humulus (acrid bitter relaxant) • Magnesium salts (in solution is best) • Mentha piperita (relaxant, diaphoretic) • Nepeta (acrid bitter relaxant, antispasmodic) • Passiflora (relaxant) • Sambucus (cooling, sedative, relaxant, slightly stimulating aromatic) • Umbellularia (acrid stimulating relaxant, entheogen; leaf, nut) • Taraxacum (muscle spasm; flower) • Valeriana (acrid relaxant) • Verbena (acrid bitter, relaxant, diaphoretic; neck tension) • Viburnum opulus (tension) • Viburnum trilobum (tension, excitation) • Zingiberis (tension, depression).

Relaxation

This is one of two states associated with excess dampness; the other is stagnation. In the former state, the tissues are moist (including the skin, since it is an excretory organ), and water readily sheds from the body. In the latter case, the water is stuck, or stagnant, inside the body cavities; it does not flow through them, but fills them and stays there. This represents another type of loss of tone, which the old doctors called "torpor," referring to heavy, waterlogged, soggy, toneless tissue.

Symptoms of (excessive) relaxation: tissues lacking in tone; collapse, prolapse, leaking fluids, free secretion of mucin, sweat; diarrhea; clear, copious urine; cool, clammy skin; pale skin with veins showing through; low energy; tongue moist, streamers between the center and the sides of the tongue, sometimes a white, yeasty coat; yeast infection (systemic or vaginal); easy vomiting in children; pulse relaxed, soft, empty, languid.

Recommended herbs for (excessive) relaxation: • Achillea (excitation, relaxation) • Aesculus hip. (relaxation, tension) • Agrimonia (tension, relaxation) • Alchemilla (relaxation) • Angelica (depression, relaxation, atrophy, tension) • Calendula (depression) • Cinnamomum spp. (depression, relaxation) • Equisetum (relaxation, depression, atrophy) • Hypericum (depression, relaxation) • Juglans nigra (relaxation; leaf) • Potentilla (astringent, slightly mucilaginous) • Rubus canadensis (nourishing and astringent) • Sanguisorba (astringent) • Myrica (astringent and stimulating) • Quercus (strongly astringent) • Rosmarinus (mild pungent warming stimulant) • Urtica (stimulating, diffusive, earthen/mineralizing, diuretic/drying) • Vaccinium spp. (astringent; leaf).

Dry/Atrophy

There are two kinds of moisture—water and oil. Nutrition requires water and oil to get from the gastrointestinal system to the tissues.

Therefore, dry/atrophy can be due to lack of water, oil, or nutrition, or the body's inability to handle one or all of these substances. The early signs of dry/atrophy are tissue dryness due to lack of fluids; later signs include withering from poor nutrition.

Symptoms of dryness: dry, wrinkled, withered, hardened tissues; poor scalp health, falling out of hair; weakness; bloating, gas, constipation, hard stool; tongue is thin (side-to-side, or upper surface to lower), dry, cracked in some cases, and withered in severe cases; pulse is narrow on one or both sides, and sometimes tense on one side.

Recommended herbs for dryness: • Althaea (atrophy, excitation) • Angelica • Aralia racemosa • Arctium (atrophy, stagnation) • Asclepias tuberosa (atrophy) • Betonica (atrophy) • Capsella (atrophy, depression) • Ceanothus (atrophy, relaxation) • Codonopsis (atrophy) • Helianthus • Ligusticum porteri • Linum (fresh ground seed or flaxseed oil) • Liriodendrum (spasm and atrophy) • Mahonia (atrophy, torpor; increases secretions) • Panax ginseng • Panax quinquefolius • Rehmannia (cooked root; nourishing blood tonic) • Ulmus (atrophy, excitation) • Sabal serrulata (sexual organs) • Salvia • Symphytum (atrophy, relaxation) • Trigonella (atrophy, depression) • Ulmus (atrophy; moistens and mineralizes) • Urtica • Verbascum (dry mucosa) • Vinca (cerebral circulation) • Withania.

Damp/Stagnation

This is the most difficult tissue state to understand. It may be visualized as a condition where the fluids can't get out through the normal channels of elimination; they back up and tend to precipitate and thicken into catarrh, phlegm, or mucus. The old doctors, back to Hippocrates, referred to this as "humors." The idea was that the "humors" were not being cooked down by digestion and metabolism, and were collecting in the body. Later this condition was called "impure blood" (German) or "bad blood" (American Indian). Today it is frequently called "toxic blood" or "toxic liver." One or more of the channels of elimination (skin, kidneys, colon, lungs) may not be open, or the metabolism may be faulty. The latter may be due to low preparatory metabolism in the liver, low thyroid, or low cellular metabolism. There may also be lymphatic congestion, with lowered immunity.

When this condition occurs, the tissues were described in nineteenth-century medicine as "torpid," or in a state of "torpor." The tissues are heavy, full of water and phlegm, with lessened activity and expression in the eyes and face. The most frequent symptom associated with this condition is skin eruption, since metabolic waste products have to leave through the skin instead of the kidneys and lymphatics, or they are not being adequately processed by either the liver or the skin.

When hypothyroidism was discovered and described in the early twentieth century, many doctors realized that it accounted for the symptoms of "bad blood" (Barnes 1976), which included thickening of the fluids into catarrh; cool, rough, inactive, expressionless skin; loss of expression in the eyes and face; fatigue; and weight gain. Hypothyroidism can, therefore, be a cause of "bad blood" or damp/stagnation. However, this is not always the case; sometimes hypothyroidism can be caused by "bad blood." There are also times when the thyroid is not involved at all.

Symptoms of dampness: catarrh, phlegm, or mucus; fluids are retained and thickened; tongue is coated white or yellow; dull expression of skin and musculature; dull facial expression; hangover-like feeling, worse in the morning or after taking food or alcohol; pulse obscure (filmy, dull edges), turgid (as if there is thickened water in the blood), or slippery.

Recommended herbs for dampness: • Arctium (atrophy, stagnation; oil metabolism) • Iris • Juglans nigra (stagnation; hull) • Berberis vulgaris • Cassia (stagnation; cathartic) • Cnicus (stagnation, tension) • Mahonia (atrophy, stagnation) • Phytolacca (stagnation, depression) • Rhamnus purshiana (laxative) • Rheum (stagnation, spasm) • Rumex crispus (excitation, stagnation, relaxation) • Scrophularia (stagnation, depression), Stellaria media (external) • Taraxacum (diuretic; water stagnation; leaf) • Taraxacum (alterative; heat stagnation; root) • Trifolium pratense (atrophy, torpor; opens skin, drains lymphatics, detoxifies) • Urtica (detoxifying, nourishing, but diuretic/drying).

I have been accused of making up these tissue states and therefore "traditional Western herbalism." This shows a complete lack of education on the part of my critics. Anyone who reads the writings of eclectic medicine and physiomedicalism, or even nineteenth-century allopathy, can find these tissue states mentioned throughout the literature. Indeed, look in the index of any contemporary neurology textbook.

Adjuvants, Accelerators, Synergists

One of the great mysteries of herbal medicine is the problem of compounding or mixture. What happens when two or more plants are combined? This question involves both pharmacology and energetics. When volatile oils are mixed they can recombine to form new compounds not found in the original herbs. Other constituents do not mix at all but their effects may harmonize in the new admixture—or not.

Herbs that *assist* the functioning of other remedies are known by many names. The term "adjuvant" is fairly broad, and can be used to refer to plants that act to "tweak" a formula, perhaps by directing it to a specific organ, changing the consistency of the herbal material, or integrating diverse effects. Adjuvants include accelorators and synergists.

When an herb *increases* the effectiveness of another plant or a formula, it is called an "accelerator" in Southern folk medicine. Many of these are "diffusives" that stimulate the nerves or circulation, or both, to help the formula "get into all the corners." Examples here are *Lobelia, Capsicum* (cayenne), and *Zanthoxylum* (prickly ash). Others help a medicine cross the small intestinal membrane. A good example here is the addition of 1 part *Piper nigra* (pepper) to 10 parts *Curcuma* (turmeric) in Ayurvedic medicine. This increases the effectiveness of turmeric many times over. Some accelerators *increase* actions in unknown ways.

Plants that *complement* each other are known as "synergists": the two plants together have more power than either one by itself. For instance, *Crataegus* (hawthorn berry) increases the coronary circulation, while hawthorn leaf and flower increase the peripheral circulation. *Achillea* (yarrow) increases the action of the veins; *Zanthoxylum* of the capillaries—so the two are synergists.

These relationships can only be learned by experience, and are difficult to identify.

Slightly different is the idea of one organ helping another. By strengthening or sedating one organ, we may affect another that depends upon or is being overshadowed by it. For instance, in order to help the heart, we might have to work with the kidneys and lungs as well. William LeSassier used the term "emissary" to describe an herb for an organ that also assists another organ.

Samuel Thomson originated the use of "diffusives"—plants that strongly stimulate the nervous system, firstly for their specific effect, and secondly to help carry a formula deeper into the system. The term diffusive was coined by Dr. John Thatcher in 1810 and not by Thomson, who was functionally and medically illiterate (Wood 2000). The Thomsonian diffusives increase circulation to the periphery or stimulate the deep organs, or both. Eastern chai spices and Chinese "spleen yang tonics" increase circulation to the stomach and center of the body, so are similar to Western herbal carminatives and diffusives.

Diffusives (Thomsonian and related Western herbs): • Achillea (diffusive to the blood and neurovascular system) • Betonica (diffusive through the nerves to head, stomach, periphery) • Capsicum (diffusive to the blood and neurovascular system, heart, and stomach) • Echinacea (diffusive to the lymph and veins) • Liriodendron (gently diffuses the pulmonary circulation and periphery by thinning the blood) • Lobelia (vagal, autonomic diffusive; directs other remedies to their appropriate place) • Myrica (diffusive to the mucosa; increases peripheral circulation) • Phytolacca (diffusive to the nerves, blood, lymph, glands) • Rosmarinus (diffusive to the neurovascular system, brain, spine) • Tsuga (diffusive to the kidneys, lower back, and down to the feet) • Turnera (diffusive to the nerves) • Zanthoxylum (diffusive to the nerves and capillary bed).

Diffusives (Chai Spices, Spleen-Warming Herbs, and Analogs from Eastern Herbalism): • Angelica • Cinnamomum (warming and astringent; bark) • Comptonia (warming, astringent, sweet; Western herb with action like a chai spice) • Elletaria (warming, stimulating) • Eugenia (the cloves are warming and stimulating) • Illicium (warming and stimulating) • Piper (black and white; opens GI pores for increased absorption) • Zingiberis (the dried rhizome is extremely warming).

Organ Affinities: • Achillea (peripheral circulation; veins) • Aesculus hip. (veins) • Acorus (trachea; brain) • Agrimonia (liver) • Alchemilla (pelvic-floor astringent) • Asclepias (synovium) • Astragalus (strengthens the periphery; not diffusive but nutritive) • BETONICA (brain and stomach nervine) • Bupleurum (liver) • Capsella (pelvic-floor stimulant) • CAPSICUM (heart-muscle and peripheral-circulation stimulant) • Carthamus (neurovascular; arterioles; congealed blood; the flowers in formulation, the oil in salves) • CEANOTHUS (broad action on the fluids and lymph system; spleen; neutral in temperature, so combines well with other herbs) • Chimaphila (lymphatics and kidneys) • Chionanthus (gall bladder) • Cimicifuga (brain and spine) • Collinsonia ("golden arc") • CRATAEGUS (berry for coronary circulation; leaves and flowers for peripheral circulation) • Eupatorium purpureum (capillary bed) • Euphrasia (eye) • Helonias (uterus) • HYDRASTIS (stomach, intestines, mucosa and autonomic nervous system)

• Illicium (maxillary sinus) • Lilium longiflorum (cervix)
• Lobelia (autonomic) • Monarda fistulosa (senses) • Panax
ginseng (male, warming) • Panax quinquefolius (female, moistening) • Podophyllum (gall bladder; very small dose) • Rosmarinus (cerebral and spinal circulation) • Smilacina (pelvic-floor
relaxant, nutritive) • Solidago (kidneys, back, feet) • Stellaria
(extracellular matrix) • Tsuga (kidneys, back, feet) • Verbascum
(lungs) • Vinca (cerebral circulation) • Withania (muscles of the
feet and calves) • Zanthoxylum (nervous system, capillary bed;
tongue, throat; small dose).

*Note: Through organ affinity, these agents help deliver the effects of other herbal
agents to an organ, tissue, or system. For example,* Hydrastis *is a neuromuscular tonic with an affinity to the autonomic nervous system, but not to the
heart. So* Capsicum *is added to* Hydrastis *(equal parts), to lead its muscle-
stimulating property to the heart. This simple formula comes from Ellingwood.*

Synergists: • Angelica (with Inula, Marrubium, Asclepias)
• Apium (Taraxacum enhances) • Agrimonia (to coordinate
GI functions) • Arctium (with Mahonia, to add water-soluble
cleansing to fat-soluble) • Cimicifuga (Lobelia enhances action
in muscular spasm) • Curcuma (add 10% Piper nigra—traditional Ayurvedic synergism) • Dipsacus (enhances Polygonatum, Smilacina) • Galium (with Viola—BHP)
• GLYCYRRHIZA (general synergist for all remedies; also
improves taste) • Gnaphalium ("brings together the ingredients
in a formula"—Donahue) • Inula (with Angelica, Marrubium,
Asclepias) • Juglans nigra (Stellaria enhances it for thyroid)
• Lobelia (Zingiberis modifies "bad behavior" of this willful
herb) • Mahonia (Arctium enhances) • Marrubium (with Inula)
• Polygonatum (Althaea enhances it for moistening joints; Dipsacus enhances for large-joint repair) • Prunus serotina (cardiovascular and pulmonary synergist) • Salvia (lemon and honey
are synergists in sage tea) • Smilacina (with Dipsacus for small
joints) • Turnera ("volatilizes the formula"—Popham)

• Verbascum (Lobelia enhances it in atrophy and spasm)
• Veronica (with Apium, for depression) • Viola (with Galium —
BHP) • Viscum (improved by addition of 5% Eleutherococcus — D. Winston) • Zanthoxylum (Achillea enhances its effects
on the capillaries — Hedley) • ZINGIBERIS (lessens griping
pains from cathartics, and moderates Lobelia).

*Note: These agents are called "accelerators" in Southern folk medicine. I am
sure there are many more synergistic plants beyond those listed here. Each
herbalist probably collects his or her own "batch," but they are seldom mentioned in literature.*

Synergistic Effects of Oils Used Externally: • Almond oil
(mildly warming; makes a good base for massage oils) • Bear
grease (slightly cooling; externally, good for injuries and arthritis; internally, used for infertility) • Coconut oil (the most cooling of commonly available oils; combines well with cooling
agents) • Emu oil (muscles, joints, nerves, skin rash) • Ghee
(clarified butter; nutritive effect) • Goose fat (slightly cooling,
watery oil traditional in old European herbalism) • Grapeseed
(the most penetrating oil besides skunk oil; beneficial for the
skin, hair, connective tissue) • Lanolin (warming, good for carrying agents through the skin, but sticky, so not good on fur or
hair) • Lard (warming; a good base for use on skin, good for
carrying agents through the skin) • Mineral oil (does not deteriorate as easily as plant oils, and does not cause hair/fur matting
in animals — Doyle) • Olive oil (mildly warming; widely available and traditional; has healing properties of its own)
• Peanut oil (very warming; an excellent remedy for arthritis,
as a warming massage oil; introduced by George Washington
Carver and recommended by Edgar Cayce; not for people with
peanut allergy) • Rabbit tallow (on the solar plexus for nutrition) • Safflower oil (a good base for a bruise liniment because it
is good in itself for clearing congealed blood — Wood) • Sesame
oil (mildly warming; nutritive and good for pulling toxins;

placed under the tongue) • Skunk oil (the lard, not from the scent glands; the most penetrating oil known) • Sunflower oil (mildly warming, detoxifying, and drawing for use in oil-pulling; placed under the tongue).

A PLANTAIN SALVE FROM EDGAR CAYCE

This very unusual recipe comes from the famous twentieth-century psychic Edgar Cayce. It is notable both because of its source and unique approach. Notice the use of clarified butter or ghee.

"Plantago—fresh root and stalk [this presumably includes the leaves]—six ounces, added to half a gallon of water, cooked down to a jelly formation, until colored black, add unsalted oil of butter fat [ghee] until it makes a salve."

—EDGAR CAYCE READING 46-1; AAWMAGAZINE.COM

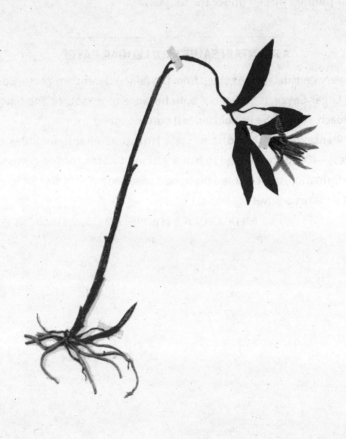

3. Organs and Systems

Mind, Emotions, Will

The old clinicians and philosophers separated the psychological functions into mind (rationality), feeling (emotion), and will (ability to act). This is a simple but useful model. It corresponds roughly with Sheldon's three types and the three doshas: *vata* (rationality), *pitta* (will), and *kapha* (emotion).

We often overlook the will today: people may get their mind and emotions in order, but they are not healthy until they can act upon their aims and desires. The section on will is shorter than the others, as I added it late in compilation.

Western herbalists often now use the Chinese term *shen*, which means "mind" or "spirit." The *shen* is "stored in the heart." *Shen* gives a sense of purpose, equilibrium of emotions and thoughts, inspiration, rationality, and yet emotional meaning, fulfillment, and balance. In a sense, the *shen* unites the mind, emotions, and will into a single effective entity. We have similar ideas in Western languages.

Psychotherapist and herbalist Trilby Sedlacek gave a good overview in a class I attended:

> My general approach to psychological treatment with herbs is to use the basic nervines (*Agrimonia, Avena, Betonica, Eschscholzia, Melissa, Piper methysticum, Passiflora, Tilia, Valeriana, Verbena hastata*, etc.), adjusting the combination for each person. Dose: 10–15 drops, 2–4 times a day. I've gotten people out of psychiatric hospitals, reduced their psych meds, stabilized relationships.

Thanks to Trilby Sedlacek, Sean Donahue, Janet Kent (see her publication *Ease Your Mind*, listed in bibliography), and Althea Northage Orr (see "The Use of Nervines and Other Herbs," also listed in bibliography) for their contributions to this section.

Mind

Concentration, Lack of Focus, Attention Deficit, ADD, ADHD, Hyperactivity: • Achillea (restlessness) • Acorus • Aesculus hip. (obsessive/compulsive) • AMYGDALUS (hyperactivity, restless mind, insomnia) • Avena (nutritive tonic; long-term use) • BACOPA (anxiety, hyperactivity; shortens learning time; increases clarity and acuity; strengthens memory in the elderly) • BETONICA (strengthens brain, increases gut-level instinct) • Ceanothus (ADHD, pupils dilated—Easley) • CENTELLA (peripheral vasodilator increasing blood to the head; for fatigue of mind and body) • Chelidonium (mental torpor from liver toxicity; dullness) • Cnicus (poor circulation to brain) • CRATAEGUS (lack of focus, restless mind; excellent for ADD/ADHD—D. Winston) • Curcuma • Eleutherococcus • Eschscholzia (overactive nervous system) • Filipendula (irritable, restless) • Gingko • Hericium (Rogers) • HYPERICUM ("herb of choice" for ADD/ADHD—Hershoff and Rotelli) • Lavandula (after prolonged concentration) • MELISSA (nervousness; combines well with Tilia) • Mesembryanthemum (ADD, PTSD, anxiety—Rogers) • Nepeta (see "Bullying" in "Will" section, below) • Ocimum (D. Winston) • Oenothera • Panax quinquefolius • Passiflora (excess mental chatter; driven personality) • Prunus serotina • Pulsatilla (emotionally labile) • RHODIOLA • ROSMARINUS (senescent vacuity of thought from blood not rising to the head; see "low blood") • SAMBUCUS (child doesn't listen, overimaginative child, in their own world) • Schisandra ("gathers scattered *shen* [mental focus], astringes consciousness, returns consciousness to the heart"—Donahue) • Scutellaria (physically overstimulated, twitchy) • Thymus (overexcited; bathe in thyme) • TILIA (hyperactivity, nervous excitability; quick speech, mind that "flits from subject to subject"—Parton) • Valeriana (anxiety-producing upset stomach in children; aggressive behavior; sub-sedating dosage) • Vinca minor • Vitis (seed extract) • Withania (overstimulation) • Urtica.

Concentration, Lack of (due to senescence): • ACORUS
• Avena ("work with that myelin sheath"—Sedlacek)
• BACOPA (Alzheimer's Disease) • BETONICA (old age, weakness; fresh leaf) • CENTELLA (senility, fatigue of mind and body) • Cnicus (poor circulation to brain; senility, lost memory or concentration) • CRATAEGUS (lack of focus, restless mind) • GINGKO • Hericium (Rogers) • LAVANDULA
• Lycopodium (premature senility) • OCIMUM • Panax ginseng • ROSMARINUS (senescent loss of concentration and memory; see "low blood") • TILIA (mind "flits from subject to subject"—Parton) • Trigonella ("loss of memory for words, confused ideas and other mental defects from functional causes"—Ellingwood) • Vinca (decreased circulation—Weiss).

Dull or Diminished Mental Function: • Betonica (senescence, weakness) • Chelidonium (mental torpor, liver toxicity)
• Dipsacus (brain fog of Lyme Disease) • Hericium (Rogers)
• Hydrastis ("dull, lethargic, melancholic and depressed type"—Parton; "sharpens the wits"—Boericke) • Mitchella (with edema before menses) • Ocimum (brain fog) • Phytolacca (apathy; "loss of personal delicacy, disregard of surrounding objects; indifferent to life"—Boericke) • Rosmarinus (mental haze)
• Salvia (fever with diminished consciousness).

Prolonged Mental Strain, Working Too Hard: • AVENA
• BORAGO • Lavandula (exhaustion from excessive practice of meditation, *qi gung*, etc.—Ryan) • Leonurus (tired brain—Parton) • Passiflora (insomnia, overwork, worry; has a quieting effect on the nervous system) • VERBENA (prolonged overapplication of will creating sickness).

Memory Lapse, Loss: • Allium ursinum • Arctium (tea of dried burs) • Avena • Bacopa • Betonica (spaciness; senescence) • CENTELLA • Collinsonia (senescence — Stacy Jones) • Crataegus • Equisetum (use with Veronica) • Euphrasia (infusion) • Gingko • Lycopodium (premature aging; can't grasp the right word) • Ocimum • Paeonia • Panax ginseng • ROSMARINUS (age, poor circulation; helps to remember good memories, and forget bad ones — LeSassier) • Salvia • SCHISANDRA • Veronica • VINCA • WITHANIA (neurasthenia, depletion, senescence).

Emotions

Depression: • Achillea ("cut to the bone") • Agrimonia • ALBIZIA (D. Winston) • Apium (languid, debilitated) • ARTEMISIA ABSINTHIUM (brutalized, deadened, insensitive; gregarious façade or flat affect; 1 drop a week to slowly work depression out of the system — Wood; confirmed — Donahue) • Artemisia vulgaris • Astragalus • Avena (with nervous exhaustion) • BUPLEURUM (repressed anger) • CALENDULA (seasonal affective disorder; worse in darkness, cloudy weather; children fear the dark) • CANNABIS (painful, spasmodic diseases) • CEANOTHUS (artistic funk, melancholy) • Centella • Chelidonium (hepatic congestion) • Chelone • Cichorium • CIMICIFUGA (stuck inside self, brooding, withdrawn; in abusive relationship; PMS; nervous exhaustion; can combine with Hypericum) • Cnicus • COLA ("depressive states associated with general muscular weakness" — BHP) • CRATAEGUS (slow-acting; despair, unforgiveness, heartache; poultice of flowers on heart — Schnell) • Equisetum (deep lack of confidence; sitz bath) • Eleutherococcus • Gentiana (self-doubt) • Gingko (in the elderly) • Humulus (flat affect in teenagers — Schnell) • Hydrastis (for the "dull, lethargic, melancholic and depressed type" — Parton) • HYPERICUM (Seasonal Affective Disorder, stuck in a rut; nervous exhaustion and depression, sadness, apathy, low self-esteem, anger, guilt, shame,

isolation, exhaustion, fear; sour disposition and sour stomach—
D. Winston) • IRIS (mood swings, depression) • LACTUCA
(harsh experience, losing track of goal) • LAVANDULA (stagnation; broken heart; "old lingering cobwebs of depression; with
digestive dysfunction" or "depressed without reason"—Schnell)
• Leonurus • Melissa (depression, nervousness, Seasonal Affective Disorder) • Nigella (hormonal imbalance) • OCIMUM
("stagnant depression ... unable to move on"—D. Winston)
• Panax ginseng • Papaver somnifera (menopausal; with arte-
riosclerotic changes in the brain—Weiss) • Piper methysticum
• Populus • Pulsatilla (emotional instability; nervousness)
• Prunus serotina (broken heart; irregular pulse) • Psilocybe
(to reawaken mind and senses) • RHODIOLA (heavy-hearted,
depressed, fatigued) • ROSA (self-judgment—Bennett)
• ROSMARINUS (stagnant depression, general debility, cardiovascular weakness) • Quercus (alcoholism; never gives up
but never succeeds; flower essence or bark) • Salvia (physiological support) • Schisandra • Scutellaria (overstimulation,
edginess) • Selenicereus (apprehension, depression, cardiac disorder, broken heart) • SILPHIUM INTEGRIFOLIUM (needs
a new vision or renewal—Schnell) • Sinapis • TARAXACUM
(manic/depressive disorder; depression; with mapped tongue;
root—Wood) • Thymus • Tilia ("major loss"—Bennett) • Turnera (loss of spirits, libido; depression in elders) • Urtica (physiological support) • Verbena (menopause) • Veronica (with
Apium) • Veronicastrum (with liver pains; 1-drop dose)
• Withania.

*Note: Curing constipation can cure depression. It is believed that this is because
more serotonin is used by the autonomic nervous system than the central nervous
system, and relieving this complaint improves the level of that neurotransmitter.*

Dysthymia, *Taedium Vitae,* **Indifference, Lack of Joy:** • Albizia
(restores capacity for joy) • Carbo vegetabilis (homeopathic;
lack of joy, neither happy nor sad) • Cinchona (apathetic,

indifferent, taciturn; loss of vital fluids, disposition to hurt others) • CRATAEGUS • Hydrastis (depression) • HYPERICUM (apathy, exhaustion, "living in the shadows" — D. Winston) • Oplopanax ("uncertain of right to be in the world" — Donahue) • PEUMUS (gall-bladder problems where "joy of life" has been lost — Welliver) • PHYTOLACCA (sense of apathy, indifference, disregard of surroundings/objects/affairs; small or homeopathic dose) • Polygonum multiflorum (deep exhaustion and indifference) • Podophyllum (depression of spirits; dose of fraction of a drop) • Rhodiola (fatigue) • Tabacum (despondent, discontented, forgetful) • Thuja • Turnera (restores sense of pleasure in the body — Donahue) • Vaccinium myrtillus (life is "empty or meaningless" — Bennett) • Zingiberis ("listless and dispirited" — Huang; dried rhizome).

Note: Characteristic symptoms of mild depression are loss of interest, sadness, tiredness, self-criticism, poor concentration, difficulty in making decisions, irritability, sleep problems, eating too much or too little — this commonly lasts from a few months to a year or two.

Restlessness, Irritability, Excitation: • CRATAEGUS (inability to concentrate, focus; ADD, ADHD — D. Winston; confirmed many times) • Melissa • Prunus serotina • RHEUM ("restless spirit, irritability, easily excited, and fever with sweating" — Huang) • Sambucus (exalted imagination) • Schisandra ("gathers scattered *shen*, astringes consciousness, returns consciousness to the heart" — Donahue) • Scutellaria (overstimulation) • TILIA ("flits from subject to subject" — Parton).

Excitement, Overstimulation: • Apium (mental debility from overstimulation) • HUMULUS (neurasthenia, debility, pain) • Hypericum • PRIMULA (nervous excitability, insomnia, anxiety) • SCUTELLARIA (prophylactic against headaches from stimulating meetings, events, nervous fear, anticipation; takes the edge off intense emotional situations).

Note: In the preceding rubric, the person is restless, while in this one they are overstimulated. The first is a deficiency state, the second an excess. In both states, heat and excitation are the issue, while in the following it is nervousness.

Nervousness, Anxiety, Hysteria: • Acorus (panic with loss of speech; dissociation) • Angelica • Apium (debilitation) • Arctium (worry, with sweaty brow) • Asafoetida • AVENA (tonic; long-term stress, frazzled nerves, hypervigilance) • Bacopa (see "Concentration" sections under "Mind," above) • BETONICA (ungrounded, hysterical, frenzied; weary of stress) • Centella (nervous breakdown) • Chamomilla • Cimicifuga • Crataegus (tonic) • Eschscholzia (agitation, overactive nervous system) • Filipendula (nervous, restless, palpitations, hyperthyroidism) • Galium (tea or tincture) • GANODERMA (nervousness, high-stress work, anger) • GENTIANA (self-doubt) • Humulus (nervous anxiety, tension) • HYPERICUM (pain and hysteria; nerve pains) • Hyssopus • Lactuca • Lavandula (sense of panic and fainting) • LEONURUS (heart palpitations, anxiety, panic; "freaked-out look"—LeSassier) • LYCOPUS (hypervigilant; looks like a hunted animal—Wood) • Majorana • Melilotus (nervous headache, nerviness, nerve pains) • MELISSA (heart palpitations, stomach anxiety) • Mesembryanthemum • Monarda fistulosa (nervousness centered in the stomach) • Monotropa (overwhelming anxiety and panic, sensory overwhelm) • NEPETA (internalizes anxiety in the stomach; menstrual) • Olea (leaf) • Passiflora • Pedicularis • Piper methysticum (social anxiety, panic attacks, anxiety after steroid drug use) • Populus (hyperthyroidism, fear, anxiety, sympathetic excess, shaky sensation in stomach) • Primula ("anxiety states associated with restlessness and irritability"—BHP) • Prunus serotina • PULSATILLA (nervousness, unease, panic attacks, fear of danger; exacerbated where there is "determination of blood to the head"—Scudder) • RHODIOLA (anxiety, nervousness, frenzy, depression, stress, insomnia, restlessness, attention deficit; can aggravate the same symptoms it cures; take in the morning) • Rosmarinus • Salvia • Satureja • Schisandra • SCUTELLARIA (muscular tension, edginess, overstimulation) • Selenicereus (nervousness, insomnia, hyperthyroidism, heart palpitations) • Tilia (restlessness) • Trifolium • Turnera (anxiety neurosis) • VALERIANA (anger and nervousness) • Verbena (neurotic, uptight, driven; "thin *vata* women that hold their head to the side; can't look at the world straight on"—Sedlacek; men too—Wood) • Viola (anxiety, panic, shyness) • Veronica • Viscum (tea) • WITHANIA (stress, worry, thin).

Anger, Irritability, Mental Tension: • AESCULUS HIP. (obsessive/compulsive disorder) • AGRIMONIA (pretends not to be angry; acts out) • Anagallis (rage) • BUPLEURUM (wiry, thin pulses) • CHAMOMILLA (over-expressed anger; whining, peevish, complaining) • Cucurbita citrullus • Ganoderma (stress, anger, anxiety) • Melissa (sunstroke with irritability and belligerence—Donahue) • Monotropa (sudden eruption of rage or affect from the unconscious—Donahue) • NEPETA (bullying; also those who are being bullied) • NUX VOMICA (homeopathic; turbulent, angry personality; indulges in anger) • Piper methysticum • Prunus serotina • Smilacina racemosa • STAPHYSAGRIA (homeopathic; repressed anger, violated, pissed off) • Valeriana (acute, chronic; holds anger inside, causing knots in stomach, low back) • Vinca (behavioral disorders—Weiss) • Viscum.

Forgiveness, Lack of: • Agrimonia • Artemisia absinthium (lack of pity, sympathy) • Borago (feels harshly judged by others—Wood) • Cimicifuga (brooding) • CRATAEGUS • ILEX ACQUIFOLIUM (flower essence) • LIRIODENDRON (feels unforgivable) • MONOTROPA (abuse issues) • Pinus spp. (guilt, shame) • Verbascum (harsh self talk, harsh on self—Popham).

Direction, Lack of, or Needing a New One: • Apocynum andro-saemifolium ("change-or-die" situation) • AGRIMONIA (can't find a solution; "put on papers or around house or office where there are unsolved problems" — Wood) • Betonica (addictions) • CEANOTHUS (artistic funk; can't think their way out of a problem) • Cichorium (self-centered, childish) • Cnicus • Crataegus (stuck in materialistic rut) • Dipsacus (feels use-less) • Eriodictyon (hidden obstructions) • Iris (petty addictions and self-indulgence) • Juglans spp. (dominated by another) • LACTUCA (aimlessness) • Phytolacca (laziness, apathy) • Polygonatum (needs something new in life) • Silphium integ-rifolium (needs a new direction — Schnell) • Quercus (broken-down, defeated, but struggles on; teaches which battles can be won) • Verbena (melancholy).

Melancholy, Creative Issues: • Acorus (writer's block) • Arte-misia vulgaris (can't translate ideas into expression) • ANGEL-ICA (blocked imagination; small dose, or inhale burning root) • CEANOTHUS (artistic funk; melancholy) • HYPERICUM ("fatigue, lethargy, indigestion, a dark outlook, ... emotional unease, and apathy" — D. Winston) • IRIS (substitutes sumptu-ous and beautiful things and addictions for creative expression) • Ledum (frustration, inability to actualize goals; with GI stress) • Ligusticum porteri (blocked imagination; small dose, or inhale burning root) • MONARDA FISTULOSA (self-judgment, blockage of artistic passions) • Nuphar (stuck creativity leading to irritated frustration — Donahue) • Psilocybe • Turnera (loss of pleasure in physical aspects of creative process — Donahue).

Note: Melancholy is not the same as "depression" or "grief" but describes the "funk" that arises from stagnation of the imagination or inability to imagine solutions to creative or life issues.

Addictions, Alcoholism, Drug Abuse, and Food Cravings:
- Acorus (brain fog from cannabis use; craving for alcohol)
- AESCULUS HIP. (specific for obsessive/compulsive disorder) • AMMI (Ayurvedic herb for alcoholism) • ANGELICA ("the writer has known this simple remedy to work wonders"; 5 drops, 3x/day, or infusion—Parton) • Apocynum androsaemifolium (last chance; "change or die"; 1-drop dose) • Arnica (homeopathic; for tobacco addiction) • AVENA (withdrawal from hard-drug addiction) • AGRIMONIA (pain hidden behind a façade; drugs and alcohol; herb or flower essence)
- Artemisia absinthium (cannabis addiction) • Betonica (dependency on alcohol, cannabis; fresh leaf) • Capsicum (classic remedy for delirium tremens from alcohol withdrawal) • Centella (drug addiction) • Chelidonium (sensitivity to alcohol; negative effects of alcohol on liver; cf. Silybum) • Chionanthes (with liver damage) • Cimicifuga (sexual addiction; delirium tremens)
- Crataegus (heroin addiction—Rogers) • Geranium maculatum (restores lost essence; people who need drugs to maintain themselves) • Humulus (withdrawal, DTs) • Hydrastis (atonic mucosa from alcoholism; bad eating habits) • Hypericum (alcohol addiction) • IRIS (hypoglycemia; addiction to sugar, shopping) • Juglans spp. (too much under the influenced of others; insufficient parenting) • Lactuca (loss of direction)
- Larrea (detoxification; toxic headache) • Lobelia • Monotropa (overwhelming psychedelic experience—Donahue) • Nepeta
- Nuphar (compulsive, unsatisfying sex for release of tension—Hale; confirmed—Donahue) • Nymphaea odorata (sex addiction, lascivious thoughts, pining, lovesickness) • Nux vomica (homeopathic standby for clearing recreational or medical drug residues from system, especially before treating chronic cases)
- OCIMUM (traditional cannabis antidote in India; neutralizes past and long-past damage to the body from cannabis use; complex hormonal dysfunction, infertility, extreme PMS aggravation, chronic structural complaints, instability, ligamentous looseness—Davis) • Panax ginseng • Passiflora (sleeplessness;

quieting effect on nervous system; opiate withdrawal, alcoholism) • Phytolacca (laziness, bad habits) • Psilocybe • Plantago • Populus tremuloides (chewing-tobacco addiction — Rogers) • Pulsatilla • QUERCUS (alcoholism, struggle against addictions; improves integrity; oft-proven remedy) • Salix nigra (lascivious thoughts and dreams) • Scutellaria (DTs, withdrawal symptoms) • SILYBUM (ill effects of alcohol on liver; *cf.* Chelidonium) • Sinapis nigra (deranged digestion due to alcoholism; seed) • Staphysagria (homeopathic; put-upon feeling) • Thymus • VERBENA (hormonal food cravings; sexual neurosis).

Infatuation, Lovesickness, Unrequited Love: • Datura stramonium (homeopathic; self-destructive obsession;) • Galium (OCD, tangled up feeling; this herb cleaves the relationship cleanly when over — Bowen, Wolff) • Geranium (helps separate energy between two people at the end of a relationship) • Hyoscamus (homeopathic; insane jealousy, stalking) • Inula (mourning a relationship that felt like home) • Juglans spp. (too much under the influence of another; Bach flower essence, or herb can be used the same way) • NYMPHAEA (pining, wasting, lovesickness; uncontrollable lascivious thoughts) • Origanum (romantic infatuation, relieved by running) • Prunus serotina (irregular pulse from stress on the heart) • Verbena hastata, Verbena (neurotic infatuation; impossible ideals; nymphomania, satyriasis).

Grief, Broken-Heartedness, Separation, Loss of Loved One: • ALBIZIA (heartbreak, loss) • Allium cepa (acute grief, setback) • Amygdalus (cup of the tea when receiving bad news, "to soften the blow" — Light) • Avena (nervous exhaustion) • Crataegus (heartbreak) • Geranium (separates one's energy from another; failed marriage, relationship, or business) • Ignatia (homeopathic; helps one get through the initial trauma of death or bereavement) • Inula (grief from lost home or lost love; "wrong-planet syndrome" — Donahue, Tucker)

• Marrubium (chronic grief) • Monarda fistulosa (self-judgment)
• Nymphaea (weakness, exhaustion, "watchings, pinings, wasting and consumption"—Salmon) • Ocimum (not recovering
from grief—D. Winston) • Prunus serotina (misuse of heart by
another; irregular pulse) • Rhodiola (fatigue from heartache,
loss of a loved one) • ROSA • SELENICEREUS (broken-
heartedness, irregular pulse) • Symplocarpus (deep grief, often
ancestral) • Viscum.

Bipolar Disorder, Manic/Depression: • Astragalus • Crataegus
• Eleutherococcus • Leonurus • Rhodiola (reported to aggravate manic/depression) • TARAXACUM (mapped tongue, neck
tension; use the tongue to monitor: as the condition gets better
the "mapping" goes away; root—Wood).

Obsessive-Compulsive Disorder (OCD): • AESCULUS HIP.
(tortured by one's own thoughts; "quick" pulse; Dr. Bach's
"White Chestnut" works as a flower essence, herb, or homeopathic remedy) • BETONICA (scattered thoughts going
around and around; obsessive thinking; worry about alien
abduction, chemtrails, invisible influences) • GALIUM (obsessive and tangled-up thoughts) • NYMPHAEA (lascivious,
obsessive, romantic, sexual thoughts, pining) • PASSIFOLIA
("quick" pulse).

**Dyspraxia (trouble dealing with people in groups; trouble with
balance):** • Phytolacca (Dowling).

Post-Traumatic Stress Disorder (PTSD): • Acorus (dissociation)
• Anagallis (rage) • Artemisia spp. (dehumanizing experiences;
deadened feeling) • Astragalus • Betonica ("out-of-the-body"
feeling) • Borago (severe, long-lasting nervous strain)
• BUPLEURUM (can bring up memories too precipitously)
• Centella • Cimicifuga (apathy after PTS; recovery of
memory and sequestered parts; use with caution for this

purpose—Donahue) • Eleutherococcus (worn out) • Ganoderma ("metabolizes experience; memories may resurface in
dreams"—Donahue) • Gentiana (self-doubt; worse from setback, shock) • Gnaphalium (ancestral or multigenerational
trauma—Native American usage) • Lactuca (prolonged emotional suffering, aimlessness) • Lobelia • Humulus • Lycopus
(anxious, feels like a hunted animal) • Melissa (combine with
Crataegus) • Monotropa (dissociation) • Nepeta (bullying
issues) • Oplopanax (restores boundaries and sense of safety)
• Ocimum • Rehmannia (uncooked; "pericardium tonic,"
restores healthy boundaries—Stickley) • Rosmarinus (to
remove bad memories—LeSassier) • Ruta • Scutellaria • Tilia.

Shame: • Berberis vulgaris (secret shame, wounds hidden even
from self) • Borago (feels judged by others—Wood) • Liriodendron (lack of self-forgiveness) • PINUS spp. (shame, guilt;
flower essence or herb).

Shock: • ACONITUM (homeopathic; deep shock, animal fear)
• Arnica (homeopathic; shock with bruising;) • Carthamus (oil-
pulling—see "Poisoning") • Ganoderma • GENTIANA (self-
doubt, setback, shock, anaphylaxis) • HYPERICUM ("nervous
shock from fright or fall"—Jones) • Panax ginseng (feeble
pulse, shortness of breath, weakness) • Schisandra.

*In thirty-five years of practice, I have only had one case of anaphylaxis from
exposure to an herb. A woman in a class sniffed corn silk and exclaimed, "I'm
gonna die!" as she turned white. Gentian flower essence (one can use the herb
too) immediately stopped the problem. I learned use of this herb as a remedy
for bee-sting and allergic reaction (from Michael Tierra's* Way of Herbs*)
via a student who had used it.*

Healing of the Soul: • Artemisia absinthium (occasional 1-drop
doses bring up old issues and heal deep wounds) • GANO-
DERMA ("restores the heart and mind connection" and

"promotes peaceful demeanor"—Sedlacek) • UMBELLU-
LARIA (contains the entheogenic substance DMT; helps a person "dream their cure"; semi-roasted nut).

Will

Bullying, Being Bullied: • Agrimony (authority issues, acting out,
making extra work for subordinates) • Borago (verbal abuse)
• Cimicifuga (sullen, withdrawn) • Gentiana (doesn't trust
instincts) • NEPETA (traditional and proven remedy for the
bully and the bullied) • Oplopanax • PULSATILLA (needs
approval of others; young women who are easily dominated,
seduced, manipulated, or bullied).

Willpower: • Acorus ("soggy will"—Donahue) • Agrimonia (sub-
verting will to higher-ups in an organization) • Artemisia absinthium (ruthless, deadened, yet life of the party) • Chamomilla
(disempowered; whining, peevish, complaining) • Chelidonium
(abuse of willpower, especially with occult, spiritual practices)
• Epilobium (flower essence and herb; balances, helps to master will; willful adults are tempered) • Pulsatilla (insecurity,
giving away power) • Rhus spp. (lacking in will, whining,
co-dependent).

FORMULARY

Acorus—with Centella (classic combination for the mind in
Ayurveda).

Albizia—with Crataegus, Rosa flos (depression, broken heart, grief,
sadness). D. Winston. Well-proven, and increasingly widely used.

Avena—with Cola, Turnera, Scutellaria (depression and exhaustion). BHP 1983, 71.

Crataegus—with Tilia, Melissa, Chamomilla (attention deficit,
hyperactivity). D. Winston.

Crataegus—with Avena, Bacopa, and Ocimum (attention deficit,
hyperactivity). D. Winston. A beautiful combination, with mild
nutritive tonic qualities.

Ganoderma—with Crataegus, Avena, Melissa, Tilia, and Scutellaria (mind and heart). D. Winston.

Ganoderma—with Schisandra (shock). Donahue.

Hydrastis—with Populus, 1:4 ratio. For the "dull, lethargic, melancholic and depressed type"—Parton.

Hypericum—with Melissa (seasonal affective disorder). D. Winston. Consider adding Calendula.

Lavandula—with Rosmarinus, Avena, Cola (depression). BHP 1983, 129.

Lavandula—with Rosmarinus, Ocimum, Damiana (stagnation depression; not recovering from a bad experience). D. Winston.

Melissa—Fresh-leaf tincture with honey and milk at night will "wash the whole hard day away"—Sedlacek.

Ocimum—with Tilia. "Formula for volatility in older people who are frustrated by their inability to be in control—like when you take away their car keys"—Sedlacek.

Rosa (thorn)—with Populus tremuloides (so badly hurt they may not recover; suicidal)—old Native American formula. Use the wild rose and aspen Bach flower essences if the herbs are not available.

ST. JOHN'S WORT *(HYPERICUM PERFOLIATUM)*

It seems natural to include a portrait of this herb in this corner of the book, due to its long association with depression. This became a "fad herb" in the 1980s for that condition. Usually I oppose fads in herbalism, but at the time I thought: "a fad could not have happened to a better herb." Then the naysayers piled on—it was said to cause high blood pressure, which it does not do—and St. John's wort was largely forgotten, except by us herbalists. Maybe that is for the best. It does enhance the breakdown of some drugs in the liver—meaning it is a liver detoxifier!—so it can't be used with many prescription drugs. It helps the body metabolize them.

In my opinion, the herbalist who has the best *Hypericum* presentation is David Winston, and I would like to quote him from his wonderful work on adaptogens:

Each herb has a personality—a range of uses, activities, and specific qualities that make it appropriate, or not, for each person.... I believe you get the best results when you treat the patient rather than the disease.... St. John's wort was used for melancholia, which to the Greeks meant that a person had an excess of the black bile. This caused fatigue, lethargy, indigestion, a dark outlook with a sense of emotional unease, and apathy. To a great degree, this describes the type of depression for which St. John's wort is most effective—mild to moderate depression with a sour disposition and "sour stomach." Think of Mr. Scrooge in *A Christmas Carol*. He goes to work every day, he eats, he goes through the motions, but he has no joy in his life. Think of this herb as being useful for people who are in the dark, living a shadow life. It opens the "emotional windows" and lets the sunlight in (Winston and Maimes 2008, 218).

Sleep and Dreams

Sleeplessness, Insomnia: • AMYGDALUS (restlessness) • Angelica (awake at night, groggy in morning) • Apium (nervous debility) • Aralia racemosa (awake at night, groggy in morning) • Artemisia absinthium (night terrors, seizures during sleep) • ARTEMISIA VULGARIS (night terrors) • Asarum canadense • Avena (long-term lack of sleep; nervousness; use long-term dosage) • Betonica (for sleep; fresh leaf) • Calendula (child afraid of the dark) • Caulophyllum (insomnia with uterine irritability) • Chamomilla (can't relax, grouchy) • Chrysanthemum (insomnia) • Cimicifuga (with muscle pain) • Cinchona (restlessness, anxiety) • CINNAMOMUM CASSIA (insomnia; shallow, dream-disturbed sleep; muscle spasms—Huang) • Citrus aurantium (insomnia—Weiss) • Crataegus (falls asleep but wakes up) • ESCHSCHOLZIA (delicate sleeper; difficulty falling asleep, staying asleep) • Filipendula (hyperactivity, hyperthyroidism) • Ganoderma (neurasthenia) • Geranium (waking to pee) • HUMULUS (insomnia; excitement and worry; hops pillow or tea) • HYPERICUM (insomnia, sleepwalking;

nightmares, night terrors, anxiety; kids imagining bad things in closets; "bad mojo"—Schnell) • LACTUCA (specific for mental overwork, negative thinking, hard, slow pulse; small doses for specificity; in large doses, it sedates most people, regardless of constitution) • Lamium • Lavendula (difficulty falling asleep) • Leonurus (nervousness, palpitations, menopausal insomnia) • Lycopodium (to calm thoughts; herb in pillow) • Lycopus (fearful, alert, hyperthyroid) • Matricaria • Melissa (difficulty falling asleep; insomnia due to nervous stomach) • Monarda fistulosa (pillow or tea) • Monarda punctata (nervous excitation) • Monotropa (from physical or mental pain) • Nepeta (restless sleep, nightmares) • Nymphaea (intense thoughts) • PASSIFLORA (circular thinking; difficulty falling asleep; menopause; grinding teeth) • Pedicularis • Piper methysticum (for sleep and dreaming) • Piscidia ("insomnia due to neuralgia or nervous tension"—BHP) • Pulsatilla • Primula (extreme restlessness, nervousness, excitability) • Rheum • Rhodiola ("lull-to-sleep root"—Iceland) • Rumex crispus (nervous stomach) • Scutellaria (sleeplessness, nightmares; with Verbena for sleepwalking) • SENECIO AUREUS (insomnia, menstrual) • Tilia (bath or tincture; insomnia from excitation) • Trifolium • UMBELLULARIA (contains the entheogenic substance DMT; improves sleep; semi-roasted nut) • VALERIANA (nonaddictive sedative) • Verbascum (waking to pee; nervous exhaustion) • Verbena (sleep-walking; with Scutellaria) • WITHANIA (habitual loss of sleep).

Grinding the Teeth: • Chamomilla • Passiflora • Scutellaria.

Dreams, Dream-disturbed Sleep: • Albizia (bad dreams) • Angelica (promotes dreaming) • Aralia racemosa (promotes dreaming) • Artemisia absinthium (night terrors, seizures during sleep) • ARTEMISIA VULGARIS (night terrors; stimulates dreaming) • Betonica (promotes sleep, dreams; fresh leaf) • Calendula (children afraid of the dark) • CINNAMOMUM

CASSIA (insomnia, dream-disturbed sleep, muscle spasms) • HYPERICUM (insomnia, sleepwalking, nightmares, night terrors, anxiety, kids imagining bad things in closets, "bad mojo"—Schnell) • Nepeta (restless sleep, nightmares) • Paeonia (nightmares) • Piper methysticum (promotes sleep and dreaming) • Ruta (see Formulary, below) • Scutellaria (sleeplessness, nightmares; with Verbena, for sleepwalking) • THYMUS (nightmares) • Tilia • UMBELLULARIA (contains the entheogenic substance DMT; promotes spiritual dreams; semi-roasted nut) • Verbena (with Scutellaria, for sleepwalking).

FORMULARY

Melissa—Fresh-leaf tincture with honey and milk at night will "wash the whole hard day away"—Sedlacek.

Passiflora—with Primula and Humulus (insomnia). BHP 1983, 171.

Tilia—with Passiflora, Ganoderma, Lavandula (insomnia, bad dreams). D. Winston.

Verbena—with Scutellaria (sleepwalking).

PEACH LEAF (AMYGDALUS PERSICA)

In addition to being a remedy for insomnia, peach leaf tea is the traditional remedy in the South to give a person when delivering bad news or discipline—to "soften the blow," as Phyllis Light told me. Everybody down there seemed to know about it, but I never heard or read about it in a book. If you don't live there, you just have to have some Southern friends.

"When we were young, we called it BOB—bringer-of-bad news," said Cherokee herbalist Sondra Boyd. "It meant a young person was going to get reprimanded by an elder."

Thomas Easley brought the story up to date: "This has degenerated in the South to a peach branch you rip off to whop somebody. That's called 'peach leaf tea.'"

Brain and Head

The brain, just like any organ, needs to assimilate nutrition and then eliminate waste. When the brain gets constipated, this blockage and subsequent back-up of waste, toxins, sludge, schmutz, goo, plaque—whatever you want to call it—causes your brain to get congested, which can then cause a thousand diseases, from Alzheimer's, senility, eye and hearing disorders to paralysis (Schulze 2011, 91).

The blood is too thick to directly feed the brain, so a sieve called the choroid plexus strains the blood, leaving the red blood cells behind and letting the rest into the ventricles of the brain, where it becomes the cerebrospinal fluid (CSF). This starlight-like substance surrounds all brain and nerve tissue in the body, following the myelin sheaths to the ends of the nerves, spilling out into the extracellular matrix, then returning to the bloodstream via the lymphatic system.

However, before the blood even gets to the choroid plexus, the arteries can sclerose, the veins congest, the capillaries become clogged or fragile, etc. Therefore, in order to eliminate waste and assimilate nutrition, as Richard Schulze says, we need to keep the blood from coagulating or thickening *(Achillea, Liriodendron);* we need to stimulate the circulation to the brain *(Rosmarinus, Gingko, Lavandula, Vinca),* stimulate the nerves *(Betonica, Acorus, Paeonia),* drain the extracellular matrix *(Ceanothus, Equisetum),* and (most of all) keep the CSF flowing without encumbrance *(Cimicifuga).* Research coming out as this book goes to press shows that the brain has a lymphatic system suffused with immune cells. (How could it not?) Therefore, we should think of remedies for these systems as acting on the brain as well *(Ceanothus, Galium, Echinacea,* etc). The benefits of chiropractic, osteopathy, acupuncture, massage, yoga, and exercise (both cerebral and physical) cannot be underestimated.

Whenever there has been a head or spinal injury or stroke, give yarrow *(Achillea)* immediately afterwards in order to prevent further nerve damage from congealed blood pressing on the nerves or blood seeping out of vessels. Congealed blood may remain for months or years after an injury; yarrow can still be used to remove it. If *Arnica* is available, it may be used instead.

Brain: • Acorus (cloudy thinking, difficulty processing language or learning new language) • Apium (exhaustion) • AVENA (exhaustion) • BETONICA (improves circulation; senility, injury, lack of groundedness) • CENTELLA (circulation) • Eleutherococcus • Gelsemium (homeopathic) • Gingko (circulation) • Ilex paraguariensis (increases oxygen to heart, brain; stimulates without causing nervousness) • Lycopodium (premature senility) • Medicago sativa (promotes mental clarity) • Panax quinquefolius (neurasthenia, loss of fluids, atrophy, debilitated habits, exhaustion of brain and nervous system) • Psilocybe (promotes neuroplasticity) • Trigonella ("loss of memory for words, confused ideas and other mental defects from functional causes"—Ellingwood) • Turnera (invigorates) • VINCA (sclerosis; increases cerebral circulation).

Note: Saturated fatty acids in the diet are also beneficial to the brain.

Head Injuries, Concussion, Stroke: • ACHILLEA (bruising, bleeding, pain, stroke, hematoma, thrombosis) • ACORUS • Aesculus hip. (concussion—Weiss) • APOCYNUM ANDROSAEMIFOLIUM (concussion, head injury, whether recent or long ago; 1-drop dose as needed) • ARNICA (homeopathic; shock, stroke) • Bacopa • BETONICA (concussion, hysteria, frenzy, stroke) • CALAMUS (mentally disjointed after head injury) • Carthamus (shock) • Hypericum (pain; convulsions following concussion) • Ocimum • PAEONIA (reorganizes the mind after head injury) • Pedicularis (strengthens cerebral vasculature—Boyd) • Ruta (blow to the head, stroke) • Scutellaria • Symphytum • Vinca (concussion) • Zanthoxylum (pain).

Headache (General): • Achillea (blood congestion) • Acorus (sinus headache, dull thinking) • Agrimonia (migraine, tension)

• Apium (debilitation) • Asarum (sinus headache; can be used with Acorus) • Avena (back of head; exhaustion) • BET-ONICA (neurasthenic, nervous) • Centaurium • CHELIDO-NIUM (migraine, cluster, sensitivity to light) • Cichorium (heat and headache in children) • Chionanthus (with indigestion; gall bladder) • Cimicifuga (ocular) • Citrus limonum
• Clematis (temples) • Cnicus (liver and digestion; frontal)
• Cola (migraine, depression, muscular exhaustion) • Cornus (from fever) • Crataegus • Echinacea (fever) • Eupatorium per-foliatum (crushing pain in head) • Filipendula (nervous, rest-less) • Gentiana (from low blood pressure) • Glechoma
• Hamamelis (from eyestrain) • Humulus • Hydrastis • Hyperi-cum • Ilex paraguariensis (psychogenic headache and fatigue)
• IRIS • Jeffersonia (with vertigo, asthenia) • LAVANDULA (oil on temples) • Leonurus • Levisticum (indigestion and hor-monal) • Lobelia (band across forehead) • Mahonia (gall blad-der, digestive dysfunction, following meals) • MELILOTUS (blood congestion) • Mentha piperita • Menyanthes (with indi-gestion, gall bladder) • Nepeta (nervous) • Passiflora (hyper-tension, nervous debility) • Pedicularis (tension) • Podophyllum (with liver stagnation, constipation; very small dose) • Polygo-natum (occipital) • Phytolacca • Populus tremuloides (dyspep-tic) • Primula vera (tea) • Prunella • Pulsatilla ("determination of blood to the head"—Scudder) • Rhodiola • Rosmarinus (hypertension, migraine) • Ruta (eyestrain) • Salvia • Satureja
• Schisandra (hormonal, liver) • Scutellaria laterifolia (tension)
• Sinapis nigra (in footbath) • Tanacetum balsamita • Tanac-etum parthenium (general nonspecific; one fresh leaf daily)
• Taraxacum • Tilia (heat, high blood pressure) • UMBELLU-LARIA (inner-orbital; inhalation of fresh leaf or tincture of leaf, but this can cause migraine too) • Verbena (tension in neck, cluster) • Veronicastrum (liver, indigestion) • Viburnum opulus (tension; PMS) • Vinca major • Viscum (hypertensive) • Vitex (frontal) • Zingiberis (with cold and cramp).

Headache (Tensive, Nervous, Neuralgic): • Agrimonia (migraine, tension) • Angelica (hypersensitive cranial nerves) • Apium • Avena (back of head; from exhaustion) • BETONICA (general headache remedy) • CHELIDONIUM (migraine, cluster, sensitivity to light; pain from back, to temples, to front of head) • Cimicifuga (ocular; with tight trapezius muscles) • CNICUS (infusion with honey) • HUMULUS • Hypericum • Ilex paraguariensis • Juglans • LAVANDULA (oil on temples) • Leonurus (hormonal) • Lobelia (band across forehead) • KRAMERIA • Mentha piperita • Nepeta • Passiflora (nervous debility, hypertension, with ringing in ears; chronic, in evenings, without hypoglycemia) • Pedicularis (tension) • Piscidia • Pulsatilla (small material dose) • Rosmarinus • Ruta (from eyestrain) • Schisandra (hormonal, liver) • Scutellaria laterifolia (starts in the eyes; tension) • Tanacetum parthenium (one fresh leaf daily) • Tilia (heat; high blood pressure) • UMBELLULARIA (inner-orbital; smell the leaf or tincture of the leaf, but this can cause migraine too) • Verbena (tension in nape of neck; cluster associated with shingles) • Veronicastrum (liver, indigestion) • Viburnum opulus (tension; PMS) • Vinca major • Viscum (hypertension) • Zingiberis (cold and cramp).

Headache (Menstrual, Hormonal): • Achillea • Acorus • Agrimonia • Avena (menopausal; occipital, reflex from uterus—Sherman) • Centaurium • Eupatorium perfoliatum (crushing pain in head) • Filipendula • Gentiana (from low blood pressure) • Glechoma • Leonurus • Levisticum (hormonal and digestive) • MELILOTUS • Mentha piperita • Nepeta (nervous) • Passiflora (nervous debility) • Pulsatilla (top of head) • Schisandra (hormonal, liver) • Tanacetum parthenium (one fresh leaf daily) • Veronicastrum (liver, indigestion) • Viburnum opulus (tension, PMS) • Vitex (frontal) • Zingiberis (cold and cramp; fresh rhizome tea or poultice).

Headache (Congestive, Unequal Distribution of Blood):
• Achillea (blood congestion) • Crataegus • Hamamelis (from eyestrain) • LAVANDULA (oil on temples) • MELILOTUS (congestion, indigestion, throbbing sensations, nervousness; fresh-plant tincture, 3–5 drops in water; or herb vinegar, one teaspoon 4x/hour — Powell) • PULSATILLA ("determination of blood to the head" — Scudder) • Rosmarinus (with excess menstrual flow) • Ruta (eyestrain) • Sinapis nigra (to draw down "high blood"; footbath) • Tanacetum parthenium (preventive, in anabolic-dominant types) • Tribulus (hypertensive).

Note: Hot footbaths are recommended for menstrual or other headaches caused by rising heat or "high blood."

Headache (Associated with Indigestion, Liver): • Acorus (sinus headache, dull thinking) • Agrimonia (migraine, tension) • BETONICA • Centaurium • CHELIDONIUM (migraine, cluster headache, sensitivity to light, back of head to temples to front; aggravated by gall-bladder stress) • Cichorium (heat and headache in children) • Chionanthus (with indigestion, following meals, gall bladder) • Cnicus (associated with liver and digestion; frontal) • Filipendula • Gentiana (from low blood pressure) • IRIS (hypoglycemic, worse from not eating; or due to leaky gut syndrome) • Mahonia (gall bladder, digestive dysfunction, following meals) • Majorana (nervous headache) • Mentha piperita • Menyanthes (migraine, indigestion, gall bladder) • Populus tremuloides (with dyspepsia; take before meals — M. Moore) • Rosmarinus • Sinapis nigra (in footbath, to draw down "high blood" or excess in upper regions) • Tanacetum balsamita (cooling; for liver/gallbladder headaches, after rich food, sometimes relieved by bowel movement) • Tanacetum parthenium (preventive, in anabolic-dominant thick types — M. Moore) • Veronicastrum (liver, indigestion).

Cerebral Circulation Impaired: • ACORUS • BETONICA • CENTELLA • Cnicus • GINGKO • LAVANDULA • Ocimum • ROSMARINUS • Salvia • Ustilago (weak innervation and circulation to the brain and spine; dizziness, unsteadiness) • VINCA (sclerosis — Weiss).

Head Lice: • Azadirachta (lice, fungus, eczema) • Delphinium staphisagria (toxic; external only) • Equisetum (wash) • Juglans nigra (leaf, wash; hull is contraindicated) • Nymphaea (needs confirmation).

Vertigo, Dizziness, Tinnitus, Ménière's Disease: • Betonica • Cimicifuga • Crataegus • Ganoderma • Gingko (dizziness, tinnitus) • Glechoma (middle-ear congestion) • Hydrastis (catarrhal deafness and tinnitus) • Leonurus • MONARDA FISTULOSA (tinnitus, Ménière's disease) • Oxydendrum • Panax ginseng • Tanacetum parthenium • Tilia • Ustilago (poor circulation and innervation; dizziness, unsteadiness) • Verbena.

Fainting: • Achillea (sniff to revive) • Aletris • Chamomilla • Lavendula (oil, applied to side of head) • Rosmarinus (oil, applied to side of head).

Hair and Scalp: • AGRIMONIA (alopecia, local and universal; "always doing something with her hair," "bad hair day"— Wood) • Apocynum cannabinum (external) • ARCTIUM (unhealthy scalp, hair loss; seed in oil externally, root internally) • Arnica (external) • Betula (external) • Capsicum (external) • Ceanothus (flowers; hair tonic, external) • Chamomilla (in rinse, for shine) • Chelidonium (external) • Cichorium (external) • EQUISETUM (thin hair, dandruff) • Juglans nigra (leaf, in lotion) • Lavendula (dry, itchy scalp, no dandruff; oil, external) • MEDICAGO (enhances hair growth) • PLANTAGO (external, on itching rash on back of head above occiput; indicates

toxins in cerebellum and is associated with toxic colon — Fenton)
• POLYGONUM MULTIFLORUM (internal) • POLYMNIA
(hair tonic, external) • Rhodiola (hair wash) • Rosmarinus (dry,
itchy scalp, no dandruff; oil, externally) • SASSAFRAS (oil for
hair lice; topical use only) • Solidago (unhealthy scalp, scabs)
• Urtica (eczema of scalp; brings back hair color and thickens;
leaves or seeds, external and internal).

Sunstroke: • Achillea • Cactus ("tight sensation from sunstroke" —
Clarke) • Chondrus • Lobelia • Hibiscus (preventive; cool tea)
• MELILOTUS (Lakota "sunstroke medicine"; face intensely
red, carotid arteries throbbing, relieved by nosebleed) • Melissa
(sunstroke with irritability and belligerence) • MENTHA
PIPERITA (sunstroke and exhaustion from heat) • Scutellaria
• Tanacetum parthenium.

Cerebrospinal: • Cimicifuga (congestion of CSF) • Ustilago (feeble innervation and circulation).

Low Blood: See "Blood."

FORMULARY

Bacopa — with Hypericum, Gingko, and Ocimum (head injury). D. Winston.

Betonica — with Scutellaria (nervous headache). BHP 1983, 42.

Betonica — with Rosmarinus and Gingko or Vinca (to increase circulation to the brain). Wood.

PERIWINKLE *(VINCA MINOR)*

Rudolf Weiss (1994) is our major modern authority on *Vinca* and its active ingredient, vincamine. Medieval herbalists, he says, considered dried periwinkle to be a remedy for headaches, vertigo, and memory, so the modern uses are sustained by tradition. Modern research and clinical results based on the use of vincamine have verified these assertions. First isolated in 1954, hundreds of papers have since been written about this substance, which has a very pronounced effect on cerebral circulation. Although the properties are well known in European phytotherapy, it is little used in North America.

Periwinkle's major uses are "primarily cerebral arteriosclerosis and the sequelae of strokes. Subjective symptoms such as poor memory, behavior disorders, irritability, restlessness, speech disorders, vertigo and headaches showed particularly good improvement. Mikus considers the main indication to be the milder forms of cerebral arteriosclerosis, with positive response seen in lack of attention and memory disorders, as well as emotional disorders" (Weiss 1994, 180).

Periwinkle has also been used for tinnitus, senescent hearing loss, Ménière's disease, and the sequelae of brain trauma. Cerebral blood flow, oxygen consumption, and blood sugar use in the brain all increase from use of vincamine. Diffuse changes in cerebral electrical activity have also been documented. Concentration and memory are particularly improved; it is believed that this is due to its influence on the cerebral arterioles. All of these uses are implied in the medieval applications. A positive effect on retinal disorders due to impaired blood flow has also been observed.

Vincamine is given orally. It usually takes three to six weeks for the effects to manifest, but it is well tolerated—gastrointestinal upset is infrequent and mild. It is considered contraindicated for brain tumors and diseases where there is intracranial pressure.

Face and Complexion

This section has been included largely to provide diagnostic information. See "Skin" section for information about skin conditions. Diagnosis from the color of the skin comes from Greek, Chinese, and eclectic medicine. Observability may depend on the race of the observer and the patient. If not visible in the skin, check the tongue for color.

Color

Blue and Red: • ACHILLEA (reddish complexion with blue veins) • ARNICA (blue and red) • BUPLEURUM (darkish, blue, red, yellowish) • Capsicum (red, darkish) • CARTHA-MUS (reddish with blue veins) • SAMBUCUS (red, dry cheeks, blue color and swelling over base of nose; marbling red, white, and blue in forearms).

Blue and Yellow: • ANGELICA (blue, green, yellow, gray) • BUPLEURUM (Huang) • CARBO VEGETABILIS (homeopathic; blue and yellow).

Blue, Red, and Yellow: • BUPLEURUM ("blood and *qi* stagnation"—Huang).

Blue and Gray: • RUBIA • SALVIA.

Pale, Fair: • Alchemilla (pale, prominent blue veins—LeSassier) • Angelica (thin and pale; poor digestion and gas with tendency to accumulate fluids) • APOCYNUM CANNABINUM (tight, smooth, glistening, usually blanched, may have pinkish streaks; cardiorenal edema; moderately toxic) • Betonica (pallor) • Carum • Celastrus (blue bands under the eyes; dry, delicate, thin, with general pallor) • CINNAMOMUM CASSIA (thin, fair, spontaneous sweating, pulse high and large) • GNAPHA-LIUM (pale, gray, tawny, yellowish; thin, pale skin from predni-sone) • Mentha piperita (dark circles under eyes, long-standing pallor, cold, anemia, amenorrhea, languor, back and loin pain, full veins) • Plantago (pallor) • REHMANNIA (pale lips, complexion, and tongue from anemia; prepared root) • ROS-MARINUS (weak digestion; cardiopulmonary edema in older persons; thin and weak skin; poor circulation to surface; cool skin; "low blood" or dark color around ankles) • (blue, pale, swollen; edema) • Senecio aureus (pallor, loss of blood, mucus,

pus; uterine prolapse, feeble appetite, backache)
• URTICA.

Yellow: • Calendula (yellowish around the eyes; boneweary—but this is a rare symptom) • BUPLEURUM (wiry pulse, liver conditions) • Ceanothus (doughy, sallow, expressionless) • CHELIDONIUM (jaundice; acute or chronically sallow complexion) • Chionanthus (dirty, sallow skin, expressionless eyes, lusterless hair, hepatic tenderness) • CNICUS (hepatitis) • Dioscorea (conjunctiva) • Euonymus (jaundice) • Nymphaea ("yellowness of the face"—Salmon) • Oenothera (sallow, dirty skin, stagnant lymphatics, torpor of the liver, spleen, mesentery, female organs) • Trigonella (aversion to exercise, overweight; slack muscle tone, stagnant lymphatics).

Note: "Sallow" means a slightly yellow color, usually long-lasting and constitutionally based.

Dirty Appearance: • Chionanthus (dirty-looking, sallow skin, expressionless eyes, lusterless hair, hepatic tenderness) • Euonymus (muddy, from sluggish liver, possibly lung and kidney ailments together) • Rheum (internal heat; reddish, oily, greasy, or dirty).

Dry: • ASCLEPIAS TUBEROSA (dry, full, and hot in fever; dry in chronic conditions) • Bupleurum (dark, reddish, yellowish) • Dioscorea (dry, yellow) • Epilobium (harsh, dirty, contracted) • Equisetum • SALVIA (dry, finely wrinkled, like a sage leaf; lichenification) • Trifolium (chronically dry) • VIOLA.

Damp, Clammy: • CINNAMOMUM CASSIA (easy sweating) • GELSEMIUM (homeopathic; in hot, damp weather) • MELISSA (clammy palms) • MONARDA FISTULOSA (entire skin clammy, cool) • RHUS SPP. (with excess urination or fluid loss; tongue may be dry, but skin moist).

Red, or Red and Pale: • Amygdalus (excitation; skin dry and sensitive; histaminic irritation) • Chamomilla (tension; sensitive skin and moods; one cheek pale, the other red-hot) • Chrysanthemum (normally pale; turning red and full with headache, fever or period) • Crataegus (excitation; meaty parts of palms and elsewhere carmine-red) • Crocus (deeply warming, for cold/depression; pallor alternating with redness; one-sided pulsation) • Grindelia (dry, red, irritable; enlarged spleen or liver with localized pain) • Prunus serotina (excitation; histaminic irritation, redness around wounds; meaty parts of palms red with general yellow tone; liver immune dysfunction—needs confirmation) • Rheum (excitation; cheeks red; yellowish around eyes, nose, mouth) • Rosa (excitation; meaty parts of palms marbled light- and dark-red, indicating heat unevenly penetrating tissues) • Rumex crispus (excitation; yellowness around eyes, nose, mouth; red cheeks) • Ruta.

Gray: • Daucus • Echinacea (dirty-gray visage of the face with chronic tendency to boils, abscesses and carbuncles, with exhaustion) • Gnaphalium (asthma) • Pinus (oxygen-poor, "smoker's complexion") • RUBIA (complexion, tongue) • SALVIA (complexion and tongue) • Urtica (face and skin).

Luminous: • Lilium longiflorum (clear, luminous skin, sometimes marred by acne on the zygomatic arch).

Trigeminal neuralgia: • Aconitum (homeopathic) • Cimicifuga • Gelsemium (homeopathic).

Location
Mouth area: • Althaea (powdery exfoliation of skin outside lips) • Rheum (yellow around mouth, nose, eyes, with red cheeks) • Rumex crispus (yellow around mouth, nose, eyes, with red cheeks).

Eyes (around or under): • Apocynum cannabinum (puffiness beginning under the eyes; pale, tumid, lucid, or wrinkled from recent swelling under the eyes; cardiorenal edema) • ARALIA RACEMOSA (dark circles under eyes; adrenal exhaustion, especially in women) • Celastrus (blue bands under the eyes; dry, delicate, thin with general pallor) • Cinchona (eyes sunken, with dark rings under) • Comptonia (dark, sunken, under eyes) • ELEUTHEROCOCCUS (dark circles under eyes; adrenal exhaustion) • Mentha piperita (dark circles under eyes, long-standing pallor, cold, anemia, amenorrhea, languor, back and loin pain, full veins) • SASSAFRAS (sooty, darkish around the eyes).

Cheeks: • Achillea (rosacea) • CRATAEGUS (red) • Rheum (yellow around mouth, nose, eyes, with red cheeks) • Rumex crispus (yellow around mouth, nose, eyes, with red cheeks).

Freckles: • Potentilla • Primula.

Pigmentation Mask: • Potentilla (over cheeks and bridge of nose) • SEPIA (homeopathic; with uterine exhaustion).

Premature Wrinkling: • Apocynum androsaemifolium (premature and sudden wrinkling) • Chondrus • Salvia (on neck).

Note: This symptom indicates changes in the extracellular matrix.

Wrinkling on Forehead: • Lavandula.

Swollen Face: • Baptisia (swollen and dusky in fevers) • GELSE-MIUM (homeopathic; swollen) • Sambucus (puffy, plethoric).

Note: Swelling of the cheeks may be due to dental infection.

Eyes

Conjunctivitis, Eye Infection, Congestion, Redness: • Acacia (leaf) • Agrimonia (gritty eyes, conjunctivitis; cooled tea eyewash) • Berberis (allergic, chronic; drops — Weiss) • Calendula (eye lotion) • Capsicum (very dilute in eyewash — Christopher) • CHAMOMILLA (compress, eyewash; catarrhal) • Cinerarea maritima • EUPHRASIA (acute infection, pain, sticky mucus, redness, ulceration, acrid tears, congestion) • Foeniculum (eyewash; blepharitis, conjunctivitis) • Fumaria (eye lotion; conjunctivitis) • HAMAMELIS (obstinate conjunctivitis with vascularity of lids) • Hydrastis • Linum (seed, under eyelid) • Lysimachia • Mahonia • PULSATILLA (mucus and redness) • Quercus (drops — Weiss) • Rubus canadensis • SOLIDAGO (allergies, clear mucus, irritation, watering, redness — Boericke; often confirmed).

Inflammation: • Acacia (leaf) • Ambrosia (bloodshot eyes, hay fever) • Berberis (chronic catarrhal, allergic: drops — Weiss) • CALENDULA (external wash) • Capsicum (very small physical doses) • Carthamus (eyelids) • Cichorium (children) • Coptis • Dicentra (corneal ulceration) • Euphrasia • Foeniculum (on eyelids) • Gnaphalium (iritis) • Hamamelis (external) • Hydrastis (acute and sub-acute; cornea, eyelids; external) • Mahonia (chronic catarrhal; external) • Polygala senega • Ruta (burning, hot, strained, easily fatigued, worse from reading or close work) • Salvia sclarea (seed considered a soothing mucilage) • Sassafras (acute) • Saxifraga • STAPHYSAGRIA (homeopathic; corneal abrasion, stye, painful eye) • Thuja (tumors on eyelids).

Stye: • Chamomilla • Commiphora myrrha (early stage; external) • Euphrasia • Hamamelis (fomentation) • Hydrastis • Mahonia (external) • Phytolacca • Pulsatilla (full-blown)

• STAPHYSAGRIA (homeopathic) • Thyme (herb, not oil)
• Xanthorrhiza (in water and salt; apply to eye using dropper).

Tear Ducts: • Achillea (chronic tearing) • Alchemilla (chronic tearing) • Althaea (dry eyes) • Asarum (lachrymitis) • Euphrasia (chronic tearing) • Pulsatilla • Rosa • Thuja.

Black Eye: • Arnica (preventive or after injury; dilution or salve, if skin is unbroken) • Hamamelis (if skin is broken) • Ledum (from a blow; external) • Symphytum (with pain in eyeball; external; root).

Note: Above remedies are from John Henry Clarke, in The Prescriber; *he used them in homeopathic dilution.*

Blepharitis: • Berberis (poultice) • Euphrasia (poultice), Foeniculum (poultice) • Juglans regia (poultice) • Quercus (poultice).

Note: The above remedies are from Rudolf Weiss, via John Sherman.

Bloodshot: • Ambrosia (prominent vessels) • Angelica ("naturopathic visine"—Sherman) • Euphrasia (in patches, burning, itching) • Hyssop (in patches; hot fomentation) • Pulsatilla • Solidago (generalized redness).

Cataract: • Arctium • Chelidonium • Cichorium • Chrysanthemum • Cineraria maritima (external) • Foeniculum ("no case should be operated upon [before this] simple remedy has been tried": use seed powder, infused several hours in 1 oz. cool water; decant and use clear liquid as an eye lotion several times a day—Parton) • Ganoderma • Glycyrrhiza • Ledum ("tonic to the eye lens"—Powell) • Melilotus • Petroselinum • Plantago • Pulsatilla • Sambucus • Saxifraga • Tilia • Vaccinium myrtillus.

Corneal Abrasions, Injuries: • Cineraria maritima (injury)
• Euphrasia (corneal ulcer; drops—Weiss) • Hamamelis (external) • Hydrastis • STAPHYSAGRIA (superb for corneal abrasions; use low homeopathic potency).

Floaters: • Iris ("usually due to liver disorder, unless former injury is the cause. If not due to the latter, use blue flag"—Parton).

Glaucoma, Intraocular Pressure: • Aesculus hip. • Argemone mexicana • Calendula • Cannabis • Capsicum • Cimicifuga • Cinerarea maritima • Clematis • COLEUS (drops in eyes, for temporary relief) • Equisetum • GINGKO • Mahonia • Myrica • PULSATILLA • Rubus canadensis • Saxifraga • VACCINIUM MYRTILLUS.

Grave's Disease (see Hyperthyroidism)

Macular Degeneration: • Vaccinium myrtillus.

Ulcerative Ophthalmia: • Eucalyptus (intense pain; steam or drop of diluted oil in the eye) • Hamamelis (distilled extract, diluted, in the eye).

Iritis: • Bryonia (homeopathic) • Cannabis • Cimicifuga • Gnaphalium • Grindelia • Pulsatilla (viral) • Saxifraga • Thuja.

Lids: • Apocynum cannabinum (wrinkled, as if they had just lost some watery swelling) • Euphrasia (acute inflammation) • Hydrastis.

Swelling Under the Eyes: • Apocynum cannabinum (kidney weakness) • Hamamelis (local treatment).

Note: Probably other diuretics are effective; swelling under the eyes occurs because there are no sweat pores there to relieve water retention from weak kidney function.

Pain: • Bryonia (homeopathic; worse from movement) • Cimicifuga • Erigeron (external) • Grindelia • Pulsatilla.

Sore, Weak, Tired Eyes: • Cimicifuga (eyestrain) • Larix (tired, sore eyes; use as ointment) • Pulsatilla • RUTA • Tilia (weak muscles).

Impaired Vision: • Bupleurum • Chrysanthemum (flower) • GINGKO (macular degeneration, decreased blood flow) • Sambucus • VACCINIUM MYRTILLUS (impaired night vision, nearsightedness, macular degeneration).

Note: Self-heal (Prunella vulgaris) is an old Native hunting remedy in Wisconsin, used to "help see the game against the background."

Retina: • Chrysanthemum (flower) • Fagopyrum (retinitis, retinal hemorrhage) • GINGKO (diabetic retinopathy) • Osmorhiza longistylis (diabetic retinopathy) • Pulsatilla • Rhus spp. (diabetic retinopathy) • Sambucus • VACCINIUM MYRTILLUS (diabetic retinopathy; *retinitis pigmentosa*) • VITIS (strengthens retinal capillaries; seed extract).

Dilation of Pupil: • Belladonna (homeopathic; for fever with dilated pupil; throbbing head and pulse; acts as if possessed by an animal) • Ceanothus (dilated pupil—Easley).

Arteriosclerosis of the Eye: • Vaccinium myrtillus • Vitis (seed extract).

Conjunctiva Yellow (Icteric): • Chelidonium • Podophyllum (small material dosage).

Strain: • Polygala (with alternating hot and cold packs) • Ruta (traditional—needs confirmation).

Dull Appearance of the Eyes: • Galium (dull eyes, poor lymphatic drainage under the chin) • Panax quinquefolius (lack of secretion from "yin deficiency").

Note: Shining eyes are due to hydration, not (I am sorry to say) the "shine of the soul." Almost always, the eyes will brighten when the right remedy is given—perhaps making the soul happier too.

FORMULARY

Borage—emollient eye drops.

Euphrasia—with Hamemelis leaf (eye lotion). BHP 1983, 114.

Fagopyrum—with Vitamin C (to reduce capillary permeability [retinopathy]). BHP 1983, 90

BILBERRY (VACCINIUM MYRTILLUS)

"Strengthens and protects veins and arteries. Helps night vision, improves short-sightedness. Maximum effect in five hours; take before visual tasks. Protects retina against macular degeneration, retinitis pigmentosa, retinal damage in diabetes (also lowers blood sugar) and arteriosclerosis. Reduces pressure in glaucoma and can halt progression of cataracts."

—HERSHOFF AND ROTELLI (2001, 160, CONDENSED)

Ears

The ear is divided into three segments—the outer (which we see), the middle ear or passage (which we don't see), and the inner ear (past the tympanum, or eardrum). The outer ear is seldom a matter for treatment, though it can be a site for eczema and occasionally inflammation. The middle ear empties into the throat, and is a common site for inflammation (otitis media, or middle-ear infection), often associated with upper respiratory tract infections.

The middle ear sometimes becomes congested and plugged, and needs to be opened; I rely on *Glechoma* for this, but other remedies are listed below. Cerumen (earwax) can build up here and cause deafness (*Verbascum*). Inside the tympanum is the inner ear, where the delicate bones capture vibrations that are turned into sounds by our sensorium. Deafness can be due to: (1) blockage of the middle ear; (2) a torn or damaged eardrum (*Alchemilla*); (3) ossification of the bone (*Eupatorium purpureum*); or (4) damage to the nerves (*Monarda fistulosa, Eschscholzia*). This is only a short list, illustrating my general lack of experience on this subject. Loss in the higher range of hearing can be due to sinus infection with swollen tissues.

Middle-Ear Infection (Otitis media), Congestion, Earache:

• Alchemilla • ALLIUM SATIVA (oil) • Ambrosia • Anthemis nobilis (severe "sticking" pains in ear) • Astragalus • Baptisia (fetid discharge from middle ear) • Calendula • Chamomilla (pain with whining and complaining in young children) • Cimicifuga (dull ache; pain in ear from cold) • Echinacea (opens Eustachian tube) • Erigeron (middle-ear infection; oil) • Eucalyptus • Euphrasia (catarrh) • Galium (old, lingering infections and swollen glands) • GLECHOMA (opens Eustachian tube) • Glycyrrhiza • Hydrastis (middle-ear inflammation, hardened wax; ceruminosis, with eczema; otorrhea) • Hypericum (pain, infection) • Larix (decreases severity) • Piper methysticum • Plantago (in equal parts glycerin and water, dropped in the ear for earache) • PULSATILLA (pressure and infection, middle-ear infection in women and children; boils in auditory canal) • Ruta (eyestrain) • Sambucus (antiviral diaphoretic) • Thuja (blocked ear) • Tussilago (juice) • Verbascum (pain and pus in ear) • Viola.

Deafness (Hearing Impaired): • Alchemilla (torn or scarred eardrum) • Allium sativa (fresh, juiced in glycerin and sweet almond oil, dropped in ear) • ESCHSCHOLZIA (damage from rock music and loud noise—Wood) • Eupatorium purpureum (calcification) • Geranium maculatum • Glechoma (middle-ear congestion) • Hydrastis (catarrhal deafness and tinnitus) • Monarda fistulosa (sharpens senses) • Plantago • Pulsatilla (after a chill; mucus congestion) • Urtica (swollen tissues) • Verbascum (removes excess wax) • Vinca (cerebral circulation, sclerosis).

Dizziness, Tinnitus, Ringing in Ears, Giddiness: • Achillea • Allium ursinum (tincture) • CIMICIFUGA (tinnitus, dizziness, vertigo) • Crataegus (tincture) • Geranium maculatum (tincture) • Hydrastis • Lycopodium • Mentha piperita (despondency and dizziness) • MONARDA FISTULOSA (specific for tinnitus and Ménière's disease; 3 drops, 3x/day) • Selenicereus • Tanacetum parthenium (tinnitus, Ménière's) • ROSMARINUS (dizziness) • Veronica (tea) • Vinca • Viscum.

Water in the Ear: • Achillea (tincture in ear). There must be more remedies for this condition.

Earwax: • Hydrastis (excess, with eczema) • Verbascum (excess, congestion; oil in ear).

Note: Ear candling can be done with herbs.

Outer Ear Canal (Eczema): • Hydrastis.

FORMULARY

Verbascum—with Hydrastis, Allium sativa, and Hypericum, in oil (ear drops).

Nose, Sinuses, and Upper Respiratory Tract

Nosebleed: • Achillea (bright-red) • Alchemilla • Ambrosia
• Calendula • Capsella (oozing) • Erigeron (oil) • Equisetum
• Hamamelis • Linaria • Lycopus (chronic) • Lysimachia
• Melilotus • Quercus (chronic) • Viscum.

Nasal Polyps: • MYRICA (powder in nose) • Sanguinaria
(sharply penetrating stimulant astringent; powder) • Thuja.

Allergies (Nose and Sinuses): • Agrimonia (chronic nasopharyn-
geal catarrh) • AMBROSIA (hay fever; bloodshot eyes, runny
eyes and nose; homeopathic, or leaf eaten directly or tinctured)
• Ammi • Angelica • ARALIA RACEMOSA (irritable cough
from wood smoke or dust; worn in the winter; from dry air,
wood stove or furnace) • ARUNDO (homeopathic; maddening
itch in ear and palate) • BIDENS ("great"—Kress) • Equisetum (cedar pollen in New Mexico; also nonspecific; susceptible
to many irritants) • Ocimum ("animal dander and mold")
• Oenothera • PLANTAGO • PROPOLIS (specific for mold,
fungus) • SOLIDAGO (conjunctiva suffused with red; injected,
watery, itchy; nose itchy and running; specific for allergy to cats
and many plants) • URTICA (nonspecific; when susceptible to
many irritants).

Adenitis: • Baptisia • CALENDULA • Galium • PHYTO-
LACCA • Stillingia.

Initial Twinge of Head Cold: • Achillea • Armoracia (opens up
sinuses) • Angelica • Capsicum • Ligusticum • Marrubium
(with salivation) • Mentha piperita • Myrica • Sambucus
(antiviral).

Rhinitis, Sinusitis, Head Cold: • ACHILLEA (hot tea) • Adiantum • Agastache foeniculum • ALLIUM CEPA (runny nose

with excoriated nostrils) • ALLIUM SATIVA • Alnus (hay
fever) • ALTHAEA (hoarseness, laryngitis, with head cold)
• AMBROSIA (chew a leaf for hay fever) • ANEMOPSIS
(swelling and congestion of nose; sub-acute, with thick mucus)
• ANDROGRAPHIS (nasal congestion, cough, sore throat,
muscle stiffness, fever) • Angelica • ARMORACIA (at onset)
• ASCLEPIAS (snuffles in children) • Asarum (dried membranes, with fever) • Astragalus (prophylactic—taken prior to
cold and flu season) • Baptisia (antiseptic; smell from nose or
mouth, swollen glands) • Betonica (catarrh) • Bidens (drippy
nose) • Calendula (raw, tender nose) • Capsicum (warming
and diaphoretic; taken at first hint of rhinitis) • Ceanothus
(chronic sinus discharge, runny) • Cetraria • Chamomilla (hot
diaphoretic, relaxing; use inhalation; sedative as tea) • Cinnamomum spp. (shivering, chilliness, dull mind, difficulty breathing
through the nose) • Commiphora myrrha • Coptis • Echinacea
(worn-out feeling) • Eleutherococcus (increases resistance to
climate stress) • Ephedra vulgaris (decongestant) • Eriodictyon
• Equisetum (hay fever, severe irritation of membrane) • Eucalyptus (inhalation) • Eupatorium perfoliatum (chill/fever, achi-
ness, stiffness, nasal catarrh) • Euphorbia (upper-respiratory
catarrh) • EUPHRASIA (sniffles in children, frontal-sinus
infection) • Filipendula (cooling, soothing) • GANODERMA
(allergic, acute, sub-acute—Hobbs) • GLECHOMA (middle-
ear infection) • GNAPHALIUM • Grindelia • Hamamelis
(catarrh; pallid, flabby mucosa, sluggish circulation) • Hedeoma
(dryness, tight membranes, with fever) • Hydrastis (thick discharge) • Hypericum (colds, flu, depression afterwards)
• HYSSOPUS • Inula (sinusitis, green mucus) • Lomatium
• Lonicera • Mahonia • Marrubium (common cold) • MEN-
THA PIPERITA (as inhalation; hot tea is diaphoretic, relaxing,
cooling) • MENTHA PULEGIUM (diaphoretic) • Myrica
(sinusitis) • Nepeta (head cold with dry skin) • Ocimum ("allergies to animal dander and mold") • PHYTOLACCA • Pinus
(sinusitis, green mucus) • PLANTAGO (mucolytic; post-nasal

drip, feeling of a string hanging down the throat) • Polemonium
• Polygonum bistorta (stimulating astringent; nasal catarrh)
• Populus • PROPOLIS • PULMONARIA • *Rhus* spp. (runny
sinuses, clear mucus) • Rubus canadensis (clear, free secretions)
• Salix alba • SAMBUCUS (antiviral; obstruction in infants;
free sweating or dry, closed skin; "chronic nasal catarrh with
deafness"—BHP; berry or flower) • Sinapis nigra (mustard
seed footbath to draw the blood down) • SOLIDAGO (allergies; "low-grade naso-pharyngeal infection with persistent
catarrh"—BHP) • Teucrium (catarrh) • Tilia • Tussilago
• Ulmus (hoarseness, laryngitis) • Urtica (tea) • Usnea • Verbascum • Verbena (chill/fever, muscle ache, sore neck) • Viola
("chronic naso-pharyngeal catarrh"—BHP) • Zanthoxylum
• ZINGIBERIS (acute rhinitis that starts with chills).

FORMULARY

Capsicum—with Armoracia, Myrica, Zingiberis, or Angelica in
vinegar (used at the beginning of a head cold). These are all variations on "Fire-Cider," introduced by Rosemary Gladstar. It is used
at the first sign of a head cold to dramatically increase circulation
to the area.

Euphrasia—fresh tincture (2 parts) with Solidago (1 part), Glechoma (1 part), and Inula (1 part). "I call this 'sinus-clearing formula.' It supports my store. Stops the swelling, tonifies the mucosa,
opens and drains the mucus"—Sedlacek (paraphrase).

Gnaphalium—(½ part) with Hyssop, Melissa, and Achillea (1 part
each); one cup of infusion when retiring (Old English sinus and
cold formula). Parton.

Sambucus flower—with Tilia flower (common cold, antiviral). BHP 1983, 214. Consider adding Prunus serotina and
Gnaphalium.

Sambucus—with Achillea, Hyssopus, Capsicum, Commiphora
myrrha (common cold). BHP 1983, 73.

Sambucus—with Achillea, Mentha piperita (common cold).

Solidago—with Gnaphalium (persistent nasal catarrh and inflammation). BHP 1983, 234.

Mouth, Gums, Teeth

Inflammation of the gums (gingivitis) occurs in nearly everyone. It is caused by bacteria that lodge between the teeth and the gums. Painless gum recession occurs first, and later inflammation, redness, swelling, tenderness, bleeding, and ultimately loosening of the teeth; this is known as "periodontal disease." If pockets of pus form, the condition is called pyorrhea. The pus pockets erode the gums below the roots of the teeth, corrode the tendons and bones, and loosen the teeth.

In addition to brushing and flossing as prevention for periodontal disease, take antimicrobial stimulants *(Asarum, Thymus, Hydrastis)* to improve circulation and remove bacteria. If the teeth are loose, use *Plantago* to pull out the infection, *Taraxacum* root to stop the decalcification and *Quercus* to tighten the tendons, astringe the gums, and regrow the bones. *Quercus* is also good for the teeth. If pyorrhea has set in (with bad breath), the antiseptic stimulants are needed *(Baptisia, Calendula, Asarum, Propolis)*.

Teeth are subject to cavitation caused by bacteria, against which they are supposedly protected *only* by brushing and flossing. In reality, they are best protected first by their environment and usage, second by care, and third by herbs. The character of the environment is largely set by the saliva, which maintains moisture to wash the teeth, and the acid/base balance. A mildly acid environment favors cavitation, while a mildly alkaline one favors plaque build-up—which hosts the bacteria that cause gingivitis; so we must walk a fine line between the two. Sugar promotes cavitation, while fiber can cause grinding down of the molars.

Bitter and sweet remedies favor salivation—*Panax quinquefolius, Trifolium pratense, Codonopsis,* and *Marrubium,* as appropriate. When the enamel is breaking down, due to either cavitation or hard grains and fibrous food, a restorative remedy is *Quercus.* Try it and watch the miracle. A healthy color for the teeth is not pure white, but faintly yellow.

Discoloration is removed by chewing on a stick of dogwood (*Cornus* spp.), which is an old Native American method. Try it. The Buddha attended to the health of his students, making sure they maintained good oral hygiene by chewing on a certain stick, although I don't know what kind. Chewing contributes to the health of the teeth because it increases saliva to protect them.

Mouth and Gums: • Acacia • Agrimonia (sores on tongue, canker sores) • Ajuga (ulcers and sores) • Alchemilla • Alnus • Alpinia (gum ulcer) • Althaea (infection in mouth, dryness, canker sores) • ASARUM (bad breath) • Baptisia (bad breath, aphthae) • Berberis (flabby, tender gums, bleeding) • Calendula (externally) • Ceanothus • Chamomilla • Cichorium • COMMIPHORA MYRRHA (spongy, sore gums, thrush, pyorrhea) • COPTIS (aphthous ulcers, pyorrhea) • Cornus florida (sore and tender gums) • Echinacea (sore and spongy gums; abscesses, boils) • Equisetum (gingivitis, canker sores) • Galium aparine (ulcers; gargle with warm tea) • Geum (bleeding, spongy gums) • Guaiacum (mouthwash) • Geranium maculatum (bleeding) • Hamamelis (sore gums) • HYDRASTIS (sores on tongue, aphthae, ulcers, gum disease) • Hypericum (gingivitis) • Iris versicolor (gums full and red) • Juglans nigra (gingivitis; leaf, as a gargle) • Krameria (pyorrhea) • Ledum • Lysimachia (bleeding gums) • Mahonia • Myrica (atony of circulation, profuse mucus discharge; pyorrhea) • Phytolacca (blisters, inflammation from low immunity) • PLANTAGO (abscessed teeth, infection after dental surgery or root canal) • Polemonium (spongy gums, ulcerated mouth and throat) • Polygonum bistorta (spongy gums) • Propolis (sores, infections, pyorrhea, bad breath) • Rhodiola (periodontosis) • Rhus spp. (canker sores) • Rumex crispus (thrush) • QUERCUS (dilapidated gums, decalcified jawbones) • Salvia (gum boils or bleeding, canker sores, bad breath) • Sambucus (oil) • Sanicula (astringent; gums, ulcers) • Taraxacum (infection in jawbones; root) • Thuja • Tsuga (aphthae) • Vaccinium (gargle) • Zanthoxylum (stimulant, in small amounts).

Canker Sores (Aphthous Stomatitis), Mouth Ulcers: • Acacia (mucilage) • Agrimonia (astringent) • Ajuga • Althaea (mucilage; flowers, roots, leaves) • Arctium (chronic) • Baptisia (antiseptic stimulant; putrescence) • Berberis (bitter tonic; mucosal stimulant) • Chamomilla (pain; hot gargle) • COMMIPHORA MYRRHA (stimulant; acute, painful) • Coptis (mucosal stimulant) • Echinacea (antiseptic diffusive) • Equisetum • Gautheria • Hydrastis (mucosal stimulant) • Levisticum (mouthwash) • Mahonia (bitter tonic, mucosal stimulant) • Myrica (diffusive stimulant; with hyperacidity and diarrhea, pale mucosa, relaxed tissue, hypersalivation) • Polygonum bistorta (stimulating astringent) • Propolis (external) • Rhus spp. (astringent) • SALVIA (astringent; gargle) • Taraxacum (root) • Thuja • Tsuga (stimulating astringent) • Vaccinium (gargle).

Lips: • Althaea (a mucilage; dry, exfoliating, fine, powdery skin; constitutional if present) • Calendula (cracked; external) • Hydrastis (cracked; external) • Phytolacca (sore, pallid) • Stellaria (cracked; external) • Trifolium pratense (dry) • Thuja (fissured) • Ulmus (mucilage).

Salivary Glands, Saliva: • Althaea (dry mouth and throat) • Capsicum (dry, scanty saliva; poor digestion) • Codonopsis • Commiphora myrrha • Hydrastis (deficient) • Iris (deficient) • Marrubium (excess) • PANAX QUINQUEFOLIUS (deficient) • Stillingia (deficient) • TRIFOLIUM (calcification in; excess or deficient saliva) • Ulmus (dry mouth and throat) • Zanthoxylum (small dose) • ZINGIBERIS (dried; for excess saliva, pale or pale-red tongue, with white or grey, greasy or slimy coating).

Palate: • SALVIA (relaxed throat, prolapsed palate—Jones).

Parotid Glands: • Chimaphila (swollen) • Cimicifuga (swollen) • Phytolacca • Trifolium pratense (swollen).

Teeth: • Achillea (root, in cavity or lost filling) • ECHINACEA (pain) • Cornus florida (brush with fresh, frayed stick to whiten) • EUGENIA (pain; oil on cotton) • Inula (loose teeth; prevents putrefaction) • JUGLANS NIGRA (prevents cavities) • LARREA (daily cup of tea to prevent cavities) • PLANTAGO (abscessed root, sensitive root) • Polygonum bistorta (loose) • QUERCUS (to prevent or cure cavities, loose teeth — Christopher; often confirmed) • Salvia (loose teeth; rub on teeth to whiten) • Solidago (loose teeth) • Urtica (gargle for ten minutes with chlorophyll or nettle concentrate, clean with dietary hydrogen peroxide) • Zanthoxylum (pain).

Note: I am not sure the daily or frequent use of Juglans *or* Larrea *for tooth care, though widely practiced, is always advisable. These are both powerful medicines that could cause side effects.* Juglans *often causes diarrhea in large or continuous doses, and may influence the thyroid.* Larrea *has caused hepatitis when dramatically overused, because it has such a stimulating effect on hepatic function.*

Tooth Abscess, Infected Root: • Arctium • Aristolochia (erosive, fistulous) • Ceanothus • Cnicus (chills and fever from blood poisoning; needs antibiotics) • Echinacea • PLANTAGO (put on tooth) • Solidago • Taraxacum (abscess eroding bone; root).

Loose Teeth: • Quercus • Rumex • Symphytum.

Dentition (Teething): • CHAMOMILLA (fretful, peevish, crying) • Scutellaria.

Breath, Offensive (Halitosis): • Anethum • Apium • ASARUM (superb mouthwash) • BAPTISIA • Carica • Cinnamomum spp. • Coriandrum • Echinacea • Eucalyptus • Eugenia (oil) • Ficus (fetid stomach) • Foeniculum • Galium • Medicago sativa • Petroselinum • Propolis • Salvia.

Mercury, Heavy-Metal Poisoning: • GLECHOMA (heavy-metal poisoning) • Guaiacum (antidote — Bartram) • Plantago (can be used with Glechoma).

Speech: • Acorus (loss of speech due to a trauma — Popham)
• Majorana (with warming herbs, for difficulty of speech due to cold or inflexible muscles — Parkinson).

FORMULARY

Asarum — a traditional American gargle for gums and mouth. This is the superior gargle in taste and effect, in my opinion. Do not overharvest.

Foeniculum — with Rosmarinus, Salvia, Hamamelis (gargle for inflammation of mouth and throat). BHP 1983, 93.

Hydrastis — with Plantago, Quercus, small dose of Zanthoxylum (gums and teeth).

Quercus — with Plantago and Taraxacum root (teeth, gums, and jawbones).

Throat

Sore Throat, Swollen Glands: • Acacia (mucilage) • Agrimonia (astringent; tea) • Althaea (mucilage; hoarseness) • Amygdalus (coolant; hoarse, dry) • Apium • Arctium • BAPTISIA (antiseptic; mononucleosis, diphtheria) • Bidens ("never-ending throat irritation" — Kress) • Calendula • CAPSELLA ("strep throat or tonsillitis cycling from tonsils to kidneys; recurrent tonsillitis in child, usually at three-week intervals" — Croft)
• Ceanothus (broad, swollen tongue, coated dirty white) • Centella • Cetraria (dry mouth, sore throat, dry cough) • Citrus limonum (sore throat, diphtheria) • Collinsonia (constriction; loss of voice, hoarse) • Commiphora myrrha (pallid membrane) • Crataegus • ECHINACEA (antiseptic stimulant; sore throat, tonsillitis, glossitis, laryngitis; with dark-blue or purplish membranes) • Equisetum • Galium (swollen throat glands,

hoarseness) • Geranium maculatum (astringent; chronic pharyngeal catarrh) • Guaiacum (acute tonsillitis) • Hamamelis (sore, red, hyperemic fauces) • Helianthemum (hard, swollen) • Hydrastis (bitter mucosal stimulant; pharyngitis, dryness, ulcers, catarrh, atony) • Hypericum • Juglans nigra (astringent; leaf) • Ledum (stimulating astringent; severe infection) • LIGUSTRUM (privet) • Myrica (diffusive astringent; sore, enfeebled, swollen tissues) • Nymphaea (mucilaginous astringent; sore) • PHYTOLACCA (glandular stimulant; swollen glands, hurts to stick out tongue) • PLANTAGO (topical; mucilaginous astringent; hoarseness) • Polygala senega • Polygonum hydropiperoides • Polygonum bistorta (stimulating astringent; gargle) • Polemonium (ulcerated) • PROPOLIS (loss of voice) • Prunella • Quercus (sore and relaxed) • Ribes nigra (inflammation) • Rubus canadensis (cankerous) • Rumex crispus (chronic sore throat with hypersecretion, swollen glands) • SALVIA ("pharyngitis, uvulitis, stomatitis, gingivitis, glossitis"—BHP; tea, gargle, mouthwash, with lemon and honey) • Sanicula • Scrophularia • Stillingia (dryness with complaints) • Thymus (sore, catarrh) • Trifolium (mumps; swollen glands in back of neck, under and around ears) • Trigonella (hot, dry, sore throat) • Tussilago (hoarseness, pharyngitis) • Verbascum (tension, sore throat).

Elongated Uvula: • Acacia • Collinsonia • Hamamelis • Salvia.

Laryngitis: • Acacia • ACORUS (loss of voice) • Agrimonia • Althaea • Aralia racemosa (chronic; runny mucus, itching throat, worse in dry and winter) • Baptisia • Calendula • Capsicum (dry throat) • Carum (gargle) • Chamomilla • Cinnamomum spp. • COLLINSONIA (laryngeal tension, inflammation with voice loss) • Commiphora myrrha • Echinacea (purulent) • Eryngium spp. • Euphorbia (laryngeal spasm) • Gnaphalium • Hamamelis • Hydrastis • Juglans nigra (catarrhal; leaf teas)

• Marrubium • Phytolacca • Panax ginseng (misuse of voice causing laryngitis) • POPULUS GILEADENSIS • PROPO-LIS (instantaneous voice-producer) • PRUNELLA • Quercus • Salvia • Stillingia (*laryngismus stridulus* or pseudocroup — BHP) • Thymus • Tussilago (tea) • Ulmus.

Pharyngitis: • Acacia (gargle) • Althaea (gargle) • Anemopsis (pale, relaxed mucosa; returns after almost healed) • Aralia racemosa (mucosa) • Castanea (gargle) • Ceanothus • Drosera • Echinacea (acute initial stage; sub-acute) • Foeniculum (gargle) • Grindelia (dried mucus) • Guaiacum (sub-acute, slow to heal; with joint pain) • Hamamelis (with swelling) • Hydrastis (pale, relaxed mucus; granular; with thick, gagging mucus; internal and external) • Ligusticum • Lomatium • Myrica (chronic; with semi-edema, over-secretion) • Nymphaea • Phytolacca (with hard, inflamed nodes in neck) • Polygala senega (thick, tenacious mucus) • Propolis • Rosmarinus • Salvia • Ulmus • Zanthoxylum.

Tracheitis: • ACORUS • Castanea • Drosera • Verbascum.

Strep Throat, Tonsillitis: • Aconitum (homeopathic; first onset) • Anemopsis (ulcerated, boggy membranes; gargle) • Arnica (peritonsillar abscess) • Baptisia (putrid, bad breath, swollen glands) • Capsicum (dry membranes, incipient) • Ceanothus • Chamomilla • Collinsonia • Commiphora myrrha (enlarged nodes; throat pale and tumid) • Echinacea (incipient; putrid) • Gnaphalium (gargle) • Guaiacum (acute, early stage; tumid, swollen) • Hamamelis (swollen, relaxed, congested) • Hydrastis (sub-acute and chronic; encrypted tonsils; catarrh) • Hyssopus • Inula • Ligusticum • Lomatium • Mentha piperita (tea) • Myrica (boggy, relaxed membranes with free secretion; ulcers) • Phytolacca • Polymnia • SALVIA • Sinapis alba (small dose) • Ulmus • Viola (dry membranes, constipation).

Note: Modern antibiotic treatment frequently leaves lingering infection, swollen glands (which the doctors call "scar tissue"), and chronic ill health. In this case, go back and treat the condition as if you were there when it originally occurred—with the appropriate remedy. Give a large dose, or extended small doses, to reproduce the original swelling and inflammation. The following remedies are particularly noteworthy here:

Strep Throat, Tonsillitis, Sore Throat (Relapsing and Chronic Sequelae): • Anemopsis (pale, relaxed mucosa; sore throat returns after almost healed) • Bidens ("never-ending throat irritation"—Kress) • Capsella (strep throat or tonsillitis cycling from tonsils to kidneys; recurrent tonsillitis in child, usually at three-week intervals—Croft) • Inula (swollen glands and irritated lymphoid tissue remain) • Phytolacca (swollen glands, pain worse from sticking out tongue; low immunity; easily gets sick; small dose or homeopathic) • Salvia (swollen glands remain; sage tea) • Solidago (relapsing respiratory conditions) • Viola (swollen glands remain).

Note: The above remedies are for chronically swollen, tender glands and low immunity, remaining years after an infection. Large doses of these remedies (small doses for Poke) stimulate a depurative lymphatic effect.

Voice: • Acorus • Allium cepa (lump in throat, with tears) • Collinsonia • Phytolacca • Pimpinella (clears mucus from throat) • Polygonatum (tension in shoulders and upper chest strains the voice) • Propolis (laryngitis) • Prunella • Verbascum • Vitex (voice changes during menstruation).

FORMULARY

Acacia—with Commiphora myrrha, Hamamelis (gargle for gingivitis, tonsillitis, pharyngitis). BHP 1983, 53.

Commiphora myrrha—with Echinacea, Capsicum, Baptisia, Gnaphalium (tonsillitis, pharyngitis, throat conditions, with septic tendency). BHP 1983, 39.

Prunus serotina—with Pimpinella and Acorus (tracheitis). Modified from BHP 1983, 160.

Salvia—with Potentilla, drops of Propolis (gargle for throat conditions). Modified from BHP 1983, 186.

Thymus serpyllum—with Commiphora myrrha, Rubus canadensis,
Echinacea (acute throat infection, gargle). BHP 1983, 212.

Tongue

The condition of the tongue body and coating has long been used in
both the East and the West as a diagnostic tool. It reveals the general
conditions of the mucosa, blood, and fluids. The various tongue indications are listed in the "Six Tissue States" section, above. A majority
of the indications are from my clinical experience, supplemented by
a half-dozen excellent descriptions by Huang, and a few by Scudder
and others.

Glossitis (Inflammation, Swelling of the Tongue): • Agrimonia
(ulcerative) • Echinacea (septic) • Hydrastis (ulcers) • Myrica
• PLANTAGO (painless, swollen tongue from dampness—
Galen) • Potentilla (ulcers) • SALVIA • Taraxacum • Trigonella • Vaccinium (as gargle, for acute glossitis—Weiss)
• Zanthoxylum (chronic, with hypersecretion, congestion not
inflammation).

Paralysis: • Cinnamomum (Jones).

Tongue Body
Carmine-Red, Elongated, and Pointed (Excitation): • ACHIL-
LEA (red on sides, blue in center; center line opened up and red
within) • Althaea (burnished, shining, reflective surface from
dryness; torn, red) • AMYGDALUS (carmine, pointed, dry,
with red tip, sometimes slightly coated) • Citrus limonum (elongated, red, with prominent papillae, thin white coat)

• Crataegus • Phytolacca (red tip) • Prunus serotina (pointed, carmine-red) • RHEUM (red, elongated tongue—Scudder; "red, tough, firm tongue body with a dry, scorched-yellow coating"—Huang) • ROSA (red, pointed, moist) • RUMEX CRISPUS (pointed, carmine-red, heavily coated white, yeasty, sometimes yellowish) • TILIA (red, pointed; autoimmune excess).

Note: The carmine- or pink-red, elongated, flame-shaped, pointed tongue shows excessive reactivity in the immune system, or a tissue state of the heat and excitation.

Dark-Red (Excitation and Depression): • Baptisia (depression; full, deep-red, brownish in coat) • BUPLEURUM (blood and *qi* stagnation; tension and depression) • BRYONIA (dark-red and dry; cracked; hot and dry membranes and tissue state) • GLE-CHOMA (beefsteak-red; intensely red, darkish, breaking up; severe heat or cancer—Eli Jones; a few confirmations, Wood) • RHEUM (internal heat with "red, tough, firm tongue body with a dry, scorched-yellow coating"—Huang) • TARAXACUM (excitation and stagnation; chronic heat in deeper tissues; adhesive, white coating with ripped-off, peeled, or mapped appearance, or dark-red tongue without any coating—Hahnemann; confirmed numerous times—Wood) • VERATRUM VIRIDE (dark-red streak down the center, with strong pulse indicating very strong fever).

Note: The dark-red tongue shows that heat has penetrated more deeply into the tissues and organs, and the condition is therefore more serious and damaging.

Pale: • Achillea (red edges, pale center; blood in the periphery, absent in the core) • Chelidonium (pale, sallow, full membranes and tongue; slight jaundice) • Chionanthus (tongue and mucosa pale) • CINNAMOMUM CASSIA (pale, or pale and dark, soft; coating thin and white; spontaneous sweating and flushed feeling—Huang) • Galium • Hydrastis (atonic; broad, slightly coated, slightly dry, pale—Boericke; confirmed—Wood) • NYMPHAEA (heavy white coat in center of pale, often dry, wide tongue—Wood) • Phytolacca (pallid, leaden, little coating) • PLANTAGO (painless swelling from dampness—Galen) • ZINGIBERIS (dried; pale or pale-red, with greasy white coating, but may be dark gray and greasy, or white and slimy—Huang).

Note: The broad, pale, moist tongue indicates excessive moisture and lack of tone in the system. The pale tongue indicates anemia or deficient blood or nutrition. The tongue almost never lies, but sometimes a pale tongue presents when heat is there but has slipped deep down into the body, leaving the surface with less blood and resulting in pallor. Yet one expects the tongue to be red from other symptoms indicating heat. This condition needs a stimulant to bring up the heat, and a coolant to sedate the heat.

Blue: • ACHILLEA (red sides, pointed red tip, blue center) • ANGELICA ARCHANGELICA, A. SINENSIS (blue underneath; indicates congested blood in pelvis; often with dysmenorrhea—often confirmed) • Bupleurum (dark red and blue—Huang) • Echinacea • Rubia (blue, grey) • SALVIA (blue, grey).

Note: The blue color is seldom found over the entire tongue body. It is usually found in spots, or in the middle but not on the sides, or in enlarged vessels on the bottom of the tongue. It always indicates stagnant blood and the need for pungent, blood-moving remedies.

Purple, Dark, Brown, or Black: • Baptisia (purple body, brownish coating) • BUPLEURUM (muscular, firm tongue with dark red or purple spots—Huang) • ECHINACEA ("purplish, or dark brown condition, or may even be black"—Massinger) • PHYTOLACCA (purple spot—Wood) • POLYGONUM PERSICARIA (black, dark, brownish, or purple spot in center).

Note: Purple in some region of the tongue indicates a stagnant, overheated condition with tendencies to sepsis. Black indicates tendency to necrosis, only common in the very senescent.

Protuberances (Inflamed Papillae): • Belladonna (homeopathic; fevers with "strawberry tongue") • CALENDULA (pink spots down area between sides and center line — Wood) • Mentha spp. (rubbed on tongue for roughness) • Rubia (strawberry tongue, but somewhat pale and dry, in anemia).

Note: In my experience, protuberances — which are inflamed and swollen papillae — indicate an overactive immune system when they are small and towards the tip. However, if they are medium-sized and in the middle, they represent lymphatic inflammation (if red), stagnation in lymphatics (if pink), or cold lymphatics (if white). Large red or pink spots in the center and back of the tongue body probably represent heat in the colon or pelvis. Enlarged spots on the very back of the tongue are considered to be normal.

Tongue Coating

Dry (Atrophy): • ACHILLEA (dry and blue in center, moist and red on sides; heat with stagnant blood blocking fluids in the center) • ALTHAEA (reddish, reflective, shiny surface with cuts; atrophy and heat driving off fluids) • Arctium (lack of oil) • LYCOPODIUM (atrophy; dry, withered, full of gas — Boericke; homeopathy) • Mahonia (dry) • Nuphar • PANAX QUINQUEFOLIUS (dried-up from lack of heat, or fluids driven off by heat — Hobbs), Rhus spp. (dry tongue with fluid loss from lower channels drying out the upper tissues; this is actually an indication for an astringent for the relaxed tissue state — Wolff).

Note: The dry tongue almost always indicates a lack of fluids and dryness in the internal tissues. A moistening and sometimes nutritive remedy is needed. However, if there is fluid loss, the inner upper areas (such as the tongue) can dry out, and in that case an astringent or warming pungent remedy is needed (see below). If there is red on the tongue body, with dryness, the fluids are being driven off by heat, and the condition needs cooling remedies.

Baked Dry in the Middle: • Bryonia (homeopathic; dark-red, very dark in center, appearing baked-dry) • Baptisia ("swollen, thick, white-coated, yellowish-white; thick fur; baked appearance in middle"—Clarke) • Veratrum viride (homeopathic; dry, red in middle).

Moist (Relaxation): • Comptonia • Geranium maculatum • Rhus spp. • Rubus canadensis • Rumex crispus (carmine-red, pointed, moist, coated), • Tilia (carmine-red, pointed, moist, with auto-immune disease).

Note: Excessive moisture on the tongue almost always indicates the relaxed tissue state, requiring astringents. As the fluids continue to flow from the tissues, they may precipitate into a white coating, which still indicates a need for astringents.

White, Not Adhesive (Relaxation): • Chimaphila (pale, coated white in center) • Geranium maculatum • Lobelia (unequal coat, fully white in back; nausea) • MYRICA • NYMPHAEA (pale, white and moist in center) • Phytolacca (white-coated, with white, foamy saliva) • Pulsatilla (creamy-white coat, nausea, taste of rancid fats) • Rumex crispus (carmine-red, pointed, elongated, with white or slightly yellow coating) • TARAXACUM (white, blotchy, adhesive, mapped; use root) • Veronicastrum (white coat with jaundice, liver pains; light-colored feces) • ZINGIBERIS (pale or pale-red tongue body with white or dark-gray and greasy, or white and slimy coating—Huang).

Note: A white coating indicates that dampness from a relaxed tissue state is precipitating into phlegm. The remedies needed are usually astringents or pungent stimulants to warm the body. When the coating is white it is usually watery, non-adhesive, and more easily washed off, and indicates tissue relaxation. When

*the coating is yellow it is usually oily, adhesive, hard to wash off, and indicates
the stagnant tissue state.*

Thick, Dry, White: • Bryonia (homeopathic) • Pulsatilla (broad,
white-coated).

Regions of the Tongue
*Based on Traditional Chinese Medicine
interpreted by Matthew Wood*

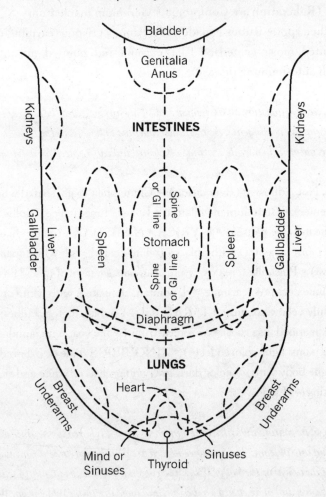

Yellow, Greasy, Adhesive (Stagnation): • Acorus (white coat on tongue matches mental fog) • Althaea (red tongue body, dry yellow coating; "smoker's tongue") • Artemisia absinthium (furred coat) • Berberis (red tongue body) • Euonymus (yellow coat with lack of appetite; liver problems) • Hydrastis (broad, pale tongue, with thin, yellow coating if any) • Mahonia (coated and dry) • Podophyllum (yellow fur, with intestinal torpor; small dose) • RHEUM (red with dried yellow coating).

Note: A yellow coating is usually due to excess oils that are not being processed correctly. They form a thick, adhesive, greasy yellow coating that is difficult to detach. This is the great indicator for what was called "humors in the blood," "canker," or "bad blood" in old-time medicine, and is the single best indicator for the use of an alterative or laxative.

A longtime smoker will usually have a dry, red tongue body with a dry, yellow coating, and a tendency to excoriated tissue. Give Althaea (marshmallow root) palliatively to moisten the mucosa.

Coating Brown (Septic Tendency): • Baptisia (yellow and brown) • Echinacea (brownish or blackish) • Mahonia (yellowish brown) • Menispermum canadense.

Note: Brown is the usual color after a person has just had coffee. If they had coffee several hours ago and the tongue is still coated brown, this indicates that the tongue is not washing itself off well, and needs lubrication (bitters). A naturally brown coating indicates putrefactive tendencies.

Coating Black (Sepsis or Mold): • Chelidonium (dull, leaden) • Echinacea • PROPOLIS (black haze mixed with clear or white coating; indicates mold allergy).

Coating Transparent: • Althaea (reflective surface) • Bryonia (translucent) • Phytolacca (clear, transparent).

Puffy (Sympathetic Deficiency) or Tremulous (Sympathetic Excess) Tongue During Menstruation: • Caulophyllum • Cimicifuga • Mitchella • Pulsatilla • Senecio • Viburnum opulus • Viburnum prunifolium.

Note: This interesting section is from Dr. E.R. Waterhouse (1908, 109). The puffy tongue indicates sympathetic deficiency or parasympathetic excess, and the tremulous tongue sympathetic excess or parasympathetic deficiency. Unfortunately, Dr. Waterhouse does not designate which remedy belongs in each category.

Mapped ("Geographical"): • Arctium (occasionally) • TARAXACUM (specific; seldom fails when the mapped or peeled tongue is present).

Note: The mapped tongue indicates that heat has penetrated deeply into some tissues and organs. The distribution of heat is unequal; according to Chinese theory, the fire is baking down the fluids into phlegm, which blocks the upward-rising heat from escaping the body. This indication for Taraxacum *came from Hahnemann's provings; I have confirmed it scores of times in practice.*

Lungs and Lower Respiratory Tract

The plant world generates oxygen (O_2) as a waste product of the production of energy by photosynthesis. This is used by the animal body to generate energy in its cells. Carbon dioxide and water (CO_2, H_2O) are released as a byproduct of this process. Photosynthesis requires carbon dioxide and generates oxygen, so there is a beautiful circle of life sustaining both plants and animals.

Chlorophyll, the molecule that takes the energy of sunlight and makes it into plant energy through photosynthesis, is responsible for the green color of leaves. It is identical to hemoglobin except that it has a magnesium ion where the latter has iron. Hemoglobin creates the red color of the blood, so the distinctive characteristics (green leaf and red blood) of these two kingdoms—plant and animal—are determined by these amazing molecules.

The respiratory process is a circuit that goes from the capillary bed in the lungs (where oxygen is picked up from the air), through the pulmonary vein, to the heart, through the arterial system, back to the capillary bed. Here the oxygen is attracted out of the blood into the extracellular fluids, and picked up by cells, who use it in "cellular respiration" to fan the fires of cell metabolism and energy production. Carbon dioxide and water, the waste products of cellular respiration, are returned to the blood and move back through the venous system, heart, and pulmonary artery to the capillary bed in the lungs. Here the carbon dioxide and water are discharged into the atmosphere, and new oxygen is picked up to continue the unending process. The exchange in the lungs is called "pulmonary respiration."

The vasculature of the lungs is the opposite of the rest of the body: oxygenated blood flows through the pulmonary *vein*, from the lungs to the heart, and then through the *arteries* to the periphery and back again through the *veins* to the heart, then through the pulmonary *artery* to the capillary bed in the lungs.

We commonly put all the emphasis on the exchange of oxygen and carbon dioxide because this is so obviously essential to life. However, there are other chemical changes of equal importance that occur as part of the respiratory circuit. The release of carbon dioxide, along with the release of uric acid by the kidneys, maintains the acid/alkaline balance of the blood, so acidosis can be caused by respiratory insufficiency. We tend not to think about the other waste product released by the lungs—water. This, however, is also very important. Every exhalation sends out a mist that clouds a mirror or piece of glass held before the mouth. If we did not remove water through the lungs, we would quickly become waterlogged.

For each structure there is an herb or herbs with an affinity to that region, tissue, or organ. The lower respiratory tract begins with the trachea (*Acorus*), descends down to the bifurcation of the tubes (*Allium sativa*), then to the bronchial tubes *(Lobelia)*, which fan out like a tree to reach the mucosa of the periphery *(Lilium)* and the alveoli *(Asclepias)*, where the exchange of O_2 for CO_2 and H_2O takes place. They are kept moist by the secretion of mucin, and open by the secretion of surfactants (*Polygala* and saponins). Mucin is secreted from the extracellular matrix, through cell walls, into the alveoli, to protect and moisten the mucosa of the tract. (*Althaea, Ulmus,* or *Verbascum* is indicated if there is too little mucin; *Rubus canadensis, Ceanothus* if too much; and *Lilium or Inula* if too thick.) The mucin is pushed upwards by cilia or mucosal hairs (*Symphytum, Verbascum* — if the hairs are worn down by prolonged coughing).

The lungs as a whole are surrounded by the pleural cavity and pleural membranes (*Asclepias, Bryonia*). Synovial fluid between the outer surface of the lungs and the inner surface of the pleural membrane, in the pleural cavity, lubricates each respiratory moment so that the lungs move smoothly within us.

Respiratory spasm can occur either in the surface muscles of the chest (*Lactuca*) or in the vagus nerve instructing the diaphragm and movements of the lungs (*Lobelia*). Lung capacity is increased when there is greater oxygen exchange. Dorothy Hall used the iron in nettles (*Urtica*) to stimulate hemoglobin production, which in turn stimulates oxygen uptake and lung capacity.

The terms "free secretion" and "free expectoration" refer to a continual discharge of clear mucin from the respiratory tract due to relaxed tissues and pores of the mucosa. It usually indicates the need for astringents or warming stimulants.

Condition

Asthma: • Achillea (heat) • Aesculus glabra (spasm; continual oppressed respiration) • Agrimonia (spasm; tortured to capture the breath; humid asthma) • Allium cepa (roasted-onion poultice or syrup on chest, to increase circulation in pneumonia) • Allium sativa (dried-out mucus on the trachea and bifurcation of the tubes; general antibiotic and tissue cleanser for the lungs) • Althaea officinalis (dry cough) • Anemopsis (moist cough) • AMMI (spasmodic cough; prevents attacks; long-term use) • Angelica (stimulating astringent and bitter; worn out, exhausted; shortness of breath; psychogenic) • Apium (debility) • Aralia racemosa (dry cough; worse at night, in winter, in dry

air) • Asclepias tuberosa ("dry above, damp below"; nonspas-modic oppression of chest) condition, Asthma, • ASTER (restor-ative, frequently profound) • Betonica (atrophy) • Ceanothus (continual discharge from lungs, sinuses) • Collinsonia
• Commiphora myrrha (moist cough; in elderly) • Convallaria (cardiac asthma) • Crataegus (emotional triggers; ears turn red at onset of attack—Donahue) • Curcuma • DROSERA (constric-tion of chest, spasmodic cough) • Ephedra • Eriodictyon (warm-ing stimulant; old, debilitated cough; free expectoration)
• EUPHORBIA (bronchitic asthma) • Foeniculum • Galium
• Ganoderma (deepens respiration, oxidation) • GECKO (TCM remedy; oppressed respiration, can't breath deeply, pro-fuse sweat) • Gingko • Glechoma • GNAPHALIUM (congenital and infantile onset, lifelong) • GRINDELIA (bronchial asthma with rapid heart action; adhesive mucus, pectoral soreness, raw throat) • Glycyrrhiza • Hieracium pilosella • HYSSOPUS (dry; short of breath; wheezing) • Inula (bronchial asthma; green mucus) • Lactuca (constriction of chest muscles) • Linum (bronchial asthma, irritated mucosa, cough, mucus) • LOBELIA (spasm; worse from tobacco smoke and exercise) • Majorana (cough, tight chest, asthma) • Marrubium (humid cough; "many kinds of coughs," psychogenic—LeSassier) • Melissa
• Mentha piperita • Monarda fistulosa (clammy skin) • Nepeta
• Oplopanax (combines well with Crataegus) • Origanum • Pari-etaria (shortness of breath) • Passiflora (preventive; long-term use) • Pimpinella (spasmodic, barking cough) • Polemonium (asthma, catarrhs, colds, pleurisy, bronchitis) • POLYGALA (children, old people, and others with weak lungs; must sit up; profuse deep mucus with much rattling and wheezing; old cases)
• Populus (panting from hyperthyroid asthma) • Prunus serotina (irritable tissue; spasmodic cough; wheezing and whis-tling in trachea and bronchi) • Ptelea (spasmodic cough, constric-tion of chest) • Pulmonaria (old, broken-down cases; wheezing)
• Sanguinaria (deep infection; dilute with other medicines)
• SQUILLA • Stellaria • Symphytum • Symplocarpus

(spasmodic, often accompanied by phlegm) • Tabebuia (humid asthma with yeast infection) • Thymus (Thyme) • Trifolium (chest tension related to psychogenic cause) • Tussilago • Urtica • Valeriana • Verbascum (cilia worn down; violent, hacking cough) • Veronica • Viburnum prunifolium • Zanthoxylum.

Bronchitis (General): • Achillea • Adiantum • ALLIUM SATIVA • Aesculus glabra (spasm) • Agrimonia (chronic) • Althaea (dry; acute) • Amygdalus (inflammatory, dry) • Anemopsis (moist) • ANGELICA (recent infection or exhaustion from old bronchitis, with exhaustion, dampness; worse from cold and damp; root, seed, internally, at the beginning and end of infection) • Aralia racemosa (irritative, from dry air; roots, berries, in honey) • Armoracia (stimulating adjuvant) • Asafoetida (chronic) • Asclepias tuberosa (acute, dry, hot) • ASTER (spasmodic, irritative) • Baptisia (septic, darkish or purplish complexion; small dose) • Carum • Cetraria (recurrent acute irritation—Weiss; senescence) • Cimicifuga (sore, bruised, stuffy sensation in chest) • Chondrus (weakness) • Cinnamomum spp. (chilliness and shivering) • Collinsonia • Commiphora myrrha (exhaustion, muco-purulence) • DROSERA ("chronic bronchitis with peptic ulceration or gastritis"—BHP) • Equisetum • Eriodictyon (chronic, exhausted cough) • Eucalyptus (steam) • EUPATORIUM PERFOLIATUM (congestion without cough reflex) • Euphorbia • Foeniculum • Galium • Ganoderma • Glechoma (chronic catarrhal) • Glycyrrhiza (catarrh) • GRINDELIA (thick, adhesive, dried-out mucus) • HIERACIUM PILOSELLA (excessive sputum, soreness, hemoptysis) • HYSSOPUS (chronic catarrhal, with anxiety— Weiss; very dry skin and lungs) • INULA (incipient bronchitis; profuse green mucus, upset stomach from swallowing mucus) • Ligusticum • Lilium longiflorum (thick, adhesive, dried mucus, whitish or brown from admixture of blood; red, congested complexion) • LINUM (inflammation; flaxseed oil) • LOBELIA • Lycopus (inflammation) • MARRUBIUM (chronic; nonproductive cough) • Melissa • Mentha piperita (inhalation of essential oil in boiling water—Weiss) • Nepeta (relax spasm) • Petasites • Petroselinum • PIMPINELLA (barking cough "like Cerberus"—Fernie) • Pinus • Plantago (children) • POLYGALA (profuse expectoration, broncho-pneumonia, rattling sound) • Polemonium • Populus gileadensis (chronic; hot, raw) • Propolis (chronic; hot, raw) • PRUNUS SEROTINA (irritation) • PULMONARIA • Sanguinaria ("asthma and bronchitis with feeble peripheral circulation"—BHP; must be diluted with other remedies) • Sanicula • Soli-dago (relapsing; kidneys not strong enough to resolve the fever) • SQUILLA (chronic; scanty sputum) • Stellaria • Stillingia • Symphytum • Symplocarpus (spasmodic; often with phlegm) • Terebintha (medicinal turpentine; 1-drop doses) • Teucrium (chronic) • Thuja (excessive and fetid mucus) • THYMUS • Trigonella (dry, "chesty" cough) • Trillium (excessive catarrh) • TUSSILAGO ("chronic spasmodic bronchial cough"—BHP) • Urtica (plus honey) • VERATRUM (strong, hard pulse with fever) • VERBASCUM (hard, racking cough; intercostal sore-ness; relapsing sub-acute bronchitis) • Viola tricolor.

Bronchitis (Acute): • Achillea • ALLIUM SATIVA • Althaea (dry; acute) • Amygdalus (inflammatory, dry) • Anemopsis (moist) • ANGELICA (at the beginning) • Armoracia (stimu-lant adjuvant) • Asafoetida (preventive) • Cetraria (recurrent acute irritation) • Cinnamomum spp. (chilliness and shivering) • Eucalyptus (upset stomach from swallowing mucus; in chil-dren, elderly; steam) • LOBELIA • MARRUBIUM • Melissa • Mentha piperita (inhale steam from oil in boiling water) • Nepeta (relaxes spasm) • Petasites • Petroselinum • PIMPI-NELLA (barking cough) • Pinus • Plantago (children) • Popu-lus gileadensis (chronic; hot, raw) • Propolis (chronic; hot, raw) • PRUNUS SEROTINA (irritation) • PULMONARIA • Stel-laria • Symphytum • Symplocarpus (spasmodic) • THYMUS • Trigonella (dry, "chesty" cough—Chevalier) • TUSSILAGO

• VERATRUM (strong, hard pulse with fever) • VERBAS-CUM (hard, racking cough; intercostal soreness; relapsing sub-acute bronchitis).

Bronchitis (Chronic): • Agrimonia • Asafoetida (spasmodic) • Cetraria (recurrent acute, irritative, in elderly) • DROSERA • Eriodictyon (weakness) • Eryngium • Eupatorium perfoliatum (nonproductive) • Ganoderma (tonic) • Glechoma (chronic catarrhal) • Grindelia • Hyssopus (dry or catarrhal, with anxiety) • Inula (infection, green mucus; semi-suppressed with antibiotics) • Marrubium • Petasites • Populus gileadensis (hot, raw) • Propolis (hot, raw) • Pulmonaria • Sanguinaria (feeble peripheral circulation) • SQUILLA (scanty mucus) • Terebintha • Teucrium • Thuja (fetid) • Thymus • TUSSILAGO ("chronic spasmodic bronchial cough"—BHP) • Verbascum (relapsing, sub-acute) • Viola (dry).

Bronchitis (Microbial): • Achillea • ALLIUM SATIVA • Anemopsis (moist) • Angelica • Armoracia (stimulant adjuvant) • Asafoetida • Baptisia • Commiphora myrrha (exhausted, muco-purulent) • DROSERA • Eucalyptus (steam) • Hyssopus • INULA (incipient bronchitis, profuse green mucus; swallowing mucus upsets stomach) • Petasites • Pinus • Polygala (profuse expectoration, bronchopneumonia, rattling) • Populus gileadensis (chronic; hot, raw) • Propolis (chronic; hot, raw) • Terebintha (medicinal turpentine—1-drop doses) • THYMUS • Tussilago.

Bronchitis (Dry): • ALLIUM SATIVA (bifurcation of the tubes; dried-out mucus) • Althaea (dry; acute) • Amygdalus (inflammatory, dry) • ARALIA RACEMOSA (irritative, from dry air; roots, berries, in honey) • Asclepias tuberosa (acute, dry, hot) • Cetraria (recurrent, irritative; senescence) • Chondrus (weakness) • EUPATORIUM PERFOLIATUM (congestion without cough reflex) • Foeniculum • Galium • Glycyrrhiza (catarrh)

• GRINDELIA (thick, adhesive, dried-out mucus) • HYS-SOPUS (dry skin and catarrh) • Lilium longiflorum (thick, adhesive, whitish, dried-out mucus) • LINUM (inflammation; fresh ground seed) • Pimpinella • Plantago (children) • Populus gileadensis (chronic; hot, raw) • Propolis (chronic; hot, raw) • PRUNUS SEROTINA (irritation) • Solidago (relapsing) • Stellaria • Symphytum • Trigonella (dry, "chesty" cough — Chevalier) • Tussilago • VERBASCUM (hard, racking cough; intercostal soreness; relapsing sub-acute bronchitis) • Viola tricolor.

Bronchitis (Moist): • Anemopsis • Angelica (internally, at the end; exhaustion, dampness) • Armoracia (stimulant adjuvant) • Commiphora myrrha (stimulant; exhaustion, muco-purulent) • Equisetum • Eucalyptus (steam) • Glycyrrhiza (catarrh) • Grindelia (thick, adhesive, dried-out mucus) • Hieracium pilosella (excessive sputum, soreness, hemoptysis) • Inula • Ligusticum • Marrubium (chronic; nonproductive cough) • Polygala (profuse expectoration, bronchopneumonia, rattling) • Pulmonaria • Symplocarpus (spasm, phlegm) • Thuja • Thymus • Trillium (excessive catarrh) • Tussilago.

Bronchitis (Spasmodic and Irritative): • Aesculus glabra • Agrimonia • Aralia racemosa (irritative) • Asafoetida • Cetraria (recurrent irritative) • Cimicifuga • DROSERA • Eryngium • Hyssopus (irritative) • LOBELIA • Marrubium • Nepeta • Petasites • Pimpinella • Polygala • PRUNUS SEROTINA (irritative) • Sambucus • Symplocarpus • Thymus (combines well with Drosera) • VERBASCUM (hard, racking cough; intercostal soreness; relapsing sub-acute bronchitis).

Bronchitis (Febrile): • Achillea • ALLIUM SATIVA • Agrimonia (chills and fever) • Amygdalus (inflammatory, dry) • Angelica (at the beginning of the chill) • Armoracia (at the beginning of the chill and congestion) • Asclepias tuberosa (to open the skin)

• Cinnamomum spp. (chilliness and shivering) • Lilium longiflorum (thick, adhesive, dried mucus, whitish or brown from
admixture of blood; red, congested complexion) • Ganoderma
• Lentinula • LINUM (inflammation; poultice of fresh-ground
seed on chest) • LOBELIA • Lycopus (inflammation) • Melissa
• Mentha piperita (inhalation of oil from boiling water)
• Nepeta (relax spasm) • Polygala (profuse expectoration, bronchopneumonia, rattling) • PRUNUS SEROTINA (irritation)
• Thymus • VERATRUM (strong, hard pulse with fever).

Bronchorrhea (free secretion of thin mucin from the lungs):
• Ceanothus • Ligusticum • Lobelia • Rubus canadensis • Salix
nigra.

Dyspnea: • Aesculus glabra (bronchial tightness, spasmodic
cough) • Aristolochia serpentaria (small dose; after chill)
• Asclepias tuberosa (oppressed respiration and pulse) • Crataegus • Gecko (with profuse sweat) • Inula • Lactuca (pressure
on chest) • Lobelia (spasm) • Passiflora (relaxes adjacent muscles) • Prunus serotina (cardiopathies, irregular or oppressed
pulse) • Schisandra.

Emphysema: • Equisetum (strengthen cartilage) • Pulmonaria
(strengthen cartilage) • Tussilago (warm tea in morning to
expectorate congealed mucus—Weiss).

Pneumonia: • Allium cepa (syrup on chest to loosen mucus)
• Alchemilla (pockets of water) • Asclepias tuberosa (dry cough
above, wet below; full, oppressed pulse) • Chelidonium (right
lung; liver origin) • Eucalyptus (steam) • Eupatorium perfoliatum (acute lobar; chronic inactive stasis, i.e., the person is congested but has no cough reflex) • Inula • Ligusticum
• Lycopodium (walking pneumonia) • Mentha piperita • Polygala (deep bronchopneumonia) • Sinapis alba, S. nigra (mustard
compress to loosen mucus) • Verbascum • Zingiberis.

Pleurisy: • Aconitum (homeopathic; acute) • ANGELICA (leaf)
• ASCLEPIAS TUBEROSA (can be acute, but usually in old
cases with adhesions in the pleura; sharp pain; oppressed pulse)
• BRYONIA (homeopathic; acute febrile pleurisy, not chronic;
dry, dark-red tongue; serrate/sharp pulse) • Eriodictyon (effu-
sion) • Harpagophytum (pleurodynia) • Linum • Polemonium
• Prunus (hectic cough, rapid breathing; irregular pulse)
• Verbascum.

Tuberculosis: • Achillea (bleeding; pulse rapid, nonresistant)
• Agrimonia (early stages) • Ajuga (pulse rapid, elevated, weak)
• Amygdalus (fever and dryness; lung abscess) • Asclepias
tuberosa • Baptisia (hectic fever and night sweats) • Bidens
(hemorrhaging) • Eriodictyon (exhausted cough, profuse discharge) • Humulus • Lactuca • Lycopus (hemorrhaging from
lungs) • Polygonatum (Occom) • Populus (dry, irritable)
• Prunus serotina (irritation) • Rosa (bleeding and fever)
• Salvia (hectic fever and night sweats) • SENECIO AUREUS
(early stages; hemorrhage, lung fever) • Symphytum (bleeding
from mucosa) • USNEA • Verbascum • Zanthoxylum.

*Note: Tubercular patients lose their civil rights, will be under the control of the
government, and cannot deviate from the prescribed course of treatment. The
above is a list of traditional remedies, perhaps still useful.*

Sleep Apnea, Snoring: • Ammi • Grindelia (breath stops when
falling asleep; waking with a start, gasping for breath)
• URTICA (swollen tissues, often confirmed).

Tobacco addiction and side effects of smoking: • Acorus (reput-
edly helps to quit) • Althaea (dried-out, irritated tissues)
• Aralia racemosa (irritation from dry air, dried-out passages)
• AVENA (reparative to tissues; helps addictions) • CAPSI-
CUM (lessens cravings, improves circulation to the lungs)
• Crataegus • Eriodictyon (weak cough) • Glycyrrhiza

• Grindelia (moistening) • Lilium longiflorum (moistening, decongesting) • LOBELIA (helps to quit and detoxifies, oft-proven) • PLANTAGO (reputedly helps to quit) • Scutellaria • Tussilago (for side effects; shortness of breath, nasty, chronic cough) • Valeriana (antispasmodic) • Zingiberis (antispasmodic).

Note: Many people smoke to relax muscles in order to relieve spasm, temporarily deepen respiration, or have a bowel movement. Attempt to identify any such physiological reason for the addiction, not just treating tobacco use wholly as a pointless addiction. Lobelia is particularly good for relaxing muscles that depend on tobacco addiction and also releasing nicotine from the tissues. Even one dose can bring on "tobacco breath." It will also release opiates and other drugs and cause "flashbacks." It was once an official drug for nicotine addiction, but was discontinued because of its capricious, unpredictable actions. It is best to combine with another herb to lessen the "wicked edge" of lobelia.

Exposure to Smoke, Particulate Matter: • Carbo vegetabilis (homeopathic; problems from exposure to smoke) • Plantago (fibers or particulates in lungs) • Verbascum (pollutants, smoke).

Lung Weakness: • Asarum (chronic cough, debility) • Asclepias tuberosa (pleuritic adhesions) • Chondrus (children and other weak persons) • Codonopsis (thin, weak, tired, dry; shortness of breath) • Commiphora myrrha (chronic cough with debility) • Eriodictyon • Eupatorium perfoliatum • Ganoderma (tonic) • Glycyrrhiza • Liquidambar (chronic debilitation; chest pains, anorexia, diminished strength) • Lobelia (exhaustion) • Marrubium • Styrax (gum benzoin; chronic weakness, debility, chest pains, diminished strength and appetite) • Symphytum • URTICA (increases iron, hemoglobin, respiration).

Cough

Acute, Initial Stages (also see following entry): • Aconitum (homeopathic) • Acorus (tracheal; worse from smoke) • Althaea (irritable fauces) • Aralia racemosa (irritable nose, throat, lungs) • Cannabis (spasmodic, paroxysmal) • Drosera (spasmodic, paroxysmal; irritable mucosa) • Eucalyptus (steam) • Glycyrrhiza • Gnaphalium • Inula (acute bronchitis) • Ligusticum (beginning and end stages) • Lobelia (sudden-onset spasm, paroxysm) • Pimpinella (dry, harsh, sharp, or weak) • Sambucus • Trifolium (irritation of fauces, throat, lungs from fluid running down) • Tussilago (irritable larynx and pharynx) • Ulmus (pharynx and larynx) • Verbascum (dry, harsh, racking; nervousness; tension in throat).

Fever with Cough: • Achillea (flushed face, fever, bronchitis; rapid, nonresistant pulse) • Aconitum (homeopathic; incipient) • Arctium (excess or lack of perspiration) • Asclepias tuberosa (dry skin) • Atropa belladonna (homeopathic; contracted pupils) • Gelsemium (spasmodic, contracted pupils; external only) • Hypericum (chronic inflammation of lungs) • LOBELIA (half of tongue red, or half-coated; high fever; asthma and bronchitis; best to combine with other agents) • Lilium (stuck mucus, with fever) • Lycium (hectic or low-grade fever with fluid loss, wheezing) • MONARDA FISTULOSA (clammy, cold sweat; bronchitis and bronchial asthma) • Polygala senega (bronchopneumonia; dry, hot cough, becoming chronic; with thick mucus at bottom of lungs) • PROPOLIS (hot, raw bronchitis) • SAMBUCUS (young children and old age; bluish complexion) • SENECIO AUREUS (lung fever).

Dry, Irritable: • ALTHAEA (irritating cough with catarrh; root tea or syrup) • Anemopsis (dry, moist, persistent — M. Moore) • ARALIA RACEMOSA (dry, irritative laryngeal cough of allergies, from dry air in winter, wood smoke, night cough) • ASCLEPIAS TUBEROSA (skin dry; after pneumonia, with difficult expectoration; pleurisy) • Betonica (weak cough reflexes) • BIDENS (moistens respiratory mucosa; antiviral — Kress, Buhner) • Bryonia (homeopathic; pleurisy; pain on movement) • Capsicum (with dry mouth) • Castanea (whooping cough/pertussis; to treat and protect other children in the family; American or European chestnut leaf) • Cetraria (recurring irritation; weakness in children and the elderly) • Cimicifuga (whooping cough; stuffy feeling in chest) • Codonopsis (dry, thin, weak, short of breath) • Commiphora myrrha (stimulant; dry, hot; in elderly) • DROSERA (irritable, persistent, explosive) • Eriodictyon (after influenza) • Ganoderma • Glycyrrhiza • Grindelia (dry, harsh; tenacious dry mucus, difficult to raise) • Guaiacum (sub-acute; moist, stubborn, recurrent) • Helianthus (irritative bronchial cough; seed or oil) • HYSSOPUS (dry skin and lungs; chronic, dried-out) • Inula • Lactuca (tightness of chest muscles, asthma without mucus) • Linum (fresh-ground seed poultice on chest) • Lobelia (spasm of the vagus with heartburn and nausea; worse from cigarette smoke) • Lycopus • Marrubium (incipient cough; hard cough with little phlegm) • Paeonia (whooping cough) • Panax quinquefolius (dried-out after febrile lung condition) • PIMPINELLA (harsh, dry, barking "like Cerberus" — Fernie) • Platanus occidentalis (whooping cough; twigs, bark, or heartwood) • Plantago (cough as if a fiber is caught in the lung; dry, irritable) • Polygala senega • Polygonatum (dry throat, thirst, cough due to dry lungs) • Pulmonaria (dry, hacking, night cough; exhaustion) • Pulsatilla • PRUNUS SEROTINA (irritative, continuous; harsh, rasping, hoarse; sore under sternum; irregular or oppressed pulse; incomplete circulation to periphery, histaminic irritation) • Pulmonaria (children's dry cough) • Rumex (dry, irritable cough) • Schisandra • Squilla (scant, tenacious mucus) • Symphytum (worn-down hairs of lungs, ulceration from chemicals, heat; under sternum) • THYMUS (dry, irritated membranes, coughing jags; whooping cough) • Trifolium (irritable, drippy mucosa with cough, hacking) • Trigonella (dry, chesty) • Tussilago (hot, dry cough; infusion of leaves to avoid extracting pyrrolizidines — Weiss) • Ulmus (weak respiration, unable to breathe deeply) • USNEA • Valeriana (when going to asleep)

• VERBASCUM (harsh, racking cough; dry membranes, worn-down hairs of lungs; nervous) • Verbena (tense, irritable cough, dried out membranes; whooping cough) • VIOLA.

Humid, Mucoid, Congested: • Angelica (congestion with influenzal symptoms; old bronchial infections with mucus) • Asclepias (pleuritic stitches from old infections; lungs dry above, wet below; pneumonia, congestive heart failure) • Capsicum • Ceanothus (runny mucus) • Cimicifuga • Eriodictyon (difficult to expel mucus; weak) • Equisetum • EUCALYPTUS (inhalation for congestion) • Eupatorium perfoliatum (lack of cough reflex) • Geum urbanum (avens; catarrhal) • Grindelia (bronchitis; clingy, dried-out mucus; scanty secretion) • Hydrastis (thick, yellow mucus) • INULA (green mucus; acute bronchitis or ripened bronchial discharge; post-nasal drip, digestive upset from swallowing mucus) • Lilium (dried-out mucus stuck in periphery of bronchial tree; with active fever) • Ligusticum • Linum (irritable mucosa) • Lomatium (hard mucus) • MARRUBIUM (congestion, wheezing, full chest, poor expectoration) • Pinus strobus (green, viscid, saplike mucus, difficult to raise) • Plantago (draws out mucus) • Polygala senega (bronchopneumonia) • Polygonum aviculare (knotgrass tea) • Populus tremuloides • Rubus canadensis (runny nose, allergies) • Sambucus (children; croup and viral infection; waking at night) • Solidago (allergies, old infections, mucus) • Squilla (scanty secretion) • Symplocarpus • Tussilago (inflamed, sensitive mucus membranes; infusion of leaves prevents uptake of pyrrolizidines — Weiss) • Urtica (congestion) • Verbascum (bronchorrhea) • Veronica (mucolytic; hot, thick mucus).

Spasmodic, Paroxysmal (Repetitive): • Agrimonia ("tortured to capture the breath," chaotic breathing; ribs bruised) • Amygdalus (dry, red tongue) • Anethum • Asarum canadense (whooping cough) • ASTER (quivery tension in lungs, aggravated by temp/humidity changes). • CASTANEA

• Caulophyllum (strangling, turns blue, hawking and vomiting)
• Chamomilla (poultice on chest) • Cimicifuga (chest tightness;
whooping cough) • Drosera (whooping cough) • Grindelia
(whooping cough) • Lactuca (tight chest) • Linum (fresh-
ground seed poultice on chest) • LOBELIA (twisted tubes)
• Marrubium (whooping cough, adhesive mucus, wheezing)
• Mentha piperita • Monarda punctata (whooping cough)
• PAEONIA (whooping cough) • Passiflora • Petasites • Pimpinella (barking cough) • Potentilla tormentilla (root) • Primula
(rattling) • Pulmonaria (whooping cough) • SAMBUCUS
(croup, suffocative night cough) • SPONGIA TOSTA (homeopathic; croup) • Stillingia • Symplocarpus • THYMUS (con-
vulsive, whooping cough; soothing for bronchitis in the elderly)
• Trifolium (drippy, sputtery; whooping cough) • Tussilago
• Verbena (dried-out, spasmodic) • Viola.

Whooping Cough (Pertussis): • Agrimonia • Asafoetida • Asarum
• CASTANEA (for prevention in other children in the
family; sometimes curative; leaves) • Caulophyllum • Cimicifuga
(5 drops in sweetened water) • DROSERA • Eryngium
• Grindelia • Hieracium pilosella • Lobelia • Marrubium
• Monarda punctata • PAEONIA • Petasites • Platanus
• Prunus serotina • Pulmonaria • Symplocarpus • THYMUS
("treatment of choice"—Weiss) • TRIFOLIUM ("only four
failures in fifty cases"—Jones) • Verbena.

Croup: • Allium sativa • Lobelia • SAMBUCUS • SPONGIA
TOSTA (homeopathic) • TRIFOLIUM.

Debilitated, Exhausted, or Absent: • Allium cepa (syrup on chest
to bring up phlegm) • Aralia racemosa (circles under eyes)
• Asarum canadense (chronic debilitated cough) • Eriodictyon
(exhausted) • EUPATORIUM PERFOLIATUM (absence of
cough with congestion; very sore, holds chest when coughing)
• Grindelia (emphysema; adhesive mucus, difficult to

expectorate) • Marrubium (non-productive) • Osmunda (chronic cough with much perspiration) • Polygala senega (rattling, wheezing, deep, hoarse; bronchopneumonia) • Pulmonaria • Squilla (emphysema) • THYMUS (chronic).

Chronic: • ASTER (quivery tension in lungs) • Aralia racemosa (irritation in throat from dry air in the winter, allergies) • Asarum canadense (debilitated) • Eriodictyon (exhausted) • Grindelia • Helianthus (irritative; seed) • Inula (infection, green mucus) • Lactuca (from tightness of chest muscles) • Osmunda (dry) • Panax quinquefolius (dry) • Tussilago • Viola (dry).

Cilia (hairs on mucosa of the lungs): • Symphytum (damage from chemicals, bleach) • Tussilago (damage from chemicals, chronic cough, lung weakness) • Verbascum (damage from dryness and chronic coughing).

Smoker's Cough: • Althaea • Vaccinium (gargle).

Inhalation Therapy (for coughs): • Chamomilla • EUCALYPTUS (oil) • Majorana • Mentha piperita (oil) • Pinus (oil) • Thymus.

Mucus

Hemoptysis (bloody expectoration): • Achillea • Bidens • Drosera • Erigeron • Lilium longiflorum (blood mixed with mucus, brown in color) • Lycopus • Verbascum.

Mucus: • Achillea (red blood in mucus) • Agrimonia (profuse, thick, sticky) • Allium cepa (small dose for clear, excoriating mucus from nose; onion syrup or pack; to increase circulation to lungs and bring up mucus in pneumonia) • Allium sativa (adherent mucus in larger tubes) • Althaea (bronchial catarrh with digestive weakness; leaf infusion) • Althaea (catarrh with irritating cough; syrup of the root) • Anemopsis (thick white/

opaque mucus; chronic conditions) • Angelica • CASTANEA
• Ceanothus (clear, runny) • Cetraria (nourishing and moistening; dried mucus) • Chondrus (dried-out) • Cinnamomum zeylanicum (bloody) • Cnicus (bitter, to increase secretion)
• Eriodictyon (abundant, easily expectorated mucus) • Eupatorium perfoliatum (congestion but no cough; atonic cough of
senescence) • Equisetum • Glechoma (respiratory catarrh)
• Glycyrrhiza (bronchial catarrh) • Grindelia (adhesive, thick,
dry) • Hieracium pilosella • Illicium (maxillary sinus congestion) • Inula (yellow to green; swallows mucus, which upsets
stomach) • Lilium longiflorum (brown mucus from admixture
of blood; dried-out and lodged in the periphery) • Lomatium
(hard) • Myrica (thick, excessive; poor expulsion) • Nymphaea
(white mucus like pastry starch) • Petroselinum (bronchial
catarrh) • Pimpinella (dried mucus with harsh, barking cough)
• Pinus (green, adhesive, viscid, sap-like) • Plantago
• Pulmonaria • Rhus spp. (clear mucin, free secretion) • Rubus
canadensis (clear mucin, free secretion) • Thymus serpyllum
• *Trigonella* • Tussilago • Veronica.

FORMULARY

Althaea—with Marrubium, Glycyrrhiza, Tussilago, and Lobelia
as an adjuvant (irritative or spasmodic cough). BHP 1983, 22–3.
Compare to the following:

Althaea—with Glechoma, Glycyrrhiza, Tussilago, and Sambucus—
"Dr. Christopher's Cough and Bronchitis Formula" (to resolve
phlegm). Les Moore 2002, 27.

Angelica—with Asclepias, Inula (traditional American formula for
bronchitis).

Asarum—with Caulophyllum (whooping cough).

Asclepias—with Lobelia, Piscidia, Glycerin (spasmodic, irritative
cough).

Chamomilla—with Thymus and Majorana (inhalation therapy for
coughs).

Drosera—with Thymus (whooping cough).

Lobelia—combine with Cimicifuga, Verbascum, or Zingiberis to reduce capricious, erratic action of this plant. Add to other formulas "to send the herbs to the right place" (paraphrasing Dr. Christopher).

Lycopus—with Prunus serotina, Bidens, Asclepias (hot, irritable, hemorrhagic lung condition). BHP 1983, 136. The original base of this formula was Lycopus and Trillium, used for bleeding in mid-nineteenth century America. I would always use Achillea for hemorrhage.

Marrubium—with Hyssopus (bronchial catarrh). BHP 1983, 117.

Marrubium—with Inula, Glechoma, Tussilago, Glycyrrhiza (cough, bronchitis). BHP 1983, 150.

Marrubium—with Pimpinella, Tussilago, Pulmonaria, Lobelia, or Capsicum (bronchitis). BHP 1983, 160, 173.

Marrubium—with Verbascum, Tussilago, Hieracium pilosella, Thymus (whooping cough). Modified from BHP 1983, 159.

Marrubium—with Zingiberis, Thymus (whooping cough). Modified from BHP 1983, 138.

Pimpinella—with Althaea, Verbascum, and Tussilago—"Weiss' Cough Formula" (dry cough). Les Moore 2002, 37.

Thymus—with Castanea, Grindelia, Marrubium, Prunus serotina, Paeonia (whooping cough). Modified from BHP 1983, 53.

Thymus serpyllum—with Prunus serotina, Marrubium, Tussilago, Lobelia (whooping cough). BHP 1983, 212.

Tussilago—with Marrubium, Verbascum, Lobelia (spasmodic, acute and chronic bronchitis). BHP 1983, 227.

NEW ENGLAND ASTER (ASTER NOVAE-ANGLIAE)

This herb was introduced into herbalism by Jim MacDonald, White Lake, Michigan. The beautiful appearance and aroma caught his attention, and he has found it to be an outstanding respiratory remedy. I was unable to include it in the repertory, so I asked Jim to share his notes with us from herbcraft.org. "Tincture of the fresh flowering tops of New England aster is indicated as a respiratory remedy. It is uniquely clearing, relaxing and decongesting to the head & lungs. This effect is readily apparent when taking a bit of the tincture; the effects aren't subtle and can be easily perceived. It seems to act very effectively to break up stuffy lungs and (to a lesser extent) sinus congestion. It's not especially astringent so it doesn't stop a drippy nose as well as, say, goldenrod. It is, however, uniquely antispasmodic for the lung tissue; it relaxes and dilates the respiratory passages. I have repeatedly (though of course not always) seen aster tincture provide a lasting (and seemingly cumulative) effect upon asthma; lessening dependence on an inhaler. As a respiratory relaxant, I think of New England aster when tension is 'quivery' and irritable, whether such a state is acute or chronic. It's less valuable in treating severe spasm states than it is in preventing them. I picture quivery, shivery, shuddery lungs which, if they shudder just enough, trigger coughing or asthma or whatever baleful respiratory woe the afflicted is predisposed to."

Herbalist Sean Donahue writes, "A tincture made from the flowering tops can immediately relieve muscle constriction around the airways. I tend to use about 15 drops in acute situations—most effective when the is tightness around the airway that signals that an attack is imminent but spasms have not begun."

The following would be Jim MacDonald's additions to *The Earthwise Herbal Repertory* for Aster novae-angliae: Asthma: • Aster (restorative, frequently profound). Bronchitis (Dry, Irritable): • ASTER (spasmodic and irritative). Cough (Spasmodic, Paroxysmal, Repetitive): • ASTER (quivery tension in lungs, aggravated by temp/humidity changes). Cough (Chronic): • ASTER (quivery tension in lungs).

Blood

The blood is the major transportation system for materials in the body. It carries glucose, lipids, proteins, and minerals from the wall of the small intestine into the interior of the organism. It also carries oxygen from the lungs to the capillary bed. As chemical forces pull the oxygen off the hemoglobin, out of the capillaries, and into the extracellular matrix, carbon dioxide bonds with the hemoglobin and is carried back with water (the other waste product produced by cellular respiration) to the lungs.

The arterial blood moves under its own power, as mentioned in the section on the heart. Researcher Gerald Pollack has determined why: the water in the blood occurs in a special form, H_3O_2, which carries a negative charge and is attracted into and through the capillaries. In addition, the arterial blood is saltier than the waters flowing out of the saturated matrix around the cells, so it is attracted to these "headwaters" to renew the salt/water balance found throughout the body. Here it discharges its load of oxygen and glucose, picking up the carbon dioxide and water that are the waste products of cellular respiration.

The journey back to the lungs, to discharge the CO_2 and water, now begins in the venous circulation. The veins do not possess the neuromuscular sheaths that the arteries do, and the blood can pool up in them if the capillary bed is congested. Though rid of oxygen and less dynamic in movement, "there is nothing exhausted or dead about the venous blood," Phyllis Light told me in a lengthy conversation we had about the "forgotten side" of the circulation. Venous blood picks up the glucose, minerals, and digested matter from the small intestine and delivers them to the liver. It drops off some of the sugar, which may be stored by the liver, carrying the rest to the arterial blood, from whence it is brought to the capillary bed around the body. It supplies blood sugar to the lungs, which are fed "in reverse" by a vein. The "blue blood" carries away the waste products of cellular respiration, which would flood and kill us without their removal.

The liver also manufactures lipids (cholesterol) and blood proteins, which regulate the blood, making it thicker or thinner, or coagulating it as needed. Traveling further, the venous blood passes the hypothalamus, where its contents are assessed. The hypothalamus, like a nurse, pulls blood for testing from a vein, not an artery. The venous blood also receives the important red, white, and platelet cells produced in the bone marrow.

The kidneys adjust salt and water levels by removing some sodium; the venous blood released from the kidneys is therefore more bland. This fine-tuning of salt levels maintains blood pressure by enlarging or reducing the size of the extracellular matrix. It is actually sodium that pulls the water from the blood in the capillary bed into the matrix or the glomerulus of the kidneys. Higher blood-sodium levels cause the blood to retain more water. (This might seem counterintuitive, since a salty mouth feels dry; yet it craves water and we drink more — taking in more water to balance the salt). Higher sodium causes higher blood pressure as the matrix plumps up and shrinks the available space for blood to circulate.

The thickening and thinning of the blood is a very important aspect of our metabolism. It is controlled by several factors. Low salt and water levels need adjustment to "plump up" the amount and con-sistency of the blood. Prostaglandins control the thickening or thin-ning of the blood through changes in lipid levels. They also control the arachadonic acid cascade that regulates the fever mechanism and influence corticosteroids, so the thickening and thinning of the blood is tied in with a lot of mechanisms regulating heat, fever, immunity, and self-healing. Thicker blood is more insulative, as oil insulates bet-ter than water. In biomedicine blood is thinned with aspirin (among other things) which act on the prostaglandins regulating blood and fever. This was the custome in Southern folk medicine, a long time before modern medicine came along. Tulip poplar bark *(Liriodendron)* has salicylates like aspirin that thin the blood.

The liver makes cholesterol and sends it into the bloodstream. All cholesterol is innately "good," until genetics or lifestyle puts it out of balance. The so-called "bad" cholesterol (LDLs) has the positive purpose of plopping patches on tears and rough spots on the vascu-lar walls — like poor-quality plaster slapped on the wall by a slum landlord. "Good" cholesterol (HDLs) acts like a "sander" to smooth out the blobs of LDLs which would, otherwise, act as a nucleous for clotting blood and attract bacterial colonies to feed off the garbage. High levels of HDLs are good; high levels of LDLs are "mischief-prone" when deposited in excess. This causes various health changes such as high blood pressure.

Anemia is usually associated with low iron, or poor assimilation or storage of iron, but can also be caused by poor nutrition in general. "Kidney anemia" occurs when the kidneys don't signal the bone marrow to produce more blood cells. In this case, the tongue is pale but moist. The bone marrow needs nourishment to manufacture good red, white, and replacement cells. Other kinds of anemia usually have a pale, dry tongue.

Blood, Congealed; Bruising: • ACHILLEA (thrombosis, bruising, hematoma; complexion red and blue) • Ajuga • Allium sativa (to lower excess fibrin through lysis) • ANGELICA (bruising or blue, green, yellow, grey complexion) • ARNICA (bruising, chronic blood coagulation; complexion red and blue; external) • BUPLEURUM (chronic; darkish, reddish complexion) • CAPSICUM (thins the blood, equalizes the circulation) • CARTHAMUS (complexion red and blue; coagulated blood) • Prunus serotina (neurovascular cause, not due to blood coagulation; slow capillary reflex; blood stuck in periphery; histaminic irritation of skin) • SASSAFRAS (thins the blood; coagulated blood, cold extremities; pulse feels thick, like oatmeal) • Scrophularia (stagnant lymphatics and blood) • SOLIDAGO (old bruises, strains, and sprains, especially of the spine, lower back; flower tops, in oil).

Blood Deficiency, Anemia: • Achillea (hemorrhagic; pernicious—Dudley) • Alchemilla (thin or watery blood, "pale complexion, blue veins show through"—LeSassier) • Aletris (uterine weakness, poor digestion, infertility) • Amygdalus (asthenic anemia or atrophy—needs confirmation) • Angelica (aplastic; iron deficiency) • Angelica sinensis • Artemisia absinthium (bitter, for appetite) • BETA (food tonic) • Ceanothus (anemia with enlarged spleen; pernicious anemia; Hodgkin's disease) • Cetraria (and seaweeds, for electrolytes and salts) • Cinchona (from blood loss; long-term exhaustion) • CODONOPSIS

(weak, thin, dried-out; *vata* people, nursing mothers) • CRA-
TAEGUS ("heart blood deficiency"; lack of concentration, waking at night, dizziness) • Eleutherococcus • Fucus (minerals)
• Gentiana (lack of appetite, poor digestion and absorption)
• Helonias (with uterine and ovarian weakness) • MEDICAGO
• Menyanthes (bitter) • Petroselinum (weakness; scanty periods
or severe dysmenorrhea; leaf) • Polygonum multiflorum (dizziness, tinnitus, poor vision, low back pain, prematurely grey
hair; prepared root) • Polymnia • REHMANNIA (excessive
menstrual bleeding, anemia in pregnancy; cooked root) • RHUS
SPP. (tongue pale but moist; "kidney anemia"—kidneys not signaling the bone marrow to produce blood cells—Light) • Rosa
(asthenic anemia) • Rubus canadensis (during pregnancy and
after) • RUMEX CRISPUS (iron assimilation, storage, release)
• URTICA (high in iron) • Silybum • Withania.

*Note: Bone-marrow stew with beets, mushrooms, and root crops is an excellent
general background tonic. MOLASSES also, as a food or the basis for a tonic.*

Hemorrhage: • ACHILLEA (bright-red, profuse) • Agrimonia
(hemorrhagic ulcer) • CAPSELLA (passive capillary bleeding;
dark, oozing) • CAPSICUM (internal or external) • CINNA-
MOMUM ZEYLANICUM • ERIGERON (from congested,
boggy mucosa; oil) • Geum urbanum (chronic, passive hemorrhage—Grieve) • Hamamelis (passive capillary bleeding)
• HYDRASTIS (passive bleeding from congested, boggy
mucosa, or active bleeding from a clean cut) • Lycopus (with
rapid, irregular pulse) • Panax ginseng (asthenic hemorrhage;
collapse from fluid loss; minute pulse) • Sanguisorba • Trillium.

*Note: "Active" hemorrhage, in the old authors, indicates bleeding from the arte-
rial circulation while "passive" means bleeding from the capillary bed or veins.
The former gives a bright red hemorrhage; the latter tends to be dark, oozing,
and clotted.*

"High Blood": • Achillea • LAVANDULA (to open the capillaries and disperse the blood; oil, on sides of head) • MELILOTUS (high blood pressure, headache) • Pulsatilla ("determination of blood to the head"—Scudder) • Rheum • Rumex crispus • Tilia • Tribulus • Verbena.

Note: "High blood" refers to a circulatory imbalance where there is "too much blood" in the head and upper part of the body. The old authors would describe it as "determination of blood to the head." This condition is characterized by mental overactivity, restlessness, hyperactivity, high blood pressure, overstimulated appetite, overeating, tendency to weight gain, diabetes mellitus type II, and mild heat conditions and is indicated by the high or large pulse.

"Low Blood": • Acorus • Capsicum • Lavandula • ROSMARINUS • Sambucus.

Note: Darkening color around the ankles past the age of fifty indicates what is called "low blood" in Southern American folk medicine. This indicates that the blood is lingering in the lower extremities and not returning to the head. It can therefore be an extremely important indicator of developing senility or mental vacuity, and it is important to head off this condition before it gets worse.

High Serum-Cholesterol Levels: • Allium sativa (reduces LDLs and triglycerides, raises HDLs, lowers blood pressure) • Arctium (uric-acid elevation; subclinical acidosis) • Capsella (high uric acid) • Centella (low T4 thyroid hormone levels) • Curcuma (strengthens blood vessels, improves blood flow, reduces LDLs, platelet stickiness, clotting, arteriosclerosis) • Cynara (lowers LDLs and triglycerides, increases HDLs) • Daucus (uric-acid elevation) • Iris (elevated LDLs, VLDLs) • Linaria (bilirubinemia, without active hepatitis) • Medicago sativa (alkalinizes the blood, prevents cholesterol absorption) • Panax quinquefolius (elevated LDLs, VLDLs; alkalosis, metabolic) • Polygonum multiflorum (lowers cholesterol, reduces arteriosclerosis, improves hormones) • Silybum (bilirubinemia, without active hepatitis) • Taraxacum (high uric acid) • Tribulus (elevated LDLs, VLDLs) • Trigonella (inhibits absorption, decreases manufacture by liver, lowers triglycerides and related high blood sugar) • Urtica (alkalinizing; subclinical acidosis) • Zingiberis (reduces cholesterol and blood pressure, thins blood, strengthens the heart, improves circulation).

Note: High acidity favors potentially harmful cholesterol absorption — hence the merit of alkalinizing remedies and foods. The above entries are largely based on Michael Moore, and Hershoff and Rotelli.

FORMULARY

Sambucus berry — with Silybum seed, honey, and brandy (blood tonic). Wood.

Prunus serotina — with Xanthorrhiza, Alnus serrulata, Goodyeara, Asarum (Cherokee Blood Tonic from Mary Chiloskey). Les Moore, 2002, 62.

Rumex crispus — with blackstrap molasses, raisins, jujubes, and/ or goji berries (blood tonic).

Rumex crispus — with Urtica, Rubus canadensis (blood tonic).

Pulse

The descriptions of pulses given in this section correspond to the definitions given in *Traditional Western Herbalism, Pulse Evaluation: A Conversation* by Matthew Wood, Francis Bonaldo Begnoche, and Phyllis Light (2015). We only have a very small number of remedies associated with specific pulses so far, but we hope this number will grow.

Rapid: • ACHILLEA (nonresistant, full, feels rapid) • Ajuga (rapid, high, weak; unequal circulation — Grieve) • Amygdalus • Convallaria (rapid, feeble; with heart problems, arrhythmia) • Crataegus • LYCOPUS (rapid and wild; during or after scarlet fever; hyperthyroid, Grave's Disease — Rafinesque)

• PRUNUS SEROTINA (rapid, strong in the liver; rapid and irregular) • Rosa • Tilia • Veratrum viride (rapid, strong, large; stressful to the heart).

Slow: • Chelidonium • CONVALLARIA (slow and weak) • Cnicus • Crataegus • Crocus (saffron) • Lactuca (slow and hard) • Prunus serotina (slow and irregular) • Selenicereus (irregular, chaotic pulse).

Note: When the pulse is rapid, friction from the blood moving through the vessels increases, and this increases blood temperature; the reverse occurs when the pulse is slow.

Large, Full, Wide: • Aconitum (homeopathic; full, with dry skin, suppressed secretions, sudden onset of fever) • Apocynum cannabinum (homeopathic; edema; full pulse with skin puffy, tight, full, and blanched) • Asclepias tuberosa (asthma, obstruction of breathing, with full, obstructed pulse) • Atropa belladonna (homeopathic; full, throbbing, with hot skin and cold extremities, in fever) • Cimicifuga (muscular and joint pain when the pulse is open and the skin not dry and constricted) • CINNAMOMUM CASSIA (large, floating, easily felt; spontaneous sweating—Huang) • Eupatorium purpureum (insufficient kidney action with large, firm pulse—Scudder) • GELSEMIUM (homeopathic; full, soft, empty pulse of exhaustion from fluid loss—Boger) • Myrica (feeble venous flow and mucosal debility; strengthens peripheral circulation; pulse full and weak—Priest and Priest) • Podophyllum (full tissues) • VERATRUM (rapid, full, strong).

Narrow, Thin: • Zingiberis (adjuvant in chronic sluggish renal function; pulse small and irritable; dried rhizome—Priest and Priest).

Note: The wide/thick and narrow/thin pulses are major indicators of the nutritional state of the body. A thick, wide, full, large pulse indicates possible overfeeding. A narrow, thin pulse (often called "small" in Western tradition) indicates inadequate nutrition. A frequent presentation is a thin pulse on one arm and a wiry one on the other, indicating lack of nutrition plus tension, a vata combination. (Though this condition is frequently encountered, I haven't made a list of remedies for it.) The wide pulse can also mean a very active fever, or blockage, bloating, edema, etc. Stimulants—like the Zingiberis mentioned above—may assist these remedies.

Wiry, Tense, Tight: • AGRIMONY (wiry; wiry and slippery)
• BUPLEURUM (wiry and thin; yellowish complexion)
• LYCOPODIUM (wiry and thin).

Note: The wiry or tense pulse is tense lengthwise, like a tendon pulled tight, while the tight pulse is tense side-to-side or top-to-bottom, and "twangs." Both are treated particularly by acrid herbs. The relaxed pulse (immediately below) is the opposite of the tense pulse; it feels like a clothesline drooping down in the middle between two poles. The relaxed pulse indicates lack of tension.

Relaxed: This indicates the need for an astringent.

Strong: • VERATRUM VIRIDE (homeopathic; strong and full; high, unyielding fever, or post-febrile condition, even after years, wearing on the constitution; tongue has red streak down the center).

Weak: • Angelica • Convallaria (slow and weak in cardiac problems) • Myrica (weak peripheral circulation — Priest and Priest) • Sanguinaria (respiratory weakness with weak peripheral circulation).

Note: A strong pulse means the heart is beating too hard, and occurs during or after a very active fever. A weak pulse indicates weak peripheral circulation.

Quick: • AESCULUS HIP. (obsessive-compulsive) • PASSI-FLORA (obsessive-compulsive).

Note: The quick pulse is "quick" in regard to the return of the systole—there is no space between beats. This indicates a lack of time for the heart to relax and—since "the heart stores the shen, or mind"—a lack of time between thoughts, hence the obsessive, compulsive behavior.

Rare, Leisurely (pauses between beats): • Rosmarinus (needs confirmation).

Note: The rare pulse has long spaces between beats, and indicates good tone from exercise and mental quiescence from medication. It is a good pulse to attain after the correct remedies have been given. However, it is not good in the elderly— especially if the pulse is also slow—as it indicates vanishing of thoughts. It is also not good in a person who feels cold and does not exercise or meditate.

Flooding: • Pulsatilla (small flooding; hormonal imbalance) • VERBENA (large flooding; "not enough yin to hold down the yang"; fire exhausting fluids).

Oppressed: • ASCLEPIAS TUBEROSA • Capsicum (capillary congestion, stagnation) • Crataegus (low capillary reflux) • PRUNUS SEROTINA (irritated arterioles block blood from entering the capillaries; low capillary reflux).

Note: The flooding pulse feels like the surf—it comes in with strength, and leaves with none. Flooding and excess indicate an approaching crisis—discharge is about to occur, with danger of bleeding or excessive fluid loss. A flooding deficient or small pulse indicates unstable personality tendencies—persons who are too much outside themselves—and stress with discharges, especially menstrual. The oppressed pulse is a flooding pulse where there is obstruction, like surf hitting the rocks on the beach. It indicates arteriolar tension, difficulty dealing with heat or cold and discharge of fluids—also, peripheral blockage in the circulation.

Irregular: • LYCOPUS (rapid, tumultuous, irregular—Rafinesque) • Melissa • PRUNUS SEROTINA (irregular, rapid or slow) • SELENICEREUS (broken-heartedness; tumbling, irregular, slow).

Even, Slow, Rare: This is the pulse of athletic tone, and indicates a person who is currently exercising; takes five years or longer to completely disappear after exercise discontinued.

Note: An even pulse always means cardiac tone, even when other, less desirable factors are present, while an irregular pulse means stress on the heart, but not actual damage unless very rapid. The even, slow pulse is equivalent to the rare pulse, above.

High: • Amygdalus • CINNAMOMUM CASSIA (floating, large, easily felt; spontaneous sweating — Huang) • Crataegus • Prunus serotina • Rhuem • Rosa • Rumex crispus • Tilia.

Low, Absent: • Apocynum cannabinum • Capsicum (depressed in acute conditions) • Cornus florida (subnormal temperature and relaxed tissues — Scudder) • Myrica (low and weak — Priest and Priest) • Salvia (low in the liver position, indicating deficient liver blood — Bonaldo) • URTICA (short pulse, absent in the proximal and distal positions — Wood).

Note: A high pulse indicates circulation is engaged towards the surface, to repel external stressors such as cold or heat; it can also indicate excess heat in the system, or a need for downwards evacuation. A low pulse indicates circulation toward the interior attempting to preserve heat and energy, or a lack of energy, blood, and circulation. These can be equivalent to high and low blood (see Blood).

Hard: • Artemisia absinthium (hard pulse in liver position) • Eupatorium purpureum (large and firm — Priest and Priest) • LACTUCA (slow and hard throughout, from external cold invasion) • Rhus toxicodendron (homeopathic; sharp, hard pulse — Scudder; skin inflammation).

Soft: • CINCHONA (full, soft, empty; after fluid loss during fever) • GELSEMIUM (homeopathic; full, soft, sometimes empty; from fluid loss; enervation, exhaustion, lethargy).

Note: A hard pulse indicates nervous tension and resistance, while soft shows nervous prostration and exhaustion. A hard pulse also means resistance due to cold, dry, heat, or wind conditions, while soft indicates lack of resistance, from damp excess or concurrent loss of fluids.

Long: Usually a good sign not needed remediation, unless there is over-consumption of food.

Short: • URTICA (specific indication).

Note: The long pulse, according to the Greeks, is long in the apex. It shows capacity in the heart, and strength, if other factors are good. The long pulse in TCM means the pulse extends further down the arm from the proximal position and indicates a well-fed system. The short pulse in Chinese medicine is short from top to bottom, so that the pulse feels like it doesn't reach the bottom — "doesn't have feet," so to speak. It feels like three little disconnected blips. Then the distal or proximal pulses disappear (one or both), showing that the circulation is no longer reaching the bottom or the top. This pulse is an excellent indication for nettles (Urtica), and can involve weak respiration and circulation (low distal pulses) and weak kidney expulsion (low proximal pulses). The Greek short pulse is sometimes called the "pencil-point pulse" because it is extremely bunched together in the apex. It means there is stress on the heart, very little capacity in the heart, and a possible incipient heart attack.

Choppy: A good indication for remedies for congealed blood.

Note: The choppy pulse is like the irregular pulse, but more forceful and oppressed; it always indicates a bruise, shock, strain, or sprain. The jolt of such injuries can cause a systemic reaction, and is weakening to the heart, which gives rise to the irregularity of the beat in time, force, and location.

Unequal: • Artemisia vulgaris (weak on the right, stronger on the left—Cowan) • Capsicum (highly unequal among the various pulse positions).

Note: Like the choppy pulse, the unequal indicate stress on the heart, from unequal distribution of the blood or impediments to circulation.

"Moving Bean," Vibrating: • Apis (homeopathic) • Gentiana (severe allergic reaction, anaphylaxis).

Note: The pulse of acute allergic reaction, occurring during pulse-taking, feels like the finger is on a bee's wing. I have used Apis several times, but the use of Gentiana needs confirmation.

Heart, Circulation, and Cardiovascular System

It has long been known that the heart does not pump the blood; the blood circulates on its own, independently of the heart. The evidence for this is well established, described in detail by Stephen Harrod Buhner in *The Secret Teachings of Plants* (2004). He quotes Robert Marinelli *et al.* (1995), "The blood is not propelled by pressure, but rather moves with its own biological momentum and with its own intrinsic flow pattern." The circulation of the blood involves many principles, the most important of which have only been discovered recently. The circulatory activity begins with the properties of water.

It turns out that when it is in contact with a hydrophilic (water-loving) surface, the properties of water change dramatically. The usual molecular structure of water, H_2O, is revised to become H_3O_2. Because of this it has a negative charge, and can hold and discharge energy. It also possesses a liquid-crystalline structure, which has been named the "fourth phase" of water—beyond solid, liquid, and gas. All of this sounds a little technical, so I just call it "super water."

There are numerous inorganic hydrophilic surfaces, and upon them sunlight creates H_3O_2. This process resembles photosynthesis in that it begins with the splitting of water molecules. Interestingly, considering the dramatic color (green) associated with the photosynthetic process, color-containing molecules more actively create super water in the presence of sunlight. (Wow—life arises from color!)

The energy emitted by the sun is now stored in the bonds of the H_3O_2 molecules, and these molecules pile up on the surface, thousands deep, creating a lot of potential energy. When the hydrophilic surface is a tube, the energized water moves. "We found that immersing tubes made of hydrophilic materials into water produces flow through those tubes similar to blood flow through blood vessels," writes Dr. Gerald H. Pollack. He continues:

> Blood eventually encounters high resistance since capillaries are often narrower than the red blood cells that must pass through them. In order to make their way through, those red blood cells need to contort. Resistance is high. You'd anticipate the need for lots of driving pressure, yet the pressure gradient across the capillary bed is negligible. The paradox resolves itself if radiant energy helps propel flow through capillaries in the same way that it propels flow through hydrophilic tubes (Pollack 2015, 19).

Since the blood moves on its own, there would be no need for the heart except the constantly changing energy and temperature demands in local areas of the body, altering literally second by second, require additional mechanisms beyond mere circulation. This is the true work of the heart. With its network of vasculature bound together by neurons (in the arteries and arterioles), the cardiovascular system coordinates and controls the local distribution of the blood, opening the vessels here, closing them there, to meet the needs of every region. The heart is like an all-seeing God to the circulatory system, watching over it from the center of the microcosm of the body.

Pumping is used not to move but to control and direct the blood— a wave going out from the heart through the arteries, to the arterioles, which open and close to shunt the blood in or out of particular areas according to systemic and local controls. The blood continues to move in the capillaries and veins under the propulsive properties of super water and salt. When there is an invasion of toxins or microorganisms, the local area needs more white cells, oxygen, water, waste removal, *and a more rapid metabolism,* in order to deal with the local invaders. This requires more blood, and to produce this, the circulation needs to move more quickly. The hypothalamus resets the "inner thermometer" to a higher grade, and a mass of physiological changes occurs. The cardiovascular system speeds up to send more blood to the area, causing an increase in temperature, because the heart has to work harder.

Once it begins moving, the blood keeps moving. Herbalist Jim MacDonald, in a conversation with the author, likened the circulation to a merry-go-round: once set moving, it only takes a little tap to keep it going. The heart does not pump the blood; rather, it "keeps pace with the blood." If the blood goes too fast or too slow, the heart is stressed; it is like pushing the merry-go-round too fast, or forgetting to give it a tap. TCM has a concept applicable here. It places an "organ" called the "heart protector" between the heart and environmental stressors, to keep it from getting banged around too much. Like the royal guard, it stands between the king and the outer world. In modern terms, the heart is largely protected through the regulation of temperature and water by the hypothalamus. However, conditions in the skin and the capillary bed are regulated by the arterioles, which are largely under local regulation. This is why attending to the condition of the surface was and is so important in traditional medicine around the world. Keep the peripheral mechanism flexible and the heart and other internal organs will be less stressed.

Through pulse readings, we can to some extent understand the difference between the circulation and the heart. It is impossible to understand the pulse to its depths without understanding these principles. Sometimes the heart is driven by the blood or circulation — then we find the *nonresistant* or *deficient slippery* pulse, which feels as if heat were driving a non-resistant heart. At other times we find the opposite: the *oppressed, tense, tight, full,* and *hard* pulses, showing opposition to the cardiovascular wave. Sometimes the circulation is wild and turbulent, with overheated tissues — and the pulse is *irregular* or *tumultuous.* The *choppy* pulse feels like "the heart has been hit by a big stick," knocking it off balance in regard to speed, timing, and location of pulse beat. The *strong* pulse shows a heart that has been working too hard to combat fever or stress, and has been ratcheted up to a strong, forceful punch that is most wearing, and can remain after the fever is gone — unless the heart or something else wears out.

Just before the bloodstream enters the heart, it picks up the comprehensive stream of lymphatic waste products and water coming through the thoracic and subclavian ducts into the subclavian veins. A quantity of this blood is taken into the expanding atrium of the right side of the heart during the diastole of the pulse (the relaxation of the heart muscle). As the blood fills the atrium, valves at the bottom (at the entry to the ventricle) are pressed shut by backwards pressure from the blood in the ventricle, which is also relaxing and expanding. Then the systolic impulse from the pacemaker of the heart (located on the right atrium) pumps the right ventricular blood into the pulmonary artery, towards the lungs. The ventricle's valves open, and the blood from the contracting right atrium moves in. As the systole fades, the right atrium relaxes again, more blood moves in, and the valves are again pressed closed by the blood in the right ventricle.

With each systole, then, the blood moves toward and through the lungs, drops off excess vapor and carbon dioxide, and picks up oxygen. The exit of water through vapor makes the remaining water saltier, which makes it "thirsty" for the capillary bed where the oxygen is headed and helps propel the arterial blood to its "goal." The systolic impulse from the pacemaker that contracts the left ventricle (forcing the blood outwards through the aorta), continues down the atrium and arteries.

The arteries are bendable, and expand during the systole, when the blood flows into them; the blood flows out during the relaxing, collapsing diastole. The arteries terminate in the arterioles, which expand and contract to shepherd the blood — not through impulses from the heart but by control mechanisms in the sympathetic nervous system (SNS). Feedback mechanisms between the capillary bed and the arterioles influence the SNS to tighten or loosen the blood entering the ever-changing micro-regions of the body, filling their capillary beds with greater or lesser amounts of blood.

Finally, the capillaries dump their oxygen in the body tissues and take up CO_2 and H_2O. These, with other small waste products, are picked up in the venules at the far end of the capillaries, and passed to the veins. The lymphatic capillaries pick up more water and larger waste products.

The vascular system is not stationary and fixed; the capillaries are generated and replaced constantly. When we lose a pound of weight, we lose a million miles of capillaries, and when we gain a pound we gain a million miles. The arteries can also regrow to some extent — hence the success of cardiac-bypass surgery.

Coordination of the circulation and all parts of the cardiovascular system is necessary for the health of the heart. Conditions in the peripheral areas pressing back on the heart cause high blood pressure, resulting in expansion of the heart cavities and enlargement of its muscles, or "cardiac compensation." Eventually, these compensatory efforts are not enough, and the heart muscles deteriorate into a floppy, ill-conditioned "decompensation." This pushback is caused by hardening of the arteries (calcification), high osmotic pressure in the kidneys (due to salt imbalance), deposition of cholesterol narrowing the arteries, deposition of fibrin and thrombocytes forming scabs or blood coagulations, bacterial infections in these depositions causing heat and swelling, imbalances in distribution of the blood, ill effects in the coronary artery, etc. The stress of high blood pressure is far worse than the stress of fever (unless the *strong* pulse is also encountered, which is a sign of high blood pressure as well as cardiac overwork). High blood pressure is the *cardiac killer;* hence the great concern of modern medicine with this problem.

The hardworking heart gets no rest except in the intervals between systoles. At the end of the diastole, there is a moment of rest when the nerve activity turns completely chaotic (in the healthy heart) and relaxation occurs. Thus, the "rare" pulse (with a long interval between beats) is the pulse of the best cardiac health — it is found in athletes and (guess what?) meditators. So we now know that heart health is improved by meditation.

Circulation

Circulation: • Achillea (capillary engorgement and venous stasis; skin red and blue; nonresistant pulse) • Aesculus hip. (mental tension; high blood pressure; venous relaxation *and* tension; quick pulse) • Agrimonia (wiry pulse—tension; or balloon pulse—tension and "phlegm") • Angelica (congested pelvis, abdomen, thorax; thins blood, increases circulation to cold hands and feet) • Baptisia (poor peripheral circulation in septic fever) • CAPSICUM (unequal distribution of blood; deficient and sluggish capillary circulation; flabby, middle-aged persons, senescence) • Cinnamomum spp. (poor peripheral circulation) • Crataegus (red, meaty parts of the palms, due to red blood cell stasis in the capillary bed) • Eupatorium purpureum (increases profusion from capillaries) • Gentiana (circulation to abdominal region) • Hydrastis (autonomic nerve weakness and poor circulation) • Lavandula (capillary congestion; heat; expands capillary bed) • Liatris ("by diffusion to the surface they maintain good capillary action"— Cook) • Lycopus (rapid and tumultuous pulse during or after fever) • Melilotus (blood congestion; full head; cold hands and feet) • Myrica (poor peripheral circulation, low and weak pulse) • Prunus serotina (rapid and irregular pulse, oppressed pulse; palms red and yellow) • Quercus (venous atony; capillary fragility) • Rheum (stagnation in colon; large and tense pulse—Huang) • Rhodiola ("balances circulation") • ROSMARINUS (poor peripheral circulation; poor return circulation; "low blood") • Ruta (venous tension and blockage) • Trillium (excited, hemorrhagic) • Vaccinium myrtillus (strengthens arteries, veins, capillaries) • VERATRUM VIRIDE (strong pulse; heart driven by fever beyond its innate strength) • VERBENA HASTATA (flooding pulse; blood driven into capillary bed without resistance; approaching disease crisis) • Zanthoxylum (poor capillary circulation).

Heart

Heart: • Alchemilla (weak atrial muscles) • Apocynum cannabinum (mitral and tricuspid regurgitation with low arterial tension; capillary effusion; debility, edema, cyanosis) • Asclepias tuberosa (congestive heart failure; water in lungs) • Avena (nervous weakness) • CAPSICUM (unequal circulation; floppy valves, weak muscles; heart attack; opens the peripheral circulation—Christopher) • Caulophyllum (heart pain) • Cimicifuga (heart pain) • COLLINSONIA (valvular insufficiency) • CONVALLARIA (rapid, feeble, irregular pulse; left ventricle failure, valvular disease, edema) • CRATAEGUS (weak and poorly nourished heart muscle; irritability and palpitations; clogged coronary circulation; high blood pressure, cholesterol; decomposition; valvular murmurs; sighing) • GANODERMA LUCIDUM (hypertension, high cholesterol) • HYDRASTIS (general weakness of nerves and muscles affecting the heart; congenital hole in heart—one case cured, Crow; external or internal) • Juniperus (chronic structural change) • LIRIODENDRON (muscular weakness and tension; thins the blood; after a heart attack, as an ongoing tonic for the damaged heart— Crow) • LYCOPUS (rapid pulse; palpitation; fever affecting the heart) • Panax quinquefolius (root in whiskey is a widespread tonic still used in the South as a tonic after a heart attack) • Phytolacca (fatty heart) • PRUNUS SEROTINA (rapid and weak pulse and heart action) • Pulsatilla (hypertrophy and dilatation of venous heart) • Quercus (lack of tone in venous circulation and heart) • Rosmarinus (cardiopulmonary edema in old people) • Sambucus (congestive heart failure; blue, swollen complexion and tissues) • Scoparium (cardiac dropsy, myocardial weakness) • Scutellaria (nervous, intermittent pulse) • Taraxacum (cardiopulmonary edema) • Tilia (high blood pressure; red, elongated tongue) • Trigonella (high cholesterol; postmenopausal tonic) • SELENICEREUS (pulse irregular; weakness; mitral and aortic regurgitation; "broken heart")

Heart Tonic: • Avena • CAPSICUM • CRATAEGUS (increases coronary circulation, lessens irritation and cholesterol deposition) • Eleutherococcus • Hydrastis (muscle tonic, directed to the heart by Capsicum) • Liriodendron (Native American tonic for lifelong use after heart attack; relaxes sympathetic nervous system, strengthens heartbeat—Crow, Boyd) • Olea (leaf) • Panax quinquefolius (tincture; Southern U.S. tonic for lifelong use after heart attack) • Prunus serotina (irregular pulse) • Quercus • Rosmarinus (collapsed circulation—Weiss) • Selenicereus • Trigonella • Trillium (lessens cardiac irritability).

Heart Palpitations (often due to hyperthyroidism): • Crataegus (weakness and irritability of cardiac muscles) • Filipendula (nervousness, restlessness, palpitations, hyperthyroidism) • Ganoderma (neurasthenia, insomnia) • Leonurus (nervous palpitations) • Lycopus (fever with wild and rapid pulse; "anxiety, heart palpitations, irregular pulse, purple heart"—Schnell) • Melissa • Passiflora • Prunus serotina (pulse rapid, irregular) • Selenicereus • Tilia (nervous palpitations) • Viscum.

High Blood Pressure: • ACHILLEA (capillary and venous fullness; essential hypertension; red face) • Agrimonia (peripheral tension) • Agropyron • ALLIUM SATIVA (very reliable palliative, but effect stops when administration of remedy stops) • Althaea (salt imbalance) • Asclepias tuberosa (oppressed feeling in chest; strong, oppressed pulse) • Betonica • Capsella (normalizes high and low) • Centaurium • Centella (high cholesterol) • Chamomilla • Chionanthus (portal hypertension) • Chrysanthemum (flower) • Cnicus • Coleus (thins blood, relaxes arteries, improves cardiac action, lowers blood pressure) • Collinsonia (portal hypertension) • Convallaria • CRATAEGUS (increases coronary circulation, reduces arterial irritation and cholesterol; normalizes high or low; for arterial hypertonicity, elevated diastole, essential hypertension) • ELEUTHEROCOCCUS (modulates high and low)

• Fagopyrum (with capillary bleeding) • Filipendula (nervousness, irritability) • Galium (with edema) • Ganoderma (hypertension, high cholesterol) • Gentiana (dizzy, exhausted, discouraged, swollen, damp, and inflamed) • Hamamelis (mild) • LAVANDULA • LEONURUS (stress-induced) • Lentinula • Lycopodium (externally, on kidneys) • Melilotus (blood rushes to the head, causes fullness, headache, HBP; heart racing, sleepless — Piorier) • Melissa • Menyanthes • Olea (oil) • Polygonatum • Primula • Prunella (blood rushes to the head) • Rumex crispus • Ruta (tension) • Salvia (Chinese or Western; thins the blood safely) • Scolopendrium • Scutellaria • Stellaria • TILIA (autoimmune irritation of arterial system causing high blood pressure) • Tribulus • Valeriana • Veratrum viride (strong, driven pulse; red streak down center of tongue; homeopathic) • VERBENA (pulmonary hypertension; "set in their ways"; diabetes; reddish checks, swelling under eyes, hands swollen and tight; increases depth of respiration) • Viburnum opulus • VIBURNUM PRUNIFOLIUM (high blood pressure during pregnancy — other times too?) • Vinca minor (episodic, mild) • Viola (flower) • VISCUM (episodic, with headache, dizziness, tachycardia; normalizes high and low) • Zingiberis (footbath, to draw the blood down from the head — Sedlacek).

Low Blood Pressure: • Allium sativa (high or low) • Angelica (asthenia, dry skin) • Apocynum cannabinum (cold, weak, edemic; skin tight, puffy, blanched) • Aristolochia (cold, weakness, sepsis; minute or homeopathic dosages) • Betonica • Capsella bursa-pastoris (normalizes high and low) • CRATAEGUS (normalizes high and low) • Eleutherococcus • Glycyrrhiza (asthenia; with frequent urination) • Leonurus (Weiss) • Panax ginseng (arterial hypotension) • Panax quinquefolius (Weiss) • Rosmarinus (Weiss) • URTICA • Viscum (normalizes high and low).

Cardiac Edema, Congestive Heart Failure: • Asclepias incarnata (with functional cardiac insufficiency) • Apium • APOCY-NUM CANNABINUM (cold extremities, pale, puffy skin; weak circulation, debility; minute or homeopathic dose) • Aralia hispida (with constipation) • Aristolochia (cold, weak, debilitated; homeopathic or minute dose) • Astragalus • Baptisia (with vascular stasis and septis) • Ceanothus (lung congestion) • Collinsonia (venous stasis in legs and pelvis) • CONVAL-LARIA (with swollen ankles) • Crataegus • Fouquieria • Lycopus (to increase cardiac force, decrease heart rate) • Myrica (elevates peripheral circulation) • ROSMARINUS (Kneipp; confirmed — Wood) • SAMBUCUS (lung congestion) • SCO-PARIUM (cardiac dropsy, myocardial weakness) • Squilla • TARAXACUM (leaf, often confirmed) • Zanthoxylum (debility; to strengthen peripheral circulation; small doses).

Heart Failure, Noncongestive: • CONVALLARIA • CRATEAGUS • LEONURUS • SCOPARIUM.

Hypertrophy: • Asclepias asperula (M. Moore) • Crataegus • Lycopus.

Angina pectoris (pains in chest around heart): • Ammi • Angelica • Astragalus • Avena • Cimicifuga • Convallaria (Weiss) • CRATAEGUS • Leonurus • Lobelia • NOTOGINSENG • Selenicereus (irregular pulse).

Pericarditis: • Aconite (homeopathic; acute) • Asclepias tuberosa • Selenicereus • Capsicum • Cimicifuga (rheumatic) • Crataegus • Lycopus.

Irregular Heartbeat: • Angelica • Crataegus (extra systoles) • Lycopus (rapid, irregular, tumultuous pulse) • Prunus serotina • Scoparium (atrial and ventricular fibrillation).

Tachycardia (extremely rapid pulse): • Convallaria (rapid, weak pulse; arrhythmia) • Crataegus (paroxysmal, comes and goes) • Ganoderma (anxiety, nervousness) • Leonurus (circulatory excitation, nervousness) • Lycopus (rapid, irregular pulse; nervous, anxious) • Prunus serotina (rapid, irregular pulse) • Scoparium (myocardial weakness) • Tilia (autoimmune excitation; high blood pressure) • Viscum.

Bradycardia (slow pulse): • Selenicereus (slow, chaotic pulse) • CONVALLARIA • Cnicus • Crataegus • Crocus (saffron) • Lycopus • Melissa • Prunus serotina (slow, irregular) • Zanthoxylum.

Anxiety with Cardiopathy: • Avena • Leonurus • Lycopus • Melissa • Scutellaria.

Anxiety without Cardiopathy: • Calendula (from swollen lymphatics causing pressure on heart—Wood) • Selenicereus

Note: Anxiety without cardiopathy frequently occurs due to indigestion, heartburn, GI spasm, or other problems that give a sensation of pain in the region of the heart. Of course, a cardiovascular specialist needs to analyze the case, and even then there may be uncertainty. Early in my career, at the little herb store in the inner city, a man in his mid-thirties came in with great concern about a pain in his heart. He had given up his regular job as a cab driver because he was afraid to drive over bridges.

"How do you support your family," I asked? (I knew his wife and children.) "Well I'm a mighty good cardplayer," he replied. I convinced him to go see a cardiac specialist, and he discovered that he only had a displaced vertebra. Thirty-five years ago, the inner-city minority communities were underserved by doctors of their own color and culture, leading to a lot of mistrust of the medical system.

Valvular Disease, Regurgitations: • APOCYNUM CANNABI-
NUM (homeopathic; mitral and tricuspid regurgitation; watery
infiltration due to valvular disease) • SELENICEREUS (asthenia; hyperthyroidism; mitral regurgitation) • COLLINSONIA
(with sense of heaviness).

Heartache, Broken Heart: See "Mind, Emotions, Will." Research
has established beyond doubt that emotions can cause heart
disease.

Vasculature

Arteriosclerosis: • Achillea • Allium cepa • Allium sativa (reduces
HBP and plaque; needs to be taken long-term) • Althaea officinalis • Ammi (coronary) • Ananas (bromelain, from pineapples;
reduces blood clotting; anti-inflammatory) • Angelica sinensis
• Arctium (lowers lipids) • Capsicum (with confusion, sluggishness, in the middle-aged and elderly) • Chrysanthemum (flower)
• Coleus • Commiphora muki (prevents, reduces; lowers cholesterol, triglycerides) • Commiphora myrrha • Convallaria (coronary) • CRATAEGUS (coronary; cheek tissues are often red)
• Curcuma • Fucus • EQUISETUM • Eleutherococcus (lowers lipids) • Gingko • Harpagophytum (lowers lipids) • Juglans
nigra • Myrica (dry membranes, skin; increases peripheral circulation) • Opuntia (lowers lipids; juice) • Panax quinquefolius
(lowers lipids) • Papaver (with depression) • Polygonum hydropiperoides • Prunus serotina (irregular pulse) • Prunus spinosa
(syrup) • Rosmarinus • Taraxacum • TILIA • Tribulus (lowers
lipids) • Vaccinium • Vinca minor (cerebral) • Viscum • Vitis
(prevents and even removes cholesterol build-up; seed extract)
• Zanthoxylum • Zingiberis (lowers cholesterol, lessens blood
clots, opens circulation; with confusion, sluggishness).

High Cholesterol: • Allium sativa (excess in serum; removes
deposits—Weiss and others) • Arctium (root) • Centella
• Commiphora muki • Crataegus • Cynara • Eleutherococcus

• Ganoderma • Gymnema • Juglans nigra (leaf) • Linum (flax-seed oil) • Medicago • Pleurotus ostreatus (oyster mushroom) • Taraxacum • Trigonella • Vitis (seed extract; prevents and even removes cholesterol build-up).

Note: Also see "Arteriosclerosis," in this section and "High Serum Cholesterol Levels" under "Blood."

Capillary Fragility: • Ceanothus (internal extravasation of blood) • Crataegus (berries) • Fagopyrum (petechiae due to capillary fragility; frostbite; hypertension) • Opuntia (juice from flowers and fruits) • Quercus • VACCINIUM MYRTILLUS • Viola tricolor • Vitis (seed extract; capillary fragility in the brain).

Varicose Veins: • ACHILLEA (skin red with blue veins; spider veins; aneurism) • AESCULUS GLABRA (legs, inner thighs; external or internal) • AESCULUS HIP. (tension and relaxation causing venous stasis; legs, inner thighs; external or internal) • Agrimonia (ulcerated; use in ointment) • Bellis • Calendula (external) • Capsicum (senescence) • Centella (strengthens connective tissue) • Chelidonium (in the right shoulder, due to liver congestion) • Cinnamomum spp. (stimulating astringent) • COLLINSONIA (venous stasis; legs, inner things; chronic poor diet, lipid digestion) • Crataegus • EQUISETUM (strengthens connective tissue) • Fagopyrum • FOUQUERIA (pelvic congestion; legs, inner thighs; chronic poor diet, lipid digestion) • HAMAMELIS (venous stasis with enfeebled circulation) • Lamium (astringent; compress) • Myrica (enfeebled circulation) • Phytolacca (ulcerated) • Potentilla • QUERCUS (blue-black and yellow, knobby, swollen, ugly) • RUSCUS • Salvia (blue/grey complexion; ulcerated) • Sanicula (relaxed tissue) • Silybum (hard, ropy) • Symphytum (sitz bath) • Vaccinium myrtillus (astringent).

Thrombosis, Phlebitis: • Aesculus hip. • Hypericum • Linum (fresh ground seed poultice) • Ruscus • Symphytum (warm root compress, continually applied—Parton).

Pulsations in Abdomen (Pulsating Aorta): • CINNAMOMUM CASSIA (feeling of upward motion or pulsation in abdomen; palpitations, insomnia; easily startled, flushed feeling, feverish— Huang) • Helianthus (pulsations in abdomen—Burnett).

Note: This is a syndrome known as "running piglet" in Traditional Chinese Medicine.

FORMULARY

Capsicum—with Hydrastis (myocardial tonic). Ellingwood.

Crataegus—with Allium sativa and Viscum album (5 parts each), and Arnica (½-part): 10 drops, 3/x day; use for long period (arteriosclerosis). Sherman.

Crataegus—with Selenicereus, Tilia, Viscum, Scutellaria, Melissa (heart tonic).

Crataegus—with Achillea, Tilia, Melissa (high blood pressure).

Fagopyrum—with Vitamin C (to reduce capillary permeability). BHP 1983, 90.

Hamamelis extract—with Calendula (varicose veins). BHP 1983, 45.

Leonurus—with Avena, Ganoderma, Rhodiola (stress-induced high blood pressure). D. Winston.

Prunus serotina—with Quercus and Populus tremuloides, or Liriodendrum (circulatory and heart tonic).

Rosmarinus—with Aesculus hip. (varicose veins; brings the blood up to torso from below).

Scolopendrium—with Agropyron, Althaea (hypertension).

Tilia—with Chrysanthemum flower, Leonurus (mild high blood pressure).

Zingiberis—with Myrica, Tsuga canadensis, Capsicum (small

amount), Eugenia (small amount), powder (Samuel Thomson's famous "Composition Powder" used to bring the circulation to the surface). Les Moore 2002, 51.

LEMON BALM *(MELISSA OFFICINALIS)*

This was used in one of the "cordials" of ancient times. The name "cordial" comes from the Latin *cor/cardio-* ("heart"), but cordials act more on the metaphorical heart than the physical. Samuel Westcott Tilke (1844) quotes one of the old Roman authors approvingly; according to Serapio, "A strong infusion, often drunk, causeth the mind to be merry, and reviveth the heart when faint. Good for those who have weak digestions."

Stomach and Upper Gastrointestinal Tract

The upper gastrointestinal (GI) tract begins with the lips and teeth, and continues to the end of the stomach. This part of the tract is concerned mainly with digestion—in particular, the breakdown of large chunks of food into a slurry ready for the ferocious digestive enzymes in the small intestine to tear into the fundamental particles that can be taken into the body through the gut wall. The main components of the upper GI are the mouth, throat/esophagus, and stomach.

Though composed of separate parts, the GI tract as a whole tends to function as a unit. Conditions in one area usually affect those in another. The mouth usually affects the stomach, and vice-versa. An imbalance may fall heavily on a single organ, but the whole tract is affected. With the GI more than anywhere else, perhaps, we need to keep our eyes on the whole and the parts.

The mouth and tongue have already been addressed as separate structures, but as part of the upper gastrointestinal tract as a whole, some additional facts can be offered. First, both are important for offering physical, observable evidence of the condition of the whole tract. Second, as the "antechamber" of the GI, they "set up" the digestive process, and if they are off-balance the whole tract will suffer.

The condition of the teeth has already been addressed.

On the tongue and throughout the mouth, we can read the general state of the mucosa of the upper GI. If we combine this knowledge with a few questions and observations, we can fairly easily understand what is going on in the stomach. Heat/excitation shows in high-red, pink-red, or carmine tongue and oral mucosa *(Rumex crispus, Amygdalus, Prunus serotina, Rheum)*. Usually there is excess activity in the tract — too much salivation, hunger, HC_1 (hydrochloric acid), and/or diarrhea. Aggravation of this condition from eating spicy food indicates a state of heat/excitation, while improvement after eating spices indicates a cold/depressed tissue state. *This is an extremely reliable differentiating symptom.* A pale or dark tongue, with lack of salivation, and improvement from eating spices, indicates cold/depression, lack of digestive juices and the need for warming stimulants for the stomach *(Angelica, Acorus, Citrus aurantium, Capsicum)*. These are often combined with bitters to provoke salivation and digestive juices in the stomach.

When gas and bloating is present, we have either dryness or tension. The differential symptom is whether the bloating comes on suddenly (in which case it is wind, tension) or comes slowly and goes slowly (dryness). Tension, again, is like wind (which it is called in TCM) — it comes suddenly and goes suddenly. This is the way a cramp happens, in contrast to how a lack of stomach acid and digestive juice manifests. The latter condition comes on slowly because the secretions are too slow to digest the meal. Low stomach acidity proceeds and ends slowly, as the prolonged digestion finally finishes.

For wind/tension we need relaxants *(Mentha piperita, Foeniculum, Fumaria, Nepeta)*. Since the tongue is the only strong muscle in the mouth, that is where neuromuscular tension shows — in a shaking tongue. For lack of secretion, we need bitters *(Carum, Gentiana, Mahonia)*. Sometimes there is a need for nerve tonics *(Lycopodium, Betonica, Hydrastis)*.

Some remedies combine properties nicely *(Angelica* and *Acorus* are bitter, pungent, and relaxing; *Pimpinella* is sweet and relaxing; *Citrus aurantium* is both sweet and bitter). Combining the cooling and stimulating with the bitter and astringent is indicated by a dark-blue tongue center with hot, red, damp edges—revealing stagnant blood in the stomach, as TCM would say, with drying-out of fluids due to poor circulation, but fluid loss appearing as dampness in the periphery *(Achillea)*.

The two excess-dampness states (relaxation and stagnation) appear in two different ways. A damp, watery tongue indicates excess saliva, drinking too much liquid with eating, a relaxed tissue state, and the need for astringents. In China, warming remedies would be used, while in the West we tend to use astringents; the two properties combine very well. As the dampness of relaxation gets colder, it congeals to a white or mild-yellow, thrush-like tongue coating, which is easily washed off *(Nymphaea, Rumex crispus, Rheum, Comptonia, Myrica)*. Damp stagnation, by contrast, is indicated by a heavy, yellow, adhesive, difficult-to-remove, oily coating. This is what Samuel Thomson called "canker." Oil, the heavier liquid, is backing up in the system. This condition is related to weak metabolism (liver, cells, thyroid) and poor elimination (gall bladder, colon). The alteratives are needed in this case; these act more on the liver/gall bladder than on the stomach. We can use *Mahonia, Taraxacum,* and *Arctium* here.

Another polarity is between the areas above and below the swallowing mechanism. The throat marks the descent from the conscious realm to the unconscious. The former is ruled by the central nervous system (CNS), the latter by the autonomic (ANS). So the stomach is controlled by the ANS, and therefore associated with unconscious processes, emotions, and instincts, rather than conscious ones. If the stomach doesn't like something, it can throw it up, so discomfort (physical and psychological) shows up as nausea and vomiting. The emotion of the stomach is animal instinct.

As a strong muscle, the stomach is much more influenced by the tissue state of tension *(Fumaria, Nepeta, Dioscorea)*. It is also the place where the ANS (autonomic) "comes to the surface," to communicate with us through "gut-level" or "animal" instincts (or "thumps on the belly"). Therefore, it is subject to both physical and psychological tension. Weak instincts need *Lycopodium, Betonica, Hydrastis, Hypericum,* and *Gentiana,* while excessive churning emotions in the stomach and excessive appetite need *Rumex crispus* and *Rheum.* Self-doubt and indecisiveness call for *Gentiana, Betonica,* and *Hypericum,* as they are associated with both the gall bladder (gall, the ego, decision-making) and the stomach.

Conditions in the esophagus usually originate in the stomach, through esophageal reflux (GERD), though poor esophagus tone requiring astringents may also occur. If stomach secretions are highly deficient, there will be fermentation and inflammation there, with esophageal reflux (requiring stimulants and bitters). Esophageal reflux from fermentation needs to be differentiated from the more common type caused by excess stomach acid. When reflux is caused by fermentation, the tongue is red at the tip and in the center, elongated, and flame-shaped, and there will probably be excess saliva *(Rumex crispus, Rheum).*

Stomach ulceration is usually due to cold/depression—lack of circulation to the stomach. This calls for strong stimulants—*Capsicum, Hydrastis, Asarum*—as well as mucilages to coat against the excess acidity and bitters to increase secretion. In European medicine, at least until a generation ago, stomach ulceration was seen as a forerunner of gastric cancer, so it is important to effectively treat this condition.

A very slight, white coating on the tongue indicates exfoliation of dead cells from the tongue that were not washed off due to lack of secretions. This is a dryness symptom, requiring bitters. A wide tongue, apathetic-looking and lacking in character, slightly dry and sometimes ulcerated, indicates a need for the great stomach-specific nervine stimulant *Hydrastis.* A red, flame-shaped tongue with a heavy coating of white or light yellow indicates heat with damp—use *Rumex crispus* or *Rheum.* Bad breath—when not due to poor hygiene—indicates putrefaction *(Baptisia, Isatis, Helianthemum, Propolis).* Cavities indicate *Panax quinquefolius* (for lack of saliva) and *Quercus* (for cavitation), adding *Plantago* and other remedies if root abscesses are also present. Treat germs like *Helicobacter heilmannii (Gastrospirillum hominis)* with antiputrefactives and tissue tonics such as *Hydrastis*.

Heartburn, Esophageal Reflux, GERD (hyperchlorhydria):
• Aloe vera (fresh gel) • Althaea • Apium • Chamomilla • CHONDRUS • Cnicus (bitter) • Crocus sativa • Dioscorea • FILIPENDULA (atonic dyspepsia with hyperacidity) • Fumaria • Gentiana • Glycyrrhiza • HYPERICUM (with anxiety, solar plexus issues) • IRIS (acidity, gastric reflux) • Mahonia • Medicago sativa (acidity) • Nepeta • Pimpinella • Rheum (excess saliva, appetite, and acid) • RUMEX CRISPUS (excess saliva, appetite, and acid) • Urtica (hypersecretion, nausea) • Viburnum prunifolium • Zanthoxylum.

Low acid (achlorhydria):
• Acorus (warming, pungent, bitter) • Agrimonia (with gallbladder problems • ANGELICA (warming, pungent, bitter) • Arctium ("lack of secretion"—Sherman) • Armoracia (stimulant adjuvant) • Artemisia absinthium (bitter) • Berberis (bitter) • CARUM (bitter) • Centaurium (after serious illness) • Cinnamomum spp. (warming astringent) • CITRUS AURANTIUM (orange peel is the best-tasting bitter, and combines well with others) • Cnicus (decoction—Weiss) • Collinsonia • Gentiana (bitter; if debilitated and discouraged) • Inula (bitter, pungent) • Mentha piperita • Menyanthes • Taraxacum (sweet and bitter) • Zingiberis (warming and relaxing).

Appetite, Lack of (Simple Anorexia):
• Achillea (tea) • Acorus (cold tea) • ALETRIS • Anemopsis • Armoracia (stimulant adjuvant) • ARTEMISIA ABSINTHIUM (bitter) • Artemisia vulgaris • Asclepias tuberosa ("with depressed autonomic and mesenteric stimulation"—M. Moore) • Cannabis • Capsicum (achlorhydria) • Carum (bitter) • CENTAURIUM (children) • Chamomilla • Chelone (convalescence; ileocecal cramps)

• Cichorium (tea) • Cimicifuga • Cinchona (bitter astringent) • Cinnamomum • CODONOPSIS (weak, thin, dried-out, lacking saliva, anorexic, bloated) • Cola (atonic digestion, exhaustion) • Coriandrum (slowness, sluggish digestion, eructations, flatus) • Cnicus (bitter) • Crataegus (internal) • Eriodictyon • Euonymus • Filipendula (nervous, uncomfortable) • Foeniculum • Frasera (after GI infections) • GENTIANA (anxious to put on weight) • Geum • Humulus • Hydrasis (bitter) • Juniperus • LEVISTICUM • Lobelia (nausea) • Melissa • Menyanthes • Myrica • Panax quinquefolius • Podophyllum (heavy head, dizziness, full feeling in stomach) • Populus (nervous) • Prunus serotina (gastric irritability) • Raphanus (gas, bloating, indigestion, lack of appetite, constipation; use sparingly when ulceration is present) • Rosmarinus (Weiss) • Salvia (tea) • Sanguisorba • Taraxacum (Weiss) • Teucrium • Thymus (bath) • Turnera (loss of pleasure in food) • TRIGONELLA • Zanthoxylum (achlorhydria) • Zingiberis (gas, spasm, contraction).

Appetite, Loss of, from Chemotherapy: • Acorus • Cannabis • Echinacea • Euonymus • Panax quinquefolius • Trifolium.

Anorexia Nervosa, Bulimia, Eating Disorders: • Acorus (aromatic bitter) • Aletris (bitter; anorexia from nervous dyspepsia) • Angelica (pale, thin, low appetite, colic, dyspepsia) • Arctium • Betonica (nerve-diffusive) • Borago • Cannabis (iatrogenic) • Carum • Centaurium • Cimicifuga (difficult or delayed puberty and afterwards; pelvic congestion) • Cinchona (bitter astringent) • Codonopsis • Cornus • Euonymus (iatrogenic) • GENTIANA (bitter) • Helonias (with dyspepsia) • Humulus • Levisticum • Oplopanax (iatrogenic) • Panax quinquefolius (uncured root) • Trigonella (promotes weight gain) • Verbena (bitter, relaxant).

Excessive Appetite; Sugar and Food Cravings: • Gentiana
(1 drop on tongue) • RHEUM (excess salivation, voluptuous
appetite, especially for meats, fats, or sweets; overactive GI
without exercise) • RUMEX CRISPUS (similar to Rheum
but less principal for this) • URTICA (sugar craving) • VER-
BENA (hormonal food-craving). This category needs further
development.

*Note: One teaspoon of maple syrup, per cup of liquid, drunk all day as desired,
is an old Ojibwa remedy used to stop sugar craving. It worked for myself and
others.*

Digestion, Weak or Atonic: • Acacia • Aceticum acidum (cider
vinegar) • Acorus calamus • Aletris • Alnus rubra (lipids)
• Anthemis nobilis • Artemisia absinthium • Artemisia vulgaris
• Asclepias tuberosa (sensitive constitution) • BETONICA
(nervous weakness, gastritis, gastralgia) • Calendula (warming)
• Capsicum (atonic debility of GI, especially in senescence)
• Carum carvi (mild bitter) • CENTAURIUM (weak stomach,
sourness, heartburn, nausea, vomiting; lack of appetite and
digestive fire; *cf.* Gentiana) • Cichorium (feeble, weak, hot stomach, with general weakness) • Cetraria • CHONDRUS
• Cinchona (bitter astringent) • CNICUS (lipids) • Codonopsis
(weak, thin, dry, lacking saliva and appetite) • Cornus florida
(bark) • Curcuma • Cynara (lipids) • Euonymus • Filipendula
(nervous, irritable) • Foeniculum • GENTIANA (physical and
mental weariness, discouragement, lack of secretion, debility,
discouragement, not enough energy to eat; in the elderly; when
"the fire has gone out"—Hueneke) • HYDRASTIS (atonic
mucosa; nervous debility, weakness; large, swollen, atonic
tongue) • Hypericum (irritable, weak stomach, hyper- and
hyposecretion) • Juglans cinerea (eructation) • Lycopodium
(weak, dry stomach; bloating; narrow, dry tongue) • Marrubium (lipids) • Melissa (nervous stomach) • Menyanthes (bitter) • Myrica (due to atonicity, catarrh) • Pimpinella anisum

• Podophyllum (lack of gastric motility; 1-drop doses) • Rheum
• Panax quinquefolius (lack of secretion) • Populus (bitter)
• Salvia (gas) • Stellaria (tonic) • Taraxacum (lipids) • Teucrium • Trigonella • ULMUS (during convalescence; can't take
much food in stomach; gruel).

Bloating, Discomfort, Eructation, Gas: • Achillea (heartburn,
heaviness, pressure; red center of tongue) • Acorus (wind;
worse from overeating) • Aletris (asthenic, slow to digest,
flatulent, gaseous) • Alnus rubra (deficient gastric secretion,
drowsiness after meals; in old people) • Alnus serrulata (relaxed
stomach walls with imperfect peptic function) • Alpinia (flatulent indigestion) • Althaea • Anethum • Angelica (bloated,
gassy, pale, cold) • Arctium • Asarum canadense (harsh, dry
skin) • Betonica (weakness, gas, sour risings, continual belch-
ing) • Bidens • Calendula • CAPSICUM (flatulent dyspepsia
without inflammation) • Carica papaya • Carum (flatulent dyspepsia and colic) • Caulophyllum (pain after taking food, from
muscular stiffness) • Chamomilla (painful distention) • Cimicifuga (with rheumatic, sore, stiff muscles) • CINNAMOMUM
SPP. • Citrus aurantium (slow digestion, large quantities of gas,
neurasthenia) • Codonopsis (weak, thin, dry, bloated, lacking
saliva and digestive juices) • Coriandrum (sluggish digestion,
eructations, flatus, anorexia) • Dioscorea • Eugenia (flatulence,
nausea, vomiting) • Filipendula (nervous irritable) • FOENIC-
ULUM (chronic flatulence) • FUMARIA (spasm) • Gentiana
• Hedeoma (flatulent colic) • Illicium (sweet stimulant; sluggish
digestion, eructation, flatus, distension) • Juglans cinerea (flatulent distention) • Juglans nigra (flatus, overeating) • Lavandula
• LEVISTICUM • Liatris (with renal inactivity) • Lycopodium
(bloating during meals; dry, withered tongue) • Mahonia • Melilotus • MELISSA (dried) • MENTHA PIPERITA
• MENTHA PULEGIUM • Monarda fistulosa • MYRISTICA
• Oenothera biennis (dirty, sallow, full, expressionless skin and
tongue, upset stomach, vomiting, frequent desire to urinate)

• PETROSELINUM • Pimpinella • Piper nigra (flatulent after meals) • Populus (nervousness in stomach) • Raphanus (gas, bloating, indigestion, lack of appetite, constipation; use sparingly if ulceration is present) • Rheum (distress after eating; heat and congestion) • Rosmarinus • Salvia • Solidago (flatulence) • Teucrium • Thymus serpyllum • Thymus vulgaris • Valeriana (fullness due to gas with nervousness; use smaller dosage) • Zanthoxylum (flatulence from overeating; berry) • Zingiberis.

Nervous Dyspepsia, Colic, Spasm: • Achillea (inflammation, stomachache, cramp) • Agastache • Aletris • Ammi • Artemisia vulgaris • Asafoetida • Asarum canadense (spasm) • Ballota • Betonica (anxiety, lack of groundedness) • Calendula (tea) • Carum • Chamomilla (whining, complaining) • Collinsonia (spasm with constipation) • Coriandrum (adjuvant) • Dioscorea (cramping pain and vomiting) • Equisetum (compress) • Filipendula • FUMARIA (spasm) • Helonias • Humulus • Hypericum • Illicium (sweet stimulating adjuvant) • Lavendula (flower tea, for nervous stomach) • Linum • Lycopodium • MELISSA • Mentha piperita (peppermint) • Mentha spicata (morbidly irritable) • Monarda fistulosa (tension held in stomach, chest, shoulders) • Monarda punctata (flatulence, flatulent colic, bowel spasm, nausea) • Myristica • Nepeta (internalizes stress into the stomach; tension causes digestive upset) • Oenothera (herb; dyspepsia and vomiting) • Pimpinella anisum • Populus tremuloides • Prunella (colic) • Prunus serotina (vomiting in children) • Rosmarinus • Thymus • Turnera • Urtica • Valeriana (smaller doses) • Verbascum (colic) • Viscum (tension in solar plexus) • Zingiberis (cramp).

Indigestion, Gastritis, Irritation, Burning, Dyspepsia: • Acacia • Achillea • Acorus • Agrimonia (indigestion) • Alcea rosea • Alchemilla • Althaea officinalis (use with a stimulant) • Anemopsis • Amygdalus (irritation; elongated, dry, carmine tongue) • Angelica (pale, appetite loss, colic, dyspepsia) • Arctium (in cachectic individuals) • Artemisia absinthium (atonic dyspepsia) • Asafoetida (flatulent colic) • Berberis (with halitosis, skin problems) • BETONICA (weakness, pain, burning, mild ulceration) • Borago • CAPSICUM (stimulant; flatulence without inflammation) • Cetraria (nutritive mucilage) • Chamomilla (acute, spasmodic, complaining of pain) • Chelidonium (biliousness) • Chondrus • Cichorium (indigestion) • Cinnamomum spp. (flatulent dyspepsia) • Collinsonia (with constipation) • Euonymus (bilious) • Filipendula (nervous, atonic, with heartburn and hyperacidity) • Foeniculum (flatulent) • FUMARIA (spasm) • GENTIANA (poor lipid digestion) • Geranium maculatum • Glechoma • GLYCYRRHIZA • Helonias • Heracleum • Hydrastis • Hypericum (irritation, gastritis, ulcers) • Iris (biliousness) • Juglans nigra (indigestion) • Lamium • Lobelia (heartburn, hiatal hernia, spasm) • Mahonia • Melissa • Mentha piperita • Myrica (inflammation) • Myristica (flatulent, nervous) • Petroselinum (flatulent dyspepsia with intestinal colic) • Polygonum bistorta • Prunus serotina • Rheum (irritation of the stomach with elongated, carmine tongue) • Rumex acetosella (tea) • Rumex crispus (red, pointed, coated tongue; bloated, short of breath; chronic—Herschoff/Rotelli) • Trigonella (fenugreek) • Ulmus (use with a stimulant).

Gastric, Duodenal, and Peptic Ulcers: • Achillea • Acorus • Agrimonia (ulceration on tongue, stomach) • Alchemilla • Aloe (gel) • ALTHAEA (root) • Anemopsis (mucus and ulceration) • Asarum (stimulates circulation, putridity) • Bidens (peptic) • Calendula (soothing) • Capsella • Capsicum (stimulant; with Althaea) • Chamomilla (acute; irritated, complaining of the pain) • Cinnamomum (bleeding) • Codonopsis • CURCUMA (combine with bromelain or pepper) • Erigeron (bleeding) • Eucalyptus • Ficus (fetid) • FILIPENDULA (peptic ulcer; for prophylaxis and treatment) • Geranium (bleeding) • HYDRASTIS (ulceration in bite marks on the tongue; peptic ulcer; 1-drop doses) • Hypericum (erosive gastritis—Weiss) • Myrica • Piper methysticum (duodenal) • Quercus • Rheum • Ulmus.

Gastric Catarrh (Mucus in Stomach): • Agrimonia (ulcerative gastric catarrh) • Alnus • ECHINACEA (gastritis, fermentative dyspepsia, ulcerative stomatitis, intestinal indigestion, duodenal catarrh; ½- to 1-dram dose—Massinger) • Frasera • GERANIUM MACULATUM (frothy, relaxed stomach; for children) • Geum urbanum (cold, phlegmatic stomach) • HYDRASTIS ("in minute doses, is the leading remedy for dyspepsia"—Jones) • Lycopodium (dry stomach and tongue) • Mahonia (with cholecystitis) • Monarda punctata • Myrica (heavy catarrh in stomach, atonicity, bad digestion, poor peripheral circulation, diabetes; low, weak pulse) • Rubus canadensis (frothy, relaxed stomach; for children).

Note: A damp, mucoid stomach is common in infants and children.

Gastroenteritis: • Acorus • Agrimonia • Alchemilla • Althaea • Anemopsis • Carum (flatulent) • Centella • Cetraria • Chamomilla • Chondrus • Commiphora myrrha • Dioscorea (spasmodic) • Epilobium • Filipendula (nervous, irritable) • Foeniculum (flatulent) • Glycyrrhiza • Hydrastis (atonic tongue) • Hypericum (Weiss) • Iris • MAHONIA • Myrica (coated tongue) • Nepeta • Panax ginseng (chronic GI disease; distention without bloating; thin abdominal muscles; debility) • Rheum (tongue elongated, firm, tough, red, dry, with scorched-yellow coating; strong heat) • Rosa • Rumex crispus (tongue elongated, red, coated) • Silybum • Thymus vulgaris • Ulmus • Veratrum viride (homeopathic; red streak down center of tongue, strong pulse).

Gastroptosis (Prolapse of the Stomach, determined by palpation): • Artemisia absinthium (with Centaurium—Sherman; tea) • HYDRASTIS.

Fermentation: • Allium sativa (crushed in wine) • Echinacea.

Nausea and Vomiting: • Achillea • Anemopsis (catarrhal)
• Amygdalus (hypersensitivity; cold tea of leaves) • Asafoetida
(food can't decide whether to go up or down) • Avena
• Capsella (hematemesis) • Carica papaya (infants) • Cetraria
(due to chemotherapy; also for cancer cachexia; vomiting in
pregnancy) • Chamomilla • Chelone • Chionanthus • Cinchona
(bitter astringent; nausea, debility, lack of appetite) • Cinnamomum cassia ("colic or dyspepsia with flatulent distention and
nausea"—BHP) • Crataegus • Filipendula (nervous, irritable)
• Dioscorea • Gentiana (anorexia; before eating) • Geranium
(frothy mucus in stomach; hematemesis; in infants) • Hamamelis
(hematemesis) • Hydrastis (in morning, from alcohol hangover)
• Iris (after breakfast, biliousness) • Lavendula • Lobelia (nausea, spasm preventing emesis) • Mahonia • Mentha arvensis
• MENTHA PIPERITA • Mentha spicata • Myrica (catarrhal
in morning; hangover) • Myristica • Nepeta • Prunus serotina
(gastric tenderness with nausea) • Solidago (nausea from weakness) • Symphytum (hematemesis) • Urtica (with hypersecretion) • ZINGIBERIS (clear, thin, odorless vomitus; abdominal
distention, pain, excess saliva, aversion to cold; pale or pale-red
tongue with a greasy white coating; dried rhizome—Huang)
• ZINGIBERIS (antispasmodic relaxant; fresh rhizome).

Motion Sickness: • ZINGIBERIS (candied).

Hiccough, Obstinate: • Anethum (tea of seeds) • Apium (tea of
seeds) • Citrus limonum • Carum carvi • Caulophyllum
• Dioscorea • Eupatorium perfoliatum (with Capsicum, manip-
ulate T6 vertebra—Sherman) • Mentha piperita (oil or spirits)
• Nepeta • SACCHARUM (hold one tablespoonful of sugar in
mouth) • SCUTELLARIA • Sinapis (seed) • Viburnum prunifolium • Zingiberis (needs confirmation).

Hiatal Hernia: • Ballota • Betonica • Chamomilla • Dioscorea • Filipendula • Lobelia • Humulus • Nepeta.

Stomach Problems from Stress: • Ballota (jolt in stomach) • BETONICA (weakness) • MELISSA (nervous stomach) • NEPETA ("headache, colic or stomach ache due to stress"— Hershoff and Rotelli; LeSassier) • VALERIANA ("queasy gut feeling of strong emotional response"—Sedlacek) • Viscum (tension in solar plexus).

FORMULARY

Althaea—with Capsicum or Hydrastis as an adjuvant (stomach ulcer)—traditional.

Angelica—with Helonias (anorexia and dyspepsia). BHP 1983, 27.

Ballota—with Cetraria (vomiting). BHP 1983, 59.

Ballota—with Filipendula (vomiting). BHP 1983, 92.

Calendula—with Geranium herb or root (duodenal ulcer). BHP 1983, 45, 101.

Cinchona—with Chamomilla, Melissa, Althaea root, Angelica root, Humulus (anorexia nervosa). BHP 1983, 67.

Cinnamomum spp.—with Filipendula, Chamomilla, Ulmus, Althaea root (flatulent dyspepsia and gastritis). BHP 1983, 68–9.

Codonopsis—with Glycyrrhiza and Aloe gel (stomach ulcer).

Filipendula—with Althaea, Melissa (gastric conditions). BHP 1983, 92.

Filipendula—with Melissa, Chamomilla, Humulus (dyspepsia). BHP 1983, 141.

Gentiana—with Zingiberis, Rheum (gastrointestinal atony, stagnant food).

Gentiana—with Valeriana (anorexia nervosa).

Gentiana—with Collinsonia, Taraxacum, Artemisia absinthium (achlorhydria). Sherman.

Gentiana—with Menyanthes, Calamus (achlorhydria, anorexia, atonicity, digestion).

Gentiana (2 parts) — with Scutellaria laterifolia (1 part). This is the "Dr. Carroll's Capsules" formula for digestive stagnation, given by Sherman.

Hydrastis — with Filipendula, Chamomilla (stomach, gastric irritability). BHP 1983, 114.

Inula — with Taraxacum, Berberis (achlorhydria). Sherman.

Mentha piperita — Artemisia absinthium (achlorhydria). Weiss.

Mentha piperita — with Melissa, Acorus, Foeniculum (gastritis). Weiss.

Petroselinum — with Althaea root, Melissa, Chamomilla, Ballota (dyspepsia with nausea and vomiting). BHP 1983, 155.

Populus — with Berberis vulgaris and Chelone (anorexia with digestive weakness). BHP 1983, 169.

Rheum (2 parts) — with Potassium bicarbonate (2 parts), Hydrastis (1 part), Cinnamomum cassia (1 part), Mentha piperita (1/32 part) in glycerin, alcohol, and water. This is the famous eclectic formula (Glyconda "Neutralizing Cordial") for indigestion, food stagnation, and constipation. "The pulse tends to be either moderate or slippery, and the tongue usually has a white, greasy coating." This version is given by Les Moore (2002, 61), but of particular help is his observation of the pulse.

The Autonomic Nervous System

The autonomic nervous system runs the functions of the body that do not need conscious oversight. We do not, for instance, need to shove little particles of food through the gut wall in full consciousness, though we need to chew in full awareness so as not to bite the side of our cheek or tongue or choke. The autonomic therefore particularly runs the digestive tract, cardiovascular system, and other largely involuntary activities. Some partially voluntary functions are ruled by the ANS and its partner, the CNS or central nervous system — overseer of conscious activity. For instance, we can control the breath when we need to, but we don't most of the time.

The ANS is massive, and as a nervous system it produces and uses more serotonin than the brain. A section of it is called the "enteric brain" because it is located in the digestive tract. Because large dinosaurs had to eat so much to feed their huge bodies they actually had enteric brains larger than their cranial brains. The autonomic is like a queen overseeing the dark world of unconscious functioning, like the moon overlooking dark waters of the night.

Not only does it rule unconscious functions in the body, but through it we experience our "animal" or "gut-level" instincts. The autonomic is, in a sense, the "inner animal," in charge not only of unconscious physiological activities, but sensory input (which is edited by the parasympathetic nervous system), pleasure and pain, perception, and instinctual understanding of life — the world of the animal, in fact. It comes to consciousness through a little nerve group atop the stomach called the "solar plexus." Although not emphasized by physiologists, it is from here that we constantly get advice from our "inner animal": safe/unsafe; pleasure/pain; "pay attention," "rest up," etc. — and no physiologist would make it through traffic to work without paying constant attention to input from the ANS. Nevertheless, the inner animal is largely ignored — by science, religion, and ordinary Muggle society.

Autonomic activities are divided into two sections, under the sympathetic and parasympathetic branches. The first is responsible for activities that require attention and consciousness (like perception and the support of the CNS), while the second oversees our needs for rest, relaxation, digestion, and repose, and also sex. These two branches are competitive — when we are in one, the other is suppressed. This helps to create the two opposite constitutional poles of asthenia (thin) and sthenia (thick). In a pathological state, the dominance of one branch over the other has become unhealthy and needs treatment.

The largest branch of the autonomic is the vagus, which innervates the diaphragm, lungs, and stomach. It also sends branches up into the head, and down throughout the digestive tract, sexual organs, and elsewhere. It comes to consciousness, or we feel it, particularly in the back of the throat. This is called the "acrid" taste, or "bilious" taste in Greek medicine. I like to call it the "vomit" taste. It is produced when the vagus nerve is irritated and is considering vomiting.

Herbs that act on the ANS leave an impression here. These remedies begin with simple relaxants, and run up into the entheogens and hallucinogens that cause vomiting as part of their "trip," such as *Ayahuasca*. The back of the throat is the meeting place between human consciousness and the inner animal. The symbol of the shaman is the theriomorph (half human/half animal), in recognition of the need to establish this relationship. Then there is the "entheogenic" aspect, the spirit world.

Of all herbs acting on the autonomic and the vagus probably none is as sudden and powerful, but unpredictable and fleeting, as *Lobelia*. It acts throughout the ANS, from one corner to another. A good preparation, placed on the skin, will be felt as a prickle in the back of the throat in seconds. The great discovery of Samuel Thomson, *Lobelia* is like a powder keg: when administered to the body, even in single drop doses, it will shoot through the ANS like electricity, relaxing whatever is tense, and empowering whatever is too relaxed. It goes where it is needed, and it *acts!* For this reason, Dr. Christopher used to say that *Lobelia* "had brains"—a statement that is virtually a proverb in herbalism today. It knows what needs to be done, and where, and it sends other herbs there; so it functions as probably the best synergist in herbal medicine. Tis Mal Crow used to tell us, "*Lobelia* likes to be planted where it can hear people talking, like along the path, or under the window where the TV is on all day."

Because of its dynamic nature, *Lobelia* never acts the same way twice. The needs of the autonomic are different, literally from second to second. When it was taken out of the US Pharmacopeia in 1951, the reason given was that its action was considered "fleeting and capricious." Wow, I thought, even those guys in the white coats really understood this plant! (Wood 2010).

Although the autonomic deserves a chapter on its own, our tradition has not developed a materia medica specific to the subject. Therefore, no repertory follows this section.

Intestines and Lower Gastrointestinal

The upper gastrointestinal tract breaks up large chunks of food into smaller pieces, so that they can be presented to the lower gastrointestinal tract in a slurry of independent pieces ready to be worked over by the digestive enzymes specifically geared to each major food group—carbohydrates, lipids, proteins. The lipids still need to be further reduced in size, so they are met in the upper small intestine with bile that emulsifies them (makes them both water- and oil-soluble) so that enzymes can reach them.

The first portion of the small intestine, the duodenum, receives the digestate from the stomach while, at the same time, bile and digestive enzymes from the gallbladder and pancreas squirt into it from the common bile duct. Here in the duodenum, the digestion really gets serious, with carbohydrates, lipids, and proteins meeting the ferocious little pancreatic enzymes specific for each of these three types of food. All the ingredients for successful digestion are present.

The remainder of the small intestine is a long tube consisting of the jejunum and ileum. This portion is elongated—and stretches out even longer when filled with digestate (up to twenty-five feet)—in order for the food/toxins and enzymes to be rolled and mixed and exposed to each other, so that every single particle of digestible material can be processed. The free enzymes in the intestines are helped by stationary enzymes and white cells studded along the gut walls. The stationary immune cells are called GALT—gut-associated lymphoid tissue.

Digestion is followed by absorption through the gut wall, for assimilation into the body. The area for absorption in the small intestine is vastly increased by the presence of villi, or minute, finger-like projections. The villi are covered with cells through which the food/toxins enter the body. Each one has a capillary and a lymphatic duct (called a lacteal); the hydrophilic carbs and proteins enter the capillaries, and the oil-soluble lipids go into the lymphatic ducts.

It is said that if the surface area of the small intestine, including all the villi, were smoothed out to make a flat surface, it would cover an area about the size of a football field. So imagine throwing a meal the size of a large bowl across the surface of a football field! And imagine, furthermore, that even with all this area, some of us have the ability to rip apart and absorb every last morsel, while others have a much more limited capacity, so that they don't get as much out of their football field! As Michael Moore so often said, some of us have "digestion a lion would envy."

As we move down the small intestine, the number of nutrient-receptor sites in the cells increases, so that more assimilation and less digestion takes place. (The process of assimilation will be discussed in the next section.) There are, however, increasing patches of lymphoid tissue on the intestinal walls, culminating in "Peyer's Patches" in the ileum, just before the ileocecal valve that separates the small intestine from the large. This, obviously, is intended to head off problems caused by a backwards reflux of feces from the colon, should the valve function inappropriately.

The jejunum and ileum are completely under autonomic governance, without any input from the central nervous system. That means their functions are completely unconsciousness, without any conscious oversight. Under ANS impulse, the intestinal movements (peristalsis) continually move digestate down the tract. Supposedly, also, the digestate is completely sanative—all unfriendly bacteria not already killed is destroyed in this "dark continent" of digestion. However, a brand-new problem has recently been acknowledged in medicine, called SIBO (small-intestine bacterial overgrowth).

Due primarily to the overuse of antibiotics, the biome—natural bacterial colonies in the large intestine and even throughout the whole organism—has in many cases become pathological, occupied by alien, unhealthy bacteria. These weaken the gut walls and derange metabolic functions. It is believed that this causes "leaky gut syndrome," or holes between the cells where incompletely digested food/toxins can get into body, forcing even stronger immune reactions and pathological fluctuations in thyroid, liver, and blood-sugar levels as the body attempts to cope with these intruders. Blue flag *(Iris)* is an excellent remedy for these side-effects.

Through inattention, we are destroying our gut walls. One of my students recently asked a butcher whether they still make sausages out of intestinal casings. "No," he replied. "The intestines of pigs today are so thin, they rip like tissues and can't hold anything." That leads to an unpleasant question: are our foods any better than pig food? Do we know?

In *Man's Presumptious Brain* (1962), Albert Simeon argued that regulation by the autonomic is so complete in the small intestine that enteric functions should be completely unconscious. It is only when something is wrong that we become aware of the small intestine; it is the most hidden from us of any developed organ. Unfortunately, many people imagine that something is wrong and attempt to over-regulate what is going in this dark, invisible continent. In a sense, therefore, there is no healthy emotion for the small intestine. However, the unhealthy emotion is hypochondriasis, or imagining ill where there is none.

Back to squishing along through the ileocecal valve with our happy digestate: suddenly we find ourselves inside a new organ—the large intestine. Here we find bacteria that are helpful to us; the symbiotic bacteria that reside in the colon assist us by breaking down the leftovers that our small intestine was not meant to deal with. They are able to release certain nutrients, such as vitamin K, that we just can't digest on our own. These are picked up by the bloodstream around the colon. Recent research also shows that the symbiotic bacteria detoxify substances in the bloodstream of the colon, so that they exert an influence inside the body itself! That makes the colon, like the kidneys, liver, and lungs, an organ of detoxification.

The main function of the colon otherwise is to maintain the appropriate water/solid balance in the stool, so that it is neither too runny nor too hard—making expulsion easy and complete. In the final segment of the large intestine, the hegemony of the ANS is lost; joint regulation with the CNS resumes so that the rectum can function appropriately (under conscious control), waiting for a good bush behind which to defecate.

The colon is a pretty tough, thick-skinned organ, with a thicker gut wall than the small intestine's, though thinner than the really tough, muscular stomach. Ulceration of the large intestine, colitis, is therefore serious and potentially life-threatening, but less so than enteritis in the small intestine.

The most common problems of the colon – constipation and diarrhea – are due to muscular spasm, poor peristalsis, crazy food choices, or water control problems in or upstream from the colon. In cases of constipation, use roughage (*Plantago psyllium* husks and other foods) to exercise the colon. If this doesn't work, use mild laxatives *(Rumex crispus, Rhamnus purshiana)* to activate the colon for a short time. If these don't work, try stronger laxatives *(Cassia)* with fresh ginger added to eliminate griping. If there is alternating diarrhea and constipation, this is a case of irritable bowel syndrome (IBS), and needs completely different treatment with nervines, relaxants, and coolants. The correct use of laxatives and cathartics is aimed at re-engaging peristalsis in a weak, atonic colon. Atonicity can be associated with atrophy, relaxation, or torpor. Very small to small doses of laxatives and cathartics should be used, as large doses can actually cause atonic colon.

The major serious problem with the colon is a poisoned or deficient symbiotic colony. It turns out that babies born through cesarean section lose out on some of this bacteria, which they would otherwise pick up in the birth canal. Modern midwives and physicians are now reenacting traditional midwifery—rubbing some of the mother's fluids on the newborn.

Even after it is established, however, we can still lose our helpful symbiotic colony through food and antibiotic abuse. Recent research shows that a course of antibiotics will impact the colony for several years—possibly even a decade. Antibiotics negatively affect weight and height gains in children. Therapy for this imbalance is complex, and beyond the scope of this book. Mild cases require probiotics, severe ones fecal implants.

Atonic Colon: • Aloe barb. (unsatisfied with self; weakness of descending colon; tiny or homeopathic doses) • Aloe vera (anal prolapse) • Asclepias tuberosa (marbly, hard feces, with no inflammation) • Berberis (with halitosis and skin problems) • Capsicum (stimulant; atonic debility, especially in senescence) • Cassia (atonicity without inflammation; hard, formed feces; small dose) • Cinnamomum (slow digestion, cold abdomen) • Euonymus (liver hypofunction; anorexia) • Gentiana • Hydrastis (mucus in feces; prolapse) • Juniperus ("weakness of the intestinal muscle"—Powell) • Mahonia • Myrica (mucus in feces) • Ptelea (after intestinal infections) • Rhamnus purshiana (difficult expulsion, mucus; small dosage; avoid using with fissures or inflammation) • Rheum (difficult expulsion of stools; with inflammation, cramp) • Rumex crispus (constipation or diarrhea with difficult expulsion, inflammation, atonicity; tongue red, elongated, coated) • Zanthoxylum (lack of secretion in upper GI).

Septic Colon (Appendicitis, Typhoid, and Peritonitis): • Agrimonia (relaxant; appendix painful but not ruptured) • Angelica (stimulating astringent; appendicitis) • Asarum (stimulant; peritonitis) • Asclepias tuberosa (moistening; peritonitis) • Baptisia (antiseptic; typhoid) • Dioscorea (relaxant; pain) • ECHINACEA (antiseptic; acute appendicitis) • Epilobium (ulceration of bowels; Civil War remedy for dysentery) • EUPATORIUM PURPUREUM (peritonitis—effective in several diagnosed cases—Wood) • Monarda fistulosa (pain, no rupture) • OLEA (leaf) • POLYGONUM HYDROPIPEROIDES • Ricinus (oil pack) • TARAXACUM • Veronicastrum.

Note: Medical attention is also required in cases of septic colon.

Spastic Colon, Colic: • Achillea (pain, spasm, inflammation) • ACORUS (flatulence; umbilical region, in children) • Agrimonia (different parts of the GI are not coordinated—Hall) • Aletris • Anemopsis (chronic, catarrhal) • ANETHUM (for infantile flatus and colic, taken by mother; increases breast milk, which

"carries antispasmodic effects to the infant"—Hershoff/Rotelli)
• Angelica (flatulence) • ANTHEMIS (flatulent, griping colic,
umbilicus downward) • Asclepias tuberosa (infants and adults)
• Asafoetida (flatulent intestinal colic) • Asarum (flatulence
in depressed tissue state) • Capsicum (distention) • CARUM
(bloating) • CHAMOMILLA (irritable, restless, sleepless,
flatulent; if the baby has been nursed while the mother is angry,
drinking coffee, and/or taking drugs) • Chelidonium (stomach
distention, gallstone colic, better from heat) • Chelone (cecum;
uneasy, distressing pain) • CINNAMOMUM SPP. (tea) • CNI-
CUS • Colocynthis (homeopathic; sudden, gripping, agonizing
pain; drops to the floor) • Curcuma (from cathartics; irritable
mucosa; combine with pepper, bromelain) • DIOSCOREA (continuous pain; twisting, sharp, cutting pain, with rumbling and
passage of flatus) • Epilobium (chronic, non-inflammatory diarrhea; pains before passing stool) • FOENICULUM (flatulence;
babies and children) • Fumaria (biliousness; spasm; poor coordination of GI functions) • Gentiana • Glechoma (lead poisoning)
• Glycyrrhiza (inflammation) • Humulus • Hydrastis (chronic,
catarrhal) • Juglans cinerea (chronic; tincture of green hull)
• Juniperus • Lavendula (flatulence; small intestine) • Levisticum • Liatris (small intestine) • Lobelia • Melilotus • Melissa
(anxiety, stress, with stomach tension, spasm) • MENTHA
PIPERITA (flatulence, spastic constipation; for short-term use;
long-term use is mildly paralytic) • MENTHA PULEGIUM
• Mentha spicata (flatulence; preferred over M. piperita for
babies) • NEPETA (babies, children; flex legs to torso)
• PETROSELINUM (flatulent dyspepsia with intestinal colic,
tormina) • PIMPINELLA (nausea, indigestion, bloating, poor
appetite; infants, children) • PIPER METHYSTICUM (spasm,
anxiety, sleeplessness, tension, sensitivity to pain) • Rheum (indigestion, gas, constipation, overeating) • SAMBUCUS • Sinapis
alba • Solidago (flatulence) • Thymus serpyllum • Valeriana
(stress-related; cramps and diarrhea after eating) • Verbena
• VIBURNUM OPULUS (painful cramps, neuralgia in

stomach, abdomen, uterus, bladder, lower back) • ZINGIBERIS (cramps anywhere; fresh rhizome).

Duodenum: • ALTHAEA (ulcer) • CALENDULA (ulcer) • Chionanthes (duodenitis) • Geranium (ulcer) • GLYCYR-RHIZA (ulcer) • Symphytum (ulcer) • ULMUS (ulcer).

Colitis, Enteritis, Crohn's Disease: • ACACIA (mucous colitis) • ACHILLEA (bleeding) • Acorus • Agrimonia (colitis, ileocolitis, proctitis; ulcerative) • Alchemilla (bleeding) • Allium sativa (mucous colitis) • ALOE VERA (soothing, restorative) • ALTHAEA (widely applicable, but usually palliative) • Anemopsis (mucus secretion) • Amygdalus (celiac disease, inflammation) • Artemisia vulgaris (Crohn's disease) • Asarum (warming stimulant, antiseptic) • Baptisia (ulcerative) • Berberis (giardia—Stansbury, Wood) • Bidens (ulcerative) • Borago • BOSWELLIA • CALENDULA • Capsella • Centaurium • Chamomilla (with Glycyrrhiza) • Chelone ("from intestinal putrefaction and liver or portal dysfunction"—M. Moore) • Cinchona (hectic and passive inflammations) • Commiphora myrrha (irritable bowel syndrome, Crohn's; catarrhal mucosa) • Cnicus • CURCUMA (anti-inflammatory and regenerative; inflammation from tissue depression; combine with a little pepper, bromelain) • Echinacea • Epilobium (gut inflammation; colic, green diarrhea, no fever) • Erigeron (ulcerative bleeding) • EUPATORIUM PURPUREUM • Foeniculum • Fouquieria • Geranium maculatum (bleeding; ulcerative) • Geum spp. (aromatic; diarrhea, catarrhal and ulcerative colitis) • Glechoma (diarrhea) • Gnaphalium (celiac disease) • HAMAMELIS • Humulus • HYDRASTIS (soothing, toning to mucosa, antihemorrhagic, antiulcerative) • Hypericum (chronic inflammation of the bowels) • Iris • Juglans cinerea • Linum (flaxseed oil) • Mentha piperita (enteric-coated oil preferred) • Mitchella (catarrhal) • MYRICA (chronic; mucous) • OLEA (antimicrobial) • PLANTAGO PSYLLIUM

• Polygonatum • Polygonum bistorta • Polygonum aviculare (tea) • Potentilla (stress-related, nervous; ulcerative, hemorrhagic) • Prunus serotina (celiac disease) • Rhamnus spp., especially purshiana (chronic constipation; ulcerative colitis) • Rheum • RUMEX CRISPUS • Quercus • Sanguisorba (ulcerative) • Scolopendrium • Stellaria • Symphytum • Tabebuia (candida) • Taraxacum (root preferred) • Trigonella (irritable bowel, diarrhea and constipation) • Tsuga • Ulmus (ulcerative) • Urtica (mucus and blood in stool) • Usnea (salmonella, typhoid — Weiss) • Valeriana • Verbascum.

Constipation: • Allium sativa (persistent constipation, with irritation; low dose — Weiss) • Alnus rubra (alternating diarrhea and constipation) • Aloe barb. (homeopathic or very small dose) • Aloe vera (constipation, fullness on right side; very small amount of the yellow part of the rind) • Apocynum cannabinum (with debility, cardiorenal edema) • Arctium (dry stool; poor secretion and lubrication) • Aristolochia (poor fat absorption, sluggish portal circulation) • Berberis • Cannabis (the seed is oily, nourishing laxative for dry, deficient persons) • Carthamus (infantile) • CASSIA (take with sugar and ginger to prevent tormina in acute conditions; chronic use causes laxative dependence) • Cetraria • Chelidonium (from inactive gall bladder) • Chelone (lack of bile) • Chionanthus • Cichorium • Euonymus (lack of bile; post-febrile, poor appetite) • Fouquieria (poor fat absorption, sluggish portal circulation) • Frasera • Glycyrrhiza (dry feces, scanty secretions) • Heracleum • Hydrastis (sedentary life; chronic) • Iris (dry, grey feces) • JUGLANS CINEREA (torpor; overloaded intestine causes lumbar pain; or from gall-bladder insufficiency) • JUGLANS NIGRA (the astringent leaf as a tea is used in chronic, atonic gastric functions) • Juniperus ("weakness of intestinal muscle" — Powell) • Linum (fresh-ground seed oil for dry colon; chronic and persistent — Weiss) • Lycopodium (homeopathic; dry constitution) • Mahonia (habitual; dry constitution, light-colored feces)

• NEPETA (infantile colic and constipation) • Olea (atonic, impacted bowels; oil) • Plantago psyllium (seed is a stool softener; hull is a peristaltic stimulant) • Podophyllum (gall-bladder stagnation; puffy, yellow complexion; sluggish portal circulation; very small dose) • Prunus (dried fruit) • Ptelea (dry feces, light color, poor appetite, post-febrile) • Rhamnus frangula, R. cathartica (dry feces, tenesmus; chronic atonic, hence a substitute for its relative—see following; small dose) • RHAMNUS PURSHIANA ("the tonic laxative par excellence; daily use will create no laxative dependency"—Tierra) • RHEUM (constipation, hemorrhoids, portal congestion, worms, bloody stool, skin eruptions from faulty elimination and heat in the blood; internal heat) • RICINUS (indurated feces; post-surgical; this is probably the safest and one of the most effective laxatives; oil, externally applied to abdomen) • RUMEX CRISPUS (sluggish bowels with lower-back pain) • Sambucus (acute constipation and fluid retention; bark, dried for a year) • Sesamum (seed is an oily, nourishing laxative) • Stillingia • Taraxacum • Ulmus (weakness) • Vaccinium myrtillus (fresh berry) • Veronicastrum (hepatic stagnation, flatulent distention; very small dose) • ZINGIBERIS (antispasmodic adjuvant, for use with strong purgatives to ease their effects).

Note: The stronger laxatives and cathartics, including Aloe barb., Cassia acutifolia, Rhamnus frangula, R. cathartica, and Rheum, are usually combined with fresh ginger rhizome to cut down on griping or cramping in the intestine. These remedies, and others like them, are usually dried to reduce their activity—but not the ginger. Some other carminative and relaxant may be added.

Diarrhea (Acute): • Achillea (bacterial) • Acorus (tea) • Agrimonia (stress-related; infantile to adult) • ALCHEMILLA (epidemic diarrhea in infants) • Allium ursinum • Althaea • Andrographis • Ballota (sudden onset, cholera—Hool) • Calendula (tea) • Capsella • Capsicum (muco-bloody stools) • Carum • Castanea • Chamomilla (greenish discharges, tenderness and pain; child restless before and after; dried herb) • CINNAMOMUM (chills, beginning of bacterial diarrhea) • Coptis (with mouth sores) • Erigeron (bacterial; bloody) • FILIPENDULA (diarrhea in children) • Fragaria (children) • Gentiana (yellow diarrhea; gallbladder infection) • Geranium (infantile, bacterial, catarrhal) • Geum spp. • Glechoma • Hamamelis (tinged with blood) • Hydrastis (imperfect recovery from) • IPECACUANHA (homeopathic; amoebic) • Iris (yellowish diarrhea from bacteria in the gall bladder) • JUGLANS NIGRA (infection, bacteria; burning, acid diarrhea) • Lycopus (hemorrhagic) • Mentha piperita (spasmodic) • Monarda punctata (nervous origin) • Olea (bacterial; leaf) • Platanus (heartwood) • Polygonum aviculare (knotgrass tea) • Potentilla (tension-related, hemorrhagic) • Pulmonaria • QUERCUS (powerfully astringent; do not use to suppress diarrhea, but for severe loss of tone; frequent, small doses) • Rheum (infantile diarrhea; burning, acid) • Rhodiola (warm astringent) • Rhus glabra (the preferred sumach for diarrhea) • Ribes (juice—Weiss) • ROSA (wild rose root) • RUBUS FRUTICOSUS (acute, infantile, epidemic, all ages; chronic; "there is perhaps no better remedy"—Tierra; leaf or root bark) • Sanguisorba • Teucrium ("acute summer diarrhea of children"—BHP) • Thymus vulgaris (infantile) • Vaccinium myrtillus (dry fruit or leaf) • ZINGIBERIS (gas, cramps, bloating, indigestion).

Note: The herbal traveler should, for protection, take a mixture of equal parts Juglans nigra *and* Rubus fruticosis *tinctures, with a pinch of* Capsicum *as an adjuvant, and* Ipecacuanha *in homeopathic form. In desperation, if diarrhea sets in and these aren't available, drink nine bottles of Coca-Cola a day. Seriously. Homeopathic remedies are often available in the First and Third Worlds. The expression "summer diarrhea," used above, is very frequent in the old books and refers to contaminated well water.*

Diarrhea (Chronic): • ACACIA (diarrhea with colitis) • Achillea (bloody) • Acorus calamus (tea) • Agrimonia (stress-related)

• Allium sativa (bacillary and amoebic) • Allium ursinum
• Althaea • Anemopsis (with mouth sores) • Andrographis
• Calendula (tea) • Capsicum (muco-bloody stools) • Chamomilla (diarrhea, indigestion, bloating) • Cimicifuga • Cola
(chronic, atonic) • Commiphora myrrha (frequent, flatulent
stool) • Coptis (with mouth sores) • Epilobium (wandering
pains; chronic, bacterial, traveler's diàrrhea) • Erigeron (bacterial; bloody) • FILIPENDULA (diarrhea in children) • Geranium (bloody) • Hamamelis (tinged with blood) • Hydrastis
(imperfect recovery from) • Juglans nigra (bacterial) • KRAMERIA • Liatris • Lycopus (hemorrhagic) • Mentha piperita
(spasmodic) • Monarda punctata (of nervous origin) • Myrica
(large, mucoid, semi-formed feces) • Myristica • Nymphaea
• Olea (bacterial; leaf) • Platanus (heartwood) • Polygonatum
• Polygonum aviculare (tea) • Polygonum bistorta (stimulating
astringent; severe, bleeding; epidemic dysentery, in the old days)
• POTENTILLA (tension-related; hemorrhagic) • Pulmonaria
• Quercus (chronic, dilapidated intestine) • Rhodiola (warm
astringent) • Rhus glabra (preferred over the other sumachs for
diarrhea) • Rosa • RUBUS FRUTICOSUS (chronic, mild to
severe; "there is perhaps no better remedy"—Tierra) • Sanguisorba (acute) • SYZYGIUM (chronic) • Teucrium ("acute summer diarrhea of children"—BHP) • Thymus vulgaris (infantile)
• TSUGA (relaxation, depression; diarrhea, dysentery; orally
or enema) • Vaccinium myrtillus (dry fruit or leaf) • Zingiberis
(thin, watery stool; bloating, distention; tongue pale, coated
white or grey, greasy or slimy; dried rhizome) • Zingiberis (gas,
cramps; fresh rhizome).

Diarrhea from Gall-Bladder Infection: • Gentiana (yellow diarrhea) • Iris (yellow diarrhea).

Dysentery: • Acacia (demulcent) • Achillea (bleeding) • Alchemilla (astringent) • ALLIUM SATIVA (amebic) • Baptisia (antiseptic) • Berberis (hard, rapid pulse) • Capsicum (adjuvant,

stimulant) • Cola (atonic, chronic) • Echinacea (antiseptic)
• Geranium (astringent) • IPECACUANHA (homeopathic;
amoebic dysentery; vomiting and diarrhea) • JUGLANS
NIGRA (bacterial) • Lycopus (hemorrhagic, with rapid,
irregular pulse) • Myristica (stimulant) • Plantago psyllium
(demulcent) • Polygonum (stimulating astringent) • TSUGA
(relaxation, depression; internal or enema).

Diverticulitis, Diverticulosis: • ACHILLEA • Althaea officinalis
• Chamomilla • Dioscorea • Humulus • Myrica • Plantago
• Symphytum • Ulmus.

Duodenum: • Echinacea (catarrh) • Chionanthus (inflammation)
• Piper methysticum (duodenal ulcers, pain shooting to navel,
spastic) • Podophyllum (duodenitis; small dose).

Edema, Abdominal (see "Liver," below): • Chelone glabra
• Chimaphila • Equisetum • Iris versicolor • Juniperus.

Rectal Fissure: • Aesculus glabra • Alchemilla (strengthens
sphincter) • Althaea (lubricates the passage) • Agrimonia (pain)
• Centella • Collinsonia • Hamamelis • Hydrastis • Hypericum
(pain) • Polygonum bistorta (stimulating astringent; ointment)
• Symphytum • Ulmus (lubricates the passage).

Flatulence: • Acorus • Achillea • Alpinia (flatulence with fermentation) • Angelica (spasmodic colic and flatus) • Anthemis
• Arctium (pain, tension, gas) • ASAFOETIDA (abdominal)
• Asclepias tuberosa • Capsicum • Carum • Chamomilla (colic,
flatus, diarrhea) • CINNAMOMUM CASSIA (cramping, nausea, looseness; worse from cold food) • Dioscorea • Foeniculum
(tympanitic) • Humulus (with fermentation and acid eructations) • Hydrastis (putrid gas) • Illicium (flatulence with colic)
• Imperatoria ostruthium • Juglans cinerea (distention and flatus) • Melilotus • MENTHA PIPERITA • Pimpinella anisum

• Piper nigrum (black pepper) • Rheum (from cramping, indigestion, gas) • Salvia (flatulence and debility) • Valeriana (with nervousness) • Zanthoxylum (tympanitic) • Zingiberis.

Hemorrhage, Gastrointestinal: • Achillea • Capsella • Cinnamomum zeylanicum • Erigeron • Trillium.

Hemorrhoids: • ACHILLEA (bleeding; external) • AESCULUS GLABRA (continuous contraction of sphincter) • AESCULUS HIP. (with mental tension; external) • Agrimonia (painful) • Anethum • Bidens (bleeding—Hool) • Calendula (external) • Capsella bursa-pastoris (sitz baths) • Capsicum (assistant to other remedies) • Ceanothus • Chamomilla (painful) • Chelidonium • COLLINSONIA • Coptis • Epilobium (flower suppositories) • Equisetum • Geranium maculatum • Glechoma • HAMAMELIS (orifices relaxed, bleeding; "best ointment"— Weiss) • Hydrastis • Hypericum (painful, irritating) • Krameria (prolapsed or bleeding) • Lavendula (reduces swelling; suppository) • Myrica • Nepeta • Paeonia • Phytolacca • Plantago • Polygonum bistorta • Polygonum hydropiperoides (anal itching) • Potentilla • Pulmonaria • Quercus (large, swollen— Weiss) • Ranunculus ficaria (internal or prolapsed piles, with or without hemorrhage; topical) • Rubus canadensis (combine with Achillea in ointment) • RUMEX CRISPUS (bleeding) • RUSCUS • Sanicula (ointment) • Scrophularia (chronic) • Silybum • Stillingia • Symphytum • Ulmus (non-bleeding external piles; lubricates passage of stool) • Verbascum (highly sensitive; specific for the veins—Edgar Cayce) • Vinca • Zanthoxylum.

Note: Consider combining with a mild laxative, anti-inflammatory, antispasmodic, astringent, and bitter tonic to tone the pelvic veins. To make a cream, coconut butter is a good medium.

Hernia (external treatments): • Achillea • Alchemilla (atonic muscle) • Althaea • Capsella (atrophic muscle) • Chamomilla (tender, strangulated) • Glycyrrhiza (in oil, external rub for internal adhesions) • Hieracium pilosella • Hydrastis (torn) • Lobelia (strangulated) • Rubus canadensis (atonic muscle) • Symphytum • Trigonella.

Ileocecal Irritability: • Fouquieria • Larrea • Plantago • Rumex crispus.

Irritable Bowel Syndrome (IBS): • Agrimonia • Carum • Chamomilla • Cynara • Dioscorea (spasm) • Erigeron • Foeniculum • Glycyrrhiza • Mentha piperita (oil; 10–20 drops in a capsule, 4x/day) • Myrica (chronic ileocecal inflammation or cramps) • Plantago psyllium (mucilage) • Ulmus.

"Leaky Gut Syndrome," Dysbiosis, Food Sensitivity, Abnormal Flora: • Agrimony • Althaea (mucilage) • Borago (seed oil) • Epilobium • Eupatorium purpureum • IRIS (thyroid and blood-sugar fluctuations after eating—Wood) • Juglans nigra (abnormal flora) • Malva neglecta (mucilage—LeSassier) • Monarda fistulosa (systemic candida) • Mentha piperita (fermentation; abnormal flora—Weiss), Myrica (inactive canal, mucus in stool) • Olea • PLANTAGO • Polygonatum (abnormal flora; needs confirmation) • Urtica (mucus in stool).

Parasites, Amebas, Worms: • ALLIUM SATIVA (ameba) • Allium ursinum (fresh) • Aloe barb. • Amygdalus (poultice or compress to draw out—Grieve) • Artemisia absinthium (small doses only; sub-active gall bladder; nematoid, pinworm, roundworm), Artemisia vulgaris (thread- and roundworm) • Berberis (long-term infestation) • Calendula (tea) • Centaurium (tea daily for 2–3 months) • CHAMOMILLA (pinworms) • Chenopodium • Cucurbita pepo (tapeworm; seed) • Euphorbia (amoebas) • Granatum (pomegranate bark) • Inula (hookworm)

• JUGLANS NIGRA (dogs will eat this to deworm themselves;
hull) • Malus (traditional preventative—needs confirmation;
vinegar) • OLEA • TANACETUM PARTHENIUM (round-
or threadworm in children; scabies, *pruritus ani;* small dose)
• Thymus (hookworm, non-intestinal) • Zanthoxylum.

Prolapse: • Alchemilla (tea) • Capsella bursa-pastoris (external)
• Juglans nigra (leaf) • Rubus canadensis (leaf).

Rectum, Anus: • Aristolochia (anal fistula, erosive) • Chamomilla
(excoriation, pinworms) • HAMAMELIS (fissure, soreness,
tender piles) • Hydrastis (eczema; *pruritus ani*) • PAEONIA
(crack, fissure, fistula, ulcer, piles) • Quercus (prolapse)
• Ruscus • SCROPHULARIA (*pruritus ani*) • STELLARIA
(*pruritus ani*) • Tanacetum parthenium (*pruritus ani* from pinworms) • Tsuga (prolapse) • Urtica (pinworms).

Spasm of Circular Muscle Fibers: • Allium sativa (Weiss)
• Dioscorea.

Stool: • Anthemis (green, slimy, with rotten-egg smell) • Baptisia
(dark, rotten) • Chamomilla (green, slimy) • Chelidonium (clay-
colored) • Chenopodium • Chionanthus (clay-colored; frothy;
green) • Collinsonia (hard, ball-like) • Iris versicolor (yellowish,
greenish from gall-bladder infection) • Veronicastrum (clay-
colored; half-digested food) • Podophyllum (clay-colored or
greenish) • Rubus canadensis (watery; in children) • Urtica
(profuse, mucoid).

Ulcers: See "Colitis, Enteritis," above.

FORMULARY

Acacia—with Acorus, Mentha piperita, Filipendula, Agrimonia,
Quercus (lower-bowel complaints). BHP 1983, 53.

Acorus—with Carum, Agrimonia, Myrica, Quercus (diarrhea). BHP 1983, 49.

Agrimonia—with Linaria, Berberis, Chamomilla, Taraxacum, Petroselinum, 1 part each (appendicitis).

Agrimonia—with Polygonum hydropiperoides, Ceanothus, and a pinch of Myrica (nutritive, astringent, and cleansing bowel tonic).

Alchemilla—with Agrimonia, Geum, or Potentilla (gastroenteritis). BHP 1983, 19.

Alchemilla—with Geranium and Castanea (infantile diarrhea). BHP 1983, 53.

Althaea—with Filipendula and Capsicum as an adjuvant (flatulence or spasm of the GI). BHP 1983, 48.

Asarum—with Hydrastis and Geranium (colitis).

Bidens—with Acorus, Agrimonia, or Zingiberis (general GI). BHP 1983, 43.

Bidens—with Achillea, Rumex crispus (bleeding hemorrhoids).

Cinnamomum zeylanicum—with Geranium, Quercus, Acorus, Acacia (diarrhea with colic or tormina). BHP 1983, 68–9.

Foeniculum—with Chamomilla, Acorus, Ginger (flatulent colic). Modified from BHP 1983, 93.

Geranium—with Geum, Agrimonia, Pulmonaria (children's diarrhea). BHP 1983, 173.

Geum urbanum—with Bidens (ulcerative colitis). BHP 1983, 103.

Gnaphalium—with coolant (Rosa, Prunus serotina, Amygdalus, or Tilia) and astringent (Geranium or Ceanothus); one part each of the three (celiac sprue).

Hamamelis—with Collinsonia, Aesculus hip. (hemorrhoids).

Hamamelis—with Plantago or Ranunculus ficaria (hemorrhoids). BHP 1983, 109. Hypericum—with Hamamelis (hemorrhoids). BHP 1983, 115.

Juglans nigra (hull)—with Rubus fruticosis leaf or root bark (equal parts), plus a pinch of Capsicum as an adjuvant, in tincture (acute bacterial diarrhea).

Mentha piperita—combines well with Pimpinella (flatulent colic). BHP 1983, 141, 160.

Myrica—with Nymphaea, Quercus (diarrhea). BHP 1983, 151.

Myristica—adjuvant in dyspepsia and diarrhea formulae.

Pimpinella—aromatic sweet adjuvant to prevent tormina and griping in cathartic formulae. BHP 1983, 160.

Polygonum bistorta—with Geranium, Agrimonia, or Quercus (diarrhea). BHP 1983, 168.

Potentilla—with Acacia (diarrhea). BHP 1983, 170.

Potentilla—with Quercus, Krameria, or Geranium (chronic diarrhea, intestinal prolapse). BHP 1983, 170.

Potentilla—with Sanguisorba, Acacia (diarrhea). BHP 1983, 189.

Quercus—with Capsicum or Zingiberis, before meals (diarrhea). BHP 1983, 175.

Ranunculus ficaria—with Pulmonaria, Calendula (hemorrhoids). BHP 1983, 173.

Rhamnus purshiana—with Berberis, Glycyrrhiza, Zingiberis (constipation).

Rhamnus purshiana—with glycerin ("the hidden treasure" for constipation). Stacey Jones.

Tsuga—with Acacia, Quercus (diarrhea). BHP 1983, 219.

Veronicastrum—with Hydrastis, Acorus (constipation "associated with flatulent distension"). BHP 1983, 229. The first ingredient is very purgative; use in a small proportion.

Zingiberis—adjuvant with cathartics, to prevent spasm.

Zingiberis—with Dioscorea, Chamomilla, Acorus (intestinal colic). BHP 1983, 79.

CANADA HEMLOCK *(TSUGA CANADENSIS)*

I heard a beautiful healing story from herbalist Margi Flint. Her grandfather was a traveling salesman, selling chocolate in northern New England. A blizzard struck, and he was stranded in a small town in Maine. He came down with bloody dysentery—usually fatal without medical attention in those days.

An Indian man came out of the forest on snowshoes saying, "I heard someone in town is sick." His treatment was successful, and Margi's grandfather offered to pay him. The man replied that what he really needed was a rifle, to take care of his family. He had been unable to get one since it was illegal to sell firearms to Indians.

Margi's grandfather returned the next year with a rifle. In gratitude, the man gave him a decorated buckskin jacket. I asked Margi's father, Putnam Flint, what the remedy was, and he said, "I know for sure it had hemlock bark in it." I have seen Margi wearing that jacket.

Assimilation

Normally this function would be included with the small intestine or lower gastrointestinal tract, but in order to explore it more thoroughly, I have given it a section of its own. This is in keeping with traditions both East and West.

William Cook was one of the most observant of the physiomedical doctors; we may rightly refer to him as "wise." He draws our attention to the differences between "tonics to the digestive and to the assimilative apparatus." This is a distinction that has "not heretofore been made; but it is one of importance." He goes on to say that agents "which act on the assimilative organs are so few as to deserve especial notice." Among these he particularly points out *Geum virginianum* and *G. rivale* (avens, water avens, chocolate root), native to North America but probably cognate with the Old World *Geum urbanum*. He writes of the chocolate root:

> In those forms of indigestion which arise from debility of the duodenum, pancreas and mesenteries—connected with pains and laxity of the bowels, curdy stools, and slow loss of flesh—it is a peculiarly valuable article; and may be used freely, especially when boiled in milk and used as a sort of chocolate. From this action, it has been set down as useful in dyspepsia, whereas it is insignificant in this malady of the stomach. Its action on the duodenum and mesenteries fits it for a class of cases to which few

articles are applicable; and I am decidedly of the opinion that it will be found useful in *tabes mesenterica,* and in those forms of scrofulous looseness of the bowels which are dependent upon defective assimilation, and which often pass roughly as chronic diarrhea (Cook 1869, 448).

Lack of absorption and assimilation not only affects nutrition but the pickup of water — hence the diarrhea. The idea of assimilation in Cook's medicine is similar to the idea of the "spleen" in Traditional Chinese Medicine, which is associated with the post-digestive process of "transportation and transformation" of food and fluids. Spleen deficiency causes malnutrition, tissue laxity, and diarrhea. It is also similar to the Greek idea of the "spleen," again associated with the nutritive function.

After the food/toxins have entered the body through the gut wall, they are met by a frenzied, stirred-up army of newly minted white blood cells ready to pounce on the innumerable "bad guys" that snuck in with the more innocent food/toxins. Each time we eat, the bone marrow is signaled to manufacture millions of new white cells expressly for this meal.

In old-time medicine, doctors and folk healers used to differentiate a certain kind of malnutrition associated with the spleen. The person was pale, sallow, had low energy, poor digestion, "slow loss of flesh" (as Cook says), and loose stools. In Maine they still say a person or cow that doesn't gain weight well is "spleeny," and in the South they used to speak of people who were "born tired." Because of the massive amount of food we have today in the First World, we don't see much of this. However, there is another problem that we do see.

We may have plenty of food — too much — but it contains many more toxins than our ancestors were confronted with, and it may be that we have to produce more white blood cells with every meal than did our forebears. When I take a leukemia case, I often find that there was some poison or toxin, possibly just a spider bite, that set off an immune reaction that perhaps overstimulated white-cell production and led to the pathological production of mutated white cells — leukemia. The increasing levels of this disease — especially in children, who have a more sensitive gut — may possibly be replacing the "spleeny" problems of the past.

Cook gives a list of remedies under the heading "assimilation," which I have reproduced exactly below, except for my addition of *Ceanothus* and *Geum urbanum*. Almost all of these remedies combine astringence, stimulation, and the sweet or nutritive taste. Where one of these properties is missing, Cook tells us to supplement it. These are exactly the kind of remedies that suit "spleen yang deficiency," in the terminology of TCM, though the Chinese do not use the astringent property as much as we do in the West, preferring the warmth or stimulation which is also found in these agents. The sweet taste is also perfect because, according to TCM, it guides the herb to the spleen.

Assimilation: • Ceanothus (sweet, astringent) • Comptonia (sweet, pungent, and astringent, this agent is more like a "spleen yang tonic" than any other in the American *materia medica;* promotes digestion gently, and assimilation strongly; diarrhea) • Filipendula ("sub-acute and chronic diarrhea, scrofulous character, where the assimilative organs are at fault" — Cook) • Geum urbanum (sweet, astringent, pungent; diarrhea, dysentery, weakness, and debility; "vinous" tincture — Grieve) • Geum virginianum (sweet, astringent, pungent; curdy diarrhea, wasting) • Gnaphalium (sweet, slightly pungent and aromatic; wasting, weakness of organs) • Myrica (pungent, astringent; atonic GI mucosa with catarrh; weak peripheral circulation) • Nymphaea (mucilaginous and astringent; GI and vaginal yeast) • Populus tremuloides (bitter, astringent, sweet) • Rheum (astringent, bitter, acrid; curdy diarrhea, lack of assimilation, tumid abdomen in children) • Rumex crispus (elongated, red tongue, with heavy white or yellow coating; yeast and heat; thrush in babies; borborygmus) • Scrophularia • Verbascum (one of the best for promoting absorption — Cook).

RHUBARB (*RHEUM* SPP.)

To the extent that rhubarb is used today in Western herbalism, it is mostly as a laxative, in small doses, in formulas, and almost never as a specific, simple, or single remedy. I thought, however, to remedy that with a portrait of its specific uses, both as a laxative for constipation, and in smaller doses as a tonic for diarrhea. A good account of the constitutional indications calling for rhubarb as a laxative is given by Huang Huang in his excellent *Ten Key Formula Families in Chinese Medicine* (1994). William Cook's *A Physiomedical Dispensatory* (1869) also gives us a wonderful account of the properties of rhubarb.

Today we can get Asiatic rhubarb *(Rheum palmatum, R. officinale)* at no great cost; but perhaps many people such as myself, who grew up with rhubarb in the garden, have wondered whether common rhubarb could be used in place of the medicinal rhubarb.

Culinary rhubarb *(Rheum rhaponticum)* was developed by English market gardeners, who had been employed by traders in herbal drugs in an attempt to grow rhubarb at home and reduce the cost of bringing it from China through Russia and Turkey. This strain grew well, but failed as a drug. The gardeners, however, found a market for it, and rhubarb became a beloved pie-plant in the northern world, where fruit is less available in early spring.

Cook wondered about this, and tried the domesticated plant in place of the expensive trade item. "The density is less than that of the Asiatic species," he wrote, "and the center of the root is sometimes even short and spongy. The odor of this species is faint, and not so agreeable as that of the foreign roots; the taste is bitterish astringent, mucilaginous, and not gritty nor always pleasant." (I would say it is more "acrid" than "bitter," and more "sour" than "astringent.") Though "less agreeable to the taste, somewhat more astringent, and distinctly mucilaginous," continues Cook, the "impression upon the system is nearly identical with the foreign species, though about twice the quantity is required" (Cook 1869).

The taste of Chinese rhubarb *(Rheum palmatum)* is "heavy, compact, oily, and fragrant, with a bitter and nonastringent taste," according to Huang Huang. He used large doses of this plant for an excess constitution. "The ancients metaphorically referred to *radix et rhizoma rhei (da huang)* as the general who has the power to knock down doors and suppress turmoil" (Huang 1994, 113). The actions of large doses are "harsh," so one needs to know how to use this agent. Dr. Huang treats us to a description of both the indicated constitutional type and the symptom presentation.

The energetic condition is one of interior full heat: excess is seen in constipation and fullness, heat in tenderness, tissue and mental irritability, fever, and the "red, tough, firm tongue body with a dry, scorched-yellow coating." Huang, in fact, calls the latter "rhubarb tongue." The complexion is full and red, the lips often dark-red, and if there is mucus it is thick and adhesive. In addition to the heat symptoms, there tend to be symptoms of blood stagnation, giving a purple cast to the dark-redness of the complexion or tongue. The heat rises and causes swollen glands, fever, headache, dizziness, mouth sores, herpes, redness in the eyes, and other symptoms.

Although it is frequently used in acute febrile conditions, Chinese rhubarb is also associated with a particular constitutional type. This person is big, with firm muscles, yet lazy, a red, oily complexion, thick lips on the dark-red side, a large, self-indulgent appetite, stuffiness in the chest, and an aversion to heat. Huang mentions a dry mouth, but these people can have excessive salivation (a symptom from the homeopathic provings).

In emphasizing the basic energetics and organ affinities, but not as much the fixed syndromes or disease names, Huang Huang's approach is very similar to that of the eclectics such as Scudder, and some of the physiomedicalists.

Cook describes the use of rhubarb, in smaller doses, for a constitution that is almost the opposite of the one described by Huang. Doses of twenty to forty grains are laxative, but in four- to eight-grain doses, three times a day, "it soothes irritability of the stomach and promotes digestion." It is especially indicated in "those forms of indigestion accompanied by acidity, laxity of the gastric structures, morning looseness of the bowels, and sallow countenance. A portion of its good effects is due to its mild stimulation of the bile ducts, leading to ejection of bile" (Cook 1869).

For diarrhea and dysentery, Cook recommends two large doses three hours apart to loosen impacted material, followed by small doses thereafter until the looseness subsides. This approach leaves a gentle tonic effect from the astringency. "It is well adapted to children of scrophulous habits, with a tumid abdomen." I remember as a child that some kids seemed to crave rhubarb stalks, and ate them raw straight out of the garden. This suggests that it possesses some kind of deep nourishing effect, and Cook hints that this is so. "It seems to improve the assimilative powers well and, like *Geum, Myrica,* and a few other agents, to give firmness and activity to lax mesenteries in scrophulous constitutions." Like *Geum, Rheum* is indicated for the "curdy diarrhea" that Cook considered a characteristic of lack of assimilation.

These two different presentations illustrate opposite profiles, and demonstrate how many herbs normalize between two opposite conditions. (This principle was introduced in Part I, in the discussion of the rebound effect, and primary and secondary symptoms.)

Liver

Food, routinely digested in the stomach and assimilated through the lymph system and portal vein, would be highly toxic for us if we injected it directly into our bloodstream. Therefore, it needs to be detoxified in order to be made safe. For this reason, I do not call it "food," but "food/toxins." The job of the liver is to shield the rest of the body from this wave of toxic material, and render it into useful nutrition and replacement parts. The liver is usually thought of as the center of detoxification, but it is also the center for producing cell food. The liver is said to be in charge of the "preparatory" metabolism, while the cells themselves perform the "secondary" or cellular metabolism.

This liver does this through the breakdown and rebuilding of chemicals in the food/toxins. The metabolic process is divided into two camps: the catabolism (breaking down) and anabolism (building up). Michael Moore used to like to talk about the "catabolic dominant" and "anabolic dominant" constitutions—the former tearing down a lot of toxins, and latter making a lot of metabolites. A big, heavy man himself, he frequently joked about the "anabolic grease-ball" who loved rich foods and overbuilt the blood, carbs, lipids, and proteins in the body.

Food/toxins enter the body through the cell walls lining the intestines. The water-soluble carbs and proteins are picked up by the capillaries feeding the portal vein and brought directly to the liver, while the oil-soluble lipids are absorbed into the lymphatic ducts and taken on a circuitous journey up to the chest, dumped into the bloodstream, and finally brought to the liver. The proteins are manufactured into substances that regulate the blood. The sugars were already broken down to glucose in the intestines; they are stored in the liver as glycogen, or sent on to the cells for use or storage. Fats and oils are processed into cholesterol—the lipid "coin of the realm" from which everything oil-soluble is made in the body.

The liver even handles some minerals. Old blood cells are broken down to extract iron-rich salts, which combine with cholesterol to form the bile. This is secreted by the hepatic cells and collected, managed, and released by the gall bladder. Much of the bile is reabsorbed so that the valuable bile salts can be reused. The liver also breaks down hormones and other metabolites made in the body after they have served their purpose.

Midway through catabolism, there is a point where metabolites need to be stabilized by an antioxidant to prevent oxidation. Antioxidants must be consumed in food, in the form of fruits and vegetables. If they are not, incompletely metabolized "free radicals" will get into the bloodstream and cause inflammation. These attract oxygen, which inserts itself into a weak molecule and "blows it up." This uncontrolled chemical activity causes the "weathering" or aging of tissues. We see, therefore, why the liver is associated with uncontrolled heat processes in the body, both in Eastern and Western herbalism. We also see why antioxidants are now a nutritional fad—they have been recognized as preventing this destructive process.

If a person consumes too much food or too many toxins, requiring lots of hepatic work and lots of antioxidants, the load of unmetabolized junk can back up down the portal vein. More arterial blood is needed in the liver to complete metabolism, and this takes it away from the brain and other organs, leading to a prolonged episode of sluggishness after the meal or drug or alcohol use—a hangover. In traditional Western herbalism, the idea of a "toxic liver" or "toxic blood" is very important. This describes the sluggish hepatic function, or acute or chronic hangover due to excessive consumption of food, drugs, or alcohol. The symptoms of a sluggish liver are like those of a hangover, but are chronic. The unresolved metabolic waste products and free radicals produce toxic heat symptoms, such as skin conditions including eczema and acne.

The liver undertakes literally thousands of jobs. building up and tearing down metabolites. We could not dream of an herb or drug for every individual pathway or enzyme—nor does biomedicine. Instead, we need to have an overview of the liver, and treat the major processes by which these thousands of operations take place.

The liver is like a furnace: it needs oxygen (from arterial blood), a valve (arterial-tension regulation), fuel (food/toxins carried in from the portal vein), fire (metabolic energy), and an outlet (bile). It also needs to be cleansed; this is done by lymph and venous blood. Liver remedies, therefore, act to: (1) increase arterial circulation to the liver by promoting capillary development (*Lavandula*), relieving arterial tension (*Agrimonia*), and thinning the blood (*Achillea, Angelica*); (2) decrease venous and portal congestion (*Collinsonia, Aesculus, Potentilla*); (3) keep lymphatic drainage clear (*Calendula, Scrophularia*); (4) promote metabolism of proteins (*Urtica*), lipids (*Arctium*), glucose (*Vaccinium myrtillus*), and poisons (*Larrea, Silybum*); (5) boost both catabolism (*Arctium, Larrea*) and anabolism (*Mahonia, Lycopodium*); (6) protect liver cells (*Curcuma, Silybum*); and (7) produce and clear bile (*Chelidonium, Hydrastis, Taraxacum*).

In addition, the general body environment needs to be kept in good order so as not to overburden the liver. "Toxic liver," "liver congestion," or metabolic disorder can occur from a low thyroid condition, but can also cause it (Wilson's Thyroid Syndrome), since the liver needs to process thyroxine. Liver congestion also occurs with toxic buildup in the extracellular matrix *(Stellaria media)*, a leaky gut sending in too many toxins *(Iris, Althaea)*, and poor elimination (by skin, kidneys, and intestine) throwing toxins back into the body.

Many liver problems in the past were due to malaria, which caused swelling of the liver and spleen. Since many of our old liver remedies *(Euonymus, Veronicastrum, Chelone)* come from this period, they are no longer as useful as they once were. I have only used *Chelone* twice in thirty-five years, for travelers who picked up malaria in Central America. At the same time, our knowledge and skill level with these herbs has dropped off, so we don't understand how to use them as well.

Toxic, Congested Liver (Low Catabolism): • Achillea (congestion; poor lipid metabolism—M. Moore) • Allium sativa (garlic) • Angelica • ARCTIUM (poor lipid metabolism, low bile production; skin rashes, acne, scalp) • Astragalus • Azadirachta (general detoxifier, immune tonic, anti-inflammatory) • BERBERIS (damp and heat; low-grade bacterial infections, chronic ill health; dull-minded, shattered physically and mentally) • BETA (poor lipid metabolism—Weiss; said to regenerate hepatocytes) • BUPLEURUM (fullness in chest, hypochondrium; mood swings; wiry and/or thin pulse) • CEANOTHUS (lymphatic support) • Centaurium (clears damp heat—Hobbs) • Chelone (pain from left side of liver down to navel) • Chionanthus (stimulating, bitter) • Cichorium (cooling; low bile production and ejection) • Citrus limonum (torpor) • COLLINSONIA (for stagnation in portal vein backing up toxins to liver and gall bladder) • CURCUMA (stimulating anti-inflammatory, protectant, regenerative, bile stimulant; combine with pepper and bromelain) • Cynara (for poor metabolism of fats) • Fumaria • Galium (lymph nodes) • Glycyrrhiza (protectant) • Helianthus (one of the best detoxification oils in Ayurvedic "oil-pulling") • Hepatica (soothing and tonic) • Hydrastis (low bile production) • IRIS (congestion; leaky gut) • Juglans cinerea (sluggish bile) • Juglans nigra (leaky gut—needs

confirmation) • LARREA (depression from excess toxins; small
dose) • Lavendula (externally, to support liver capillary bed —
Gümbel) • Linaria (jaundice) • MAHONIA (dry skin, constipation; low catabolism and anabolism) • Menispermum (when
Smilax "proves ineffective, invariably yellow parilla [Menisper-
mum] will take over and relieve — possibly cure — it" — Bartram)
• Nux vomica (homeopathic) • Oplopanax • Picraena (regenerates, tones) • Plantago (protectant) • Polygonatum • Prunella
(liver fire, sore throat) • Raphanus • Rehmannia (impaired
function, hepatitis, liver damage, poisoning; uncooked root)
• Rhamnus (torpor, congestion, constipation) • Rumex crispus
(red and yellow complexion) • Schisandra (protectant) • Scolopendrium • Silybum • Smilax • Solidago (skin rashes, acne;
scalp) • Stellaria (on hot spots; swollen nodes; external)
• TARAXACUM (heat, swollen tissue; mapped tongue)
• VERONICASTRUM (depression; small dose) • Withania.

Hangover: • Larrea (dark circles under eyes) • Linaria (dark
circles under eyes) • Mahonia (dark circles under eyes) • Nux
vomica (homeopathic; grumpy).

Low Anabolism ("Liver Blood Deficiency"): • AGRIMONIA
(pale-yellowish complexion) • Artemisia absinthium (hard
liver pulse — Wood) • BETONICA (wan, leaden complexion)
• LYCOPODIUM (withered, full of gas, dry) • MAHONIA
(constipation, dry skin, acne, eczema, unhealthy scalp) • Polygonatum (to protect liver, treat fatty liver, bring down high blood
pressure) • SALVIA (senescence; low in the liver pulse — Bonaldo) • WITHANIA.

*Note: This condition, different from normal blood deficiency, is called "liver
blood deficiency" in TCM, or "liver not breeding blood" (Culpeper). Typical
symptoms when the liver is involved are: sallow, pale, dry complexion, with
atrophy and wasting.*

Liver Swelling, Pain: • Agrimonia (cirrhosis; dark, sallow skin; low anabolism) • Angelica (low metabolism—needs confirmation) • BUPLEURUM (pain in hypochondrium and chest) • Calendula (hepatitis, jaundice) • Chelidonium (hepatitis, jaundice) • Chelone • Chionanthus (sallow, dirty-looking skin, with hepatic tenderness, expressionless eyes; fats in stool) • CNICUS (intermittent chills of hepatitis) • Collinsonia • CURCUMA (anti-inflammatory, regenerative; combine with pepper) • Echinacea (abscess) • Euonymus (stomach upset with hepatic torpor) • Galium (fatty liver; hepato-protective) • Hydrangea (inactive liver associated with irritated kidneys) • Hydrastis • Iris versicolor (abscess, fatty liver) • LARREA • Lycopodium (dry, thin; low anabolism; cirrhosis) • Mahonia (stomach upset with hepatic torpor) • PEUMUS • Podophyllum (full, bloated, sallow complexion with inactive liver, or chills; full pulse; tiny dose) • Polemonium (chronic liver disease) • Polymnia (rub ointment over liver or spleen) • Senecio aureus (very small dose) • SILYBUM (mushroom poisoning, alcoholism, hepatitis, abscess) • Taraxacum (heat and swelling) • Veronicastrum (full, inactive liver, hepatitis, pain, depression) • Vitis (leaf tea).

Note: These symptoms are usually associated with hepatitis or cirrhosis.

Jaundice (Liver, Gall Bladder): • Agrimonia (tense, pinched, yellow-grey complexion) • Artemisia absinthium • Artemisia vulgaris • Berberis (with Agrimonia and Taraxacum) • Betonica (wan, leaden complexion with weakness of gall-bladder reflexes) • Bupleurum • Centaurium • Chelidonium (yellow complexion, gall-bladder congestion; pain under right shoulder blade) • Chelone (malarial) • Chionanthus (cramp on right side, stoppage of bile ducts, constipation) • Cichorium • Citrus limonum (acute jaundice, hepatic torpor, red tongue, alkaline urine) • Cnicus benedictus • Curcuma • Euonymus • Galium • Hydrastis (infection, weakness and congestion in the gall bladder) • Juglans nigra (leaf tea) • Veronicastrum (pale, dry skin,

thick-coated tongue, moderate hepatic pain) • Linaria • Mahonia • Marrubium (yellowness of the eyes) • Monarda fistulosa
(bloated and yellow complexion with gall-bladder congestion)
• Myrica (infantile jaundice) • Nux vomica (homeopathic;
infantile jaundice) • Podophyllum (catarrhal, bloated, sallow;
clay-colored stool; very small dose) • Prunella • Taraxacum
(long-term gall bladder congestion) • Veronica.

Hepatitis: • Achillea (poultice over liver) • Agrimonia (acute
viral) • Andrographis • Arctium • Artemisia absinthium (acute
viral) • Asperula • BERBERIS • BUPLEURUM (yellowish,
dark, reddish complexion) • Bryonia (pain on movement)
• Calendula • Chelidonium • Chelone • Chionanthus (light,
frothy stools, scanty urine, pain in right hypochondrium)
• Cichorium • CNICUS (deep chills, terrible flu feeling, jaundice) • CURCUMA (combine with pepper) • Cynara
• Dioscorea • Fouquieria ("chronic abdominal pain and hemor-
rhoidal aching after acute symptoms have disappeared" — M.
Moore) • Galium • Ganoderma • Glycyrrhiza • Hyssopus
(acute viral) • Iris (acute viral) • Isatis • LARREA (massive
doses have caused hepatitis, appropriate small doses help)
• Lentinula (chronic) • Leonurus • Linaria • Mahonia
• Melissa (acute viral) • MENYANTHES (acute viral)
• Prunella • Rehmannia (uncooked root) • Salvia miltorrhiza
(scar tissue) • Schisandra • Silybum (acute, chronic) • Taraxacum • Veronicastrum.

*Note: Bacteria, viruses, or poisons can cause hepatitis (liver inflammation).
The major diagnostic indication is elevated liver enzymes in the blood from
hepatic-cell die-off. Today there are specific drugs that can completely eliminate
hepatitis. There may be cases, however, where herbs are still needed to completely eliminate disease and the enzymes in the blood (from personal clinical
experience).*

Cirrhosis: • Acorus • Agrimonia • Berberis • Chelone • Dioscorea • Euonymus • Fouquieria • Iris • Menyanthes • Silybum • Taraxacum.

Ascites: • Apocynum cannabinum ("whenever the ascites is the principle trouble, if the symptoms indicate no other remedy"— Clarke; small doses) • Juglans nigra • Liatris.

FORMULARY

In the following formulas, dandelion root *(Taraxacum)* should be used.

Beta—Silybum, Taraxacum, Lavandula, Petroselinum (tonic). Wood.

Chionanthus—with Berberis, Peumus (liver and gall bladder). BHP 1983, 156.

Mahonia—with Arctium, Salvia, Silybum (liver, dry skin, eczema). Wood.

Taraxacum—with 10% Podophyllum (laxative, cholagogue). BHP 1983, 167.

Taraxacum—with Berberis, Veronicastrum (hepatic, cathartic). BHP 1983, 229.

Taraxacum—with Chelidonium, Berberis (gall-bladder disease). BHP 1983, 62.

Taraxacum—with Petroselinum, Hydrastis, Berberis (hepatic disease). BHP 1983, 155.

Taraxacum—with Silybum (liver) widespread formula.

Gall Bladder

When the liver has finished making the bile, it secretes it into the bile ducts. The bile leaves the liver in many little rivulets, which conjoin into a single channel that runs all the way down into the duodenum, where it is secreted to emulsify fats and oils. Bile is both hydrophilic and lipophilic, so it conjoins with water and oil, emulsifying the dietary lipids into a slurry that can be more easily digested.

Stationed partway down this duct is the gall bladder, a sac in which the bile is collected between meals for use during digestion. When the pyloric valve of the stomach opens to send food into the duodenum, it sends a signal to the gall bladder and gall duct to open and dump bile. Just before the sphincter where it opens into the duodenum, the gall duct is joined by a channel from the pancreas, full of pancreatic enzymes ready to jump on the digestate and tear it down. So the bile and digestive enzymes are released together.

The main function of the gall bladder is therefore a fairly simple one—to store and release bile. Problems with the gall bladder are likewise fairly simple. The gall ducts and bladder are innervated by the autonomic nervous system, which controls the digestive tract as a whole. Unconscious autonomic nervous tension causes spasms and mistimings of the release of bile—but these unpleasant symptoms can become very conscious.

Gall bladder problems were once much more common than today. Due to the prevalence of malaria, many people suffered from chills running through the autonomic. This resulted in "biliousness"—nausea, diarrhea alternating with constipation, and a taste of bile in the throat—one of the most common ailments of our ancestors, mentioned here because it helps us understand the older literature. Biliousness may be equated with GERD—gastric esophageal reflex disease—except that we commonly get the symptoms from eating heavy, greasy food, not the malaria mosquito.

Migraine headaches follow the "gall bladder meridian" of TCM from the gall bladder up over the scapula to the occiput, across the right (sometimes left) side of the head, to the eye, and sometimes down an inch below the eye. The suffering person sometimes notes indigestion or even pain in the gall bladder before the advent of the headache. This was called "bilious headache" by the old Western authors and "gall bladder headache" in Traditional Chinese Medicine. For remedies, see the "migraine" entry in the "Headache" sections (under "Brain and Head").

The other major gall bladder problem is stone formation caused by condensation of bile in the gall ducts and bladder. Mucus, calcification, heat, spasm, torpor, and inactivity can cause the bile to thicken and turn into "stones" (which may not be entirely stone-like or even made of bile). This leads to more inflammation, pain, spasm, and ultimately gall bladder removal. Many times, however, the pain continues even after the gall bladder is removed. This is because the conditions are not limited to the gall bladder itself but run back up into the gall ducts draining out of the liver, which is also under autonomic control and subject to the same pathological influences — mucus, heat, spasm, etc. Therefore, in order to cure the underlying problems of the gall bladder and related system, we need to correct the tissue imbalance by cooling or warming, toning or relaxing, drying or moistening.

Biliousness: • Agrimonia (gall bladder unsynchronized with digestion; alternating diarrhea and constipation; chills; stress) • Artemisia absinthium • Berberis (acute and chronic conditions from food or drug excess) • Chelidonium (sallow complexion; pain in right side to scapula or occiput on either side; migraine—any or all of these) • CHIONANTHUS (bilious colic) • CINCHONA (exhaustion and biliousness after chills—Scudder) • Cornus florida • Cynara • DIOSCOREA (headache, nausea, vomiting, cramps; skin dry and husky) • Euonymus (bilious indigestion) • EUPATORIUM PERFOLIATUM • Gillenia trifoliata (intermittent; bilious fevers) • IRIS (bilious attack; headache, diarrhea, cramps) • Larrea (chronic, with symptoms of "toxic liver") • Linaria • Liriodendron (tension and weakness) • Menyanthes • MAHONIA (acute and chronic, from food or drug excess) • Nux vomica (homeopathic) • PEUMUS (gall-bladder problems, where people have lost the "joy of life"—Welliver) • Podophyllum (full, puffy, sallow face, complexion, and liver area; very small dose) • Potentilla (analogue to Agrimonia) • Tilia • Veronicastrum (headache, pain in right hypochondrium; very small dose).

Bile, Insufficient (constipation with light-colored stools): • Achillea • Alnus rubra • Andrographis • Apocynum androsaemifolium (grey stool; no willpower; minute or grey stools) • Arctium • Artemisia absinthium • Artemisia vulgaris • Berberis • Chelidonium (warming, bitter) • Chionanthus (gallstone caught in duct, blocking bile; fatty stools) • Cnicus • Crataegus • Curcuma • CYNARA • Euonymus • Fumaria (spasm of bile duct) • Iris (chronic obstruction of bile duct) • JUGLANS CINEREA • Juglans nigra • Larrea • Leptandra • Mahonia (fatty stools, nausea, sick headache) • Petasites (neurodystonia) • Podophyllum (grey or whitish stool, lack of bile; very small dose) • Rhamnus • Rumex crispus • Salvia • Taraxacum (root) • Veronicastrum (torpid liver and bowels; small dose, with Zingiberis to prevent spasm).

Bile, alternating insufficiency and excess: • Agrimonia (needs confirmation) • Betonica ("autonomic nervous system mis-signaling gall bladder; alternates between biliousness and lack of appetite"—Donahue).

Inflammation of the Gall Bladder (Cholecystitis): • Achillea • Agrimonia (gastric sub-acidity; tea) • Berberis (cold tea) • Chamomilla (concentrated decoction of dried herb, to increase bitterness) • Chelidonium (heating and stimulating; depressed tissue state; pain in right hypochondrium to scapula) • Chelone • Chionanthus (sharp, cutting pain in right hypochondrium; bile-duct catarrh; with acute liver congestion) • Cichorium • Dioscorea • EUONYMUS • Gentiana • IRIS (profuse yellowish, sometimes greenish diarrhea) • Linum (flaxseed oil) • Mahonia (with catarrhal gastritis) • Mentha piperita (between attacks, to relax) • Myrica • PEUMUS • PODOPHYLLUM (miniscule or homeopathic doses) • Rumex crispus • Silybum • TARAXACUM (long-term usage; root) • Veronicastrum (acute; small doses).

Gallstones, Gallstone Colic: • AGRIMONIA (tension, gasping for breath) • Alchemilla arvensis • Ajuga reptans • Anisum (mucus congestion of gall bladder) • Apium (debilitated) • BERBERIS (acute pain radiating to all parts of the abdomen) • Betonica (weak gall-bladder reflexes) • Chamomilla (with poppy seeds, poultice on gall-bladder area for the pain) • CHELIDONIUM (thins bile, stimulates and warms gall bladder) • Chelone (pain downwards from xiphoid process to umbilicus) • CHIONANTHUS (preventative and active) • Cichorium • Collinsonia (combine with Eupatorium purpureum) • CURCUMA (anti-inflammatory; combine with a little pepper) • DIOSCOREA • Equisetum (compress) • Eupatorium purpureum • Euonymus • FUMARIA • Hydrastis (anti-inflammatory) • IRIS (sharp pains, congestion, constipation) • JUGLANS CINEREA (preventive; purges the gall bladder of stones and bile very effectively) • Linum (flaxseed oil and apple used as a flush) • Malus (softens stones) • Monarda fistulosa (colic with nervous tension) • PEUMUS (pain in liver or gall bladder) • Pimpinella anisum (mucus mixed with stones) • Podophyllum (full, sallow, puffy, congested face, skin, and gall bladder; very small dose) • Polymnia (congestion) • Rubia • Rumex crispus (in hot conditions) • Silybum (enlargement, uneasiness, nausea, distention) • TARAXACUM (slowly cleans heat and congestion in liver and gall bladder) • Verbascum • Veronicastrum (pain under right hypochondrium and scapula) • VERBENA (pain).

Neonatal Jaundice: • Myrica (breastfeeding mother should take) • Nux vomica (homeopathic; breastfeeding mother should take).

Jaundice: • Anisum (mucoid—Light) • Chelidonium • Chelone (with inflammation) • Chionanthus (liver enlargement) • Fumaria (spasmodic) • Hydrastis • Iris (clay-colored stool) • Juglans cinerea • Myrica • Podophyllum (full, sallow, puffy, congested face, skin, and gall bladder; very small dose) • Rumex crispus • Taraxacum • Veronicastrum.

FORMULARY

Betonica—with Chamomilla, Dioscorea, "for autonomic mis-signaling of the gall bladder"—Donahue.

Chionanthus—with Chelidonium, Podophyllum (½-part). This is "Dr. Carroll's Liver Formula," given by Les Moore 2002, 21. This and the following are really gall bladder remedies, not liver formulae.

Chionanthus—with Hydrastis, Gentiana, and a fraction of Rhamnus purshiana ("Clymer's Liver Formula"). Les Moore 2002, 25.

Chionanthus—with Chelidonium, Hydrastis (gall bladder stimulant). Old pharmacy recipe.

Cynara—with Artemisia absinthium ("all kinds of cholecystopathies"). Sherman.

Peumus—with Ceanothus (gallstones). Sherman.

The Golden Arc

The duodenum, liver, gallbladder, pancreas, and portal vein work in harmony to form a functional unit providing the necessary inputs for healthy operation of the stomach and intestines. The liver receives the food/toxins assimilated from the small intestine through the portal vein, and makes the bile, which is in turn supplied in a timely fashion back to the intestines by the gall bladder. The bile is joined in the common bile duct by digestive enzymes manufactured in the pancreas. The portal vein drains all these structures to make sure that toxins (their name is Legion) in the tract are attended to by the liver.

These functions are coordinated through the autonomic nervous system, with hormonal assistance here and there, so that they function as a unit (underneath the radar of consciousness), though not as a single organ or system. I call this "the golden arc." We need to learn to think of this group of organs as a unit, and attend to it wisely to keep it functioning smoothly and harmoniously.

The gall bladder is a sort of "flagship" for the golden arc—perhaps the "meeting of the ways" where all these organs and their influences and disharmonies come to bear. When there is trouble in the autonomic the problem usually shows up in the gall bladder and ducts.

Pancreas and Sugar Metabolism

The pancreas is both an exocrine and an endocrine gland, excreting digestive enzymes and secreting the hormones insulin and glucagon, which control blood-sugar levels. Diabetes type I occurs when the pancreas no longer secretes insulin; it is therefore treated by insulin supplementation, and known as "insulin-dependent diabetes." This condition is incurable (except by surgery), and no herbal practitioner should ever interfere with biomedical treatment.

Diabetes type II occurs when cells no longer take up insulin and blood sugar, even if they are in adequate supply; it is therefore called "insulin resistance." This type of diabetes can be improved by exercise, diet, and herbs. Type I diabetics often become type II diabetics after many years, because of the cells' difficulty in assimilating artificial insulin. These symptoms can be treated—but patients must not be taken off their type-I drug regimen.

Pre-diabetes precedes diabetes type II. People experiencing the former often need cooling and sedative remedies to bring down the exaggerated metabolism brought on by the excess glucose; for the latter, stimulants and astringents to control excess urination. Stevia may be used as a sugar substitute.

Hyperglycemia (temporary high blood sugar, usually after a meal), Pre-diabetes: • CINNAMOMUM (dietary or medicinal) • GALEGA (before meals; moderates sugar spikes; long-term use) • Glycyrrhiza (stabilizes blood-sugar levels) • Grifola • IRIS (blood sugar fluctuates up and down, often from leaky gut) • Ocimum • Olea • Oplopanax • Panax quinquefolius (lowers sugar spike after meals; root or leaf) • Taraxacum (root) • Trigonella • VACCINIUM MYRTILLUS (fruit).

Hypoglycemia: • IRIS (sugar-craving, hypoglycemic headaches, depression, blood sugar ups and downs, sometimes due to leaky gut) • Myrica (stimulant to increase receptor-site availability, peripheral circulation) • OPLOPANAX • Panax ginseng (cured root) • RUBUS CANADENSIS (drop in blood sugar causes shakiness, desire to eat; tea — Trilby).

Diabetes Mellitus type I (Insulin Dependence): • GYMNEMA (regenerates beta cells, increases insulin levels, decreases blood-sugar levels) • VACCINIUM MYRTILLUS (reduces blood-sugar levels; reduces insulin dependency in type I diabetics; adjunctive to insulin; fruit).

Note: This condition should not be treated by alternative medicine; do not discontinue biomedical treatment under any circumstances. However, after many years, type I diabetics may also become insulin-resistant, and can be helped by the remedies above. But, again, do not change the biomedically prescribed regimen.

Diabetes Mellitus type II (Insulin Resistance): • Aceticum acidum (cider vinegar) • Achillea • Acorus (bath — Weiss) • Allium cepa (Weiss) • Arctium • Baptisia (externally, on parts that turn black) • Curcuma (tissue regenerative; tissue depression) • Daucus • Eleutherococcus (to reduce stress) • GALEGA (before meals; moderates sugar spikes; long-term use — Dowling) • Gingko (increases cerebral circulation) • Glycyrrhiza (stabilizes blood-sugar levels) • Grifola • Gymnema (palliates by elevating insulin levels, so may worsen underlying condition) • Helonias • Hydrastis (stimulant used externally on ulcers and neuropathy of extremities; "functional hypergluconeogenesis" — M. Moore) • Hydrangea • Inula • Juniperus • Lycopus • Mahonia (see Hydrastis) • MOMORDICA CHARANTIA (traditional in Asia, Africa; reduces taste for sweets; lowers blood-sugar levels) • Myrica (increases circulation) • Ocimum (lowers blood-sugar levels) • OPLOPANAX (overweight, with high triglycerides,

cholesterol, and blood pressure) • Opuntia (juice) • OSMO-
RHIZA LONGISTYLIS (stabilizes sugar levels and reduces
symptoms; usually does not cure; for deterioration of eyesight,
neuropathy) • Panax quinquefolius (moderates sugar spikes
after meals; root, leaf) • Phaseolus (dried pod tea) • RHUS
SPP. (diabetic retinopathy, neuropathy, excessive urination and
sweating: lowers blood-sugar levels—traditional and proven)
• Rubus canadensis • SYZYGIUM ("In all cases of diabetes,
10–15 drops in a little water, 3–4x/day. If the blood sugar is very
high, 30 drops may be given every 3 hours. This should be given
along with any other medicines given to tackle the disease"—A.K.
Bhattacharya; beginning type-II cases) • Taraxacum (maintains
sugar levels) • TRIGONELLA (daily tea to reduce blood-sugar
levels) • Urtica (for the kidneys; seed) • VACCINIUM MYR-
TILLUS (reduces blood-sugar levels; to reduce insulin use in
type I; adjunctive to insulin) • Vaccinium macrocarpon • VER-
BENA (congestion in abdomen, high blood pressure of diabetes)
• Vinca • VITIS (diabetic retinopathy; seed extract).

Pancreatitis: • Belladonna (low homeopathic dose) • Chelidonium
• Chionanthus • Iris versicolor • Juniperus • Silybum.

Lymph and Immune Systems

The immune system operates through innumerable mechanisms, not
all of which are probably known at the present time. It operates
largely through the lymphatics, and therefore I treat these as a single
system.

In olden times, the lymphatic system was unknown, and its diseases were associated with the spleen and "scrofula." Scrofula starts
as glandular swelling and ends in tuberculosis, but at first it is entirely
a lymphatic problem. The term can also refer to poorly nourished
states where the skin is sallow and pale; these conditions were also
associated with the spleen. In the classification below, "spleen" refers
only to actually swelling or changes in the spleen itself.

Swollen, Congested Lymphatics: • Aesculus hip. • Alnus rubra (enlarged nodes) • Alnus serrulata • ARCTIUM (under arms, groin; chronic swelling) • Baptisia (with putrid discharges) • CALENDULA (chronically enlarged, inflamed nodes; where a mild warming agent is needed) • CEANOTHUS • Celastrus • Centella (improves condition of matrix, source of lymph) • Chimaphila (hardened glands with sluggish kidney function) • Chionanthus • Conium (homeopathic; hardened glands) • Daucus (poultice, for "lack of lymph flow"—Sherman) • Echinacea (good as an activator in lymphatic formulae) • Eryngium yuccifolium (hardening; proteins set up in extracellular matrix) • Fagopyrum (congestion) • FOUQUIERIA (especially pelvic) • GALIUM (small swollen nodes and cysts; neck and axilla, tonsils) • Hedeoma • Helianthemum • IRIS (soft, enlarged nodes; chronic illness—Martin) • Lamium (swollen nodes) • Melilotus • Menispermum • Oplopanax (root and bark poultice) • Petroselinum (fresh parsley poultice) • PHYTOLACCA (pale mucosa; hard, swollen and inflamed nodes; induration; mastitis; small dose or homeopathic) • Polemonium • Polymnia (swollen nodes) • Prunella • Quercus (induration—Sherman) • Rumex crispus • Saponaria • Sassafras (as an adjunct to lymphatics and alteratives) • SCROPHULARIA (enlarged, indurated nodes) • Smilax • Stillingia (chronic) • Thuja • Tilia • Trifolium (singular, hard, swollen, encysted nodes) • Trigonella • VIOLA (dry conditions) • Verbascum (dry conditions) • Verbena hastata (moves lymphatic congestion up from bottom of feet; decoction—Light), • Vitex (in young girls).

Spleen: • BAPTISIA (very specific for *polycythemia vera*) • CEANOTHUS (swollen; melancholy) • Cinchona (swollen; exhaustion from malaria) • Cnicus • Eupatorium cannabinum • Galium (stitch in side) • Iris versicolor (swollen, soft, yielding to pressure) • Lonicera • Mahonia • Polymnia (swollen spleen) • Rubia (hemolytic anemia) • Scolopendrium (mild astringent; swollen spleen) • Silphium integrifolium • Silybum • Taraxacum • Trifolium • Viscum.

Axilla (Underarms): • ARCTIUM • CALENDULA • GALIUM.

Lymphedema: • Aesculus hip. • Arctium • CEANOTHUS • Centella • GALIUM • Phytolacca • QUERCUS • Scrophularia • Viola.

Hyperimmunity: • AMYGDALUS (sensitive skin, mucosa) • GNAPHALIUM (normalizer) • Nigella (normalizer) • PRUNUS SEROTINA (histaminic excitation; wounds and scratches immediately get red; in redheads) • Rosa • TILIA (red tissues; red, elongated, pointed tongue).

Hypoimmunity: • Althaea • Aristolochia serpentaria (small dose) • ASTRAGALUS (to consolidate the surface, reduce sweating; in preparation for outdoor, winter work) • Baptisia • Codonopsis (weak, thin, dried-out, tired, bloated, short of breath) • CORDYCEPS • Commiphora myrrha • ECHINACEA • Eupatorium perfoliatum • Fouquieria • GNAPHALIUM (normalizer) • GRIFOLA • Iris • Lentinula • Nigella (normalizer) • Panax (all) • Phytolacca (lingering infections, low immunity, swollen nodes) • SCHISANDRA • Stillingia • Thuja • Viola • WITHANIA (exhausted, depleted, senescent).

Note: Essential fatty acids (EFAs) regulate immunity.

White Blood Cells: • Commiphora myrrha (leukopenia) • Echinacea (suppression from chemotherapy, leukocytosis, leukopenia) • Ligusticum porter (leukocytosis, leukopenia).

Note: Because lymphatic and spleen problems are frequently localized, remedies can be used externally. Mix with castor oil for best effect.

FORMULARY

Immune

Astragalus—with Codonopsis (nutritive immune tonic).

Lymph

Calendula—with Arctium (axillary lymphatics). Wood.

Calendula—with Scrophularia (stagnation in thoracic outlet). Wood.

Ceanothus—with Calendula, Galium, Trifolium Scrophularia, Viola, Echinacea (general lymphatic cleanser). Wood.

Galium—with Trifolium, Ceanothus, Echinacea (cooling lymphatic cleanser).

Iris—with Phytolacca (general lymphatic cleanser). Iris is for soft nodes, Phytolacca for hard—Martin.

Viola—with Arctium, Baptisia, Phytolacca (lingering lymph node inflammation). BHP 1983, 39.

DEEP IMMUNE TONIC

This stew goes by many names, and has many variants. It is largely based on Chinese tonic stews; the formula used below comes from David Winston, and has long by used and confirmed many others. Ganoderma (3 parts), Atractylodis (2 parts), Burdock root (2 parts), Astragalus (1½ parts), Codonopsis (1½ parts), Lentinula (1 part), and Trametes (1 part). Add to water with soup bones, and simmer for three days; at the end add carrots, celery, potatoes, beets, or other short-cooking vegetables.

Kidneys

The cells of our body have the same garbage-removal philosophy as we do: dump it in the river. However, the cells are environmentally responsible, and have a filtration unit to purify the "river" (our blood). After cellular waste products are dumped in the extracellular waters, they are removed by the lymphatic capillaries and, to some extent, the capillary venules. They end up in the bloodstream and are filtered out through the kidneys.

In a clean-burning system, the liver, cells, and regulatory system are healthy, and the main waste products arriving at the kidneys are protein fragments. Twenty per cent of the blood in the circulation is taken up by the renal capillary system in the kidneys for filtration. The blood cells are left behind while the serum is cleansed in the kidneys. Almost ninety-nine per cent of this serum will be reabsorbed back into the bloodstream. Therefore, only a small amount of the water, proteins, and electrolytes are removed. The kidneys balance the water and electrolyte levels in the blood and body fluids; this includes balancing the acid and alkaline. For this reason, much uric acid from protein waste is returned to the blood.

While they are filtering the blood, the kidneys "read" the levels of red blood cells; if these are receding, they send a hormone (erythropoietin) to the bone marrow to tell it to make more red blood cells.

This helps us picture the basic disease conditions of the kidneys: (1) lack of filtration (renal failure); (2) insufficient diuresis (inadequate water elimination); (3) insufficient reabsorption (excessive urination); (4) imbalanced blood and urine (which can result in kidney-stone formation); (5) renal anemia; (6) excess sodium not being removed from the blood (resulting in high blood pressure); and (7) inflammation from high rate of function. In addition, of course, there may be (8) bacterial infection, which can come up from the urethra and bladder or be caused by overuse of the kidneys from excessive stress or dietary protein.

Anatomically, the kidneys consist of "nephron units," each of which is an independent little filtration system. Blood flows into the capillaries there and is taken by an osmotic sodium pump through the glomeruli into the tubules. These nephron tubules are surrounded by capillaries that reabsorb almost ninety-nine per cent of the blood, electrolytes, and protein waste products. If there is no need in the body for a particular (waste) product, it will not be picked up, so we can assume that some chemical waste products from the environment are also eliminated this way. The resulting urine contains water, uric acid or protein waste products, and electrolytes, including enough sodium to make it relatively salty.

The emotion associated with the kidneys is fear, timidity, or worry, according to TCM. Here we see the kidney and adrenal functions merged together. It is true that fear does influence the kidneys. Long, drawn-out disputes, weighty legal cases, divorces, child-custody battles, or just the trivial pursuits of the day can also wear out the kidneys. Here the feeling is not fear or judgment-related but exhaustion, with a tired lower back and feet. Maria Treben says the kidneys process our emotions, which leads to their exhaustion; for this she recommends *Solidago*. It is excellent as a tea, salve, or tincture—and its efficacy is often confirmed in clinical practice.

There are of course some diseases of the kidneys that are better described by pathophysiology than as tissues states. This is true of diabetes type I or II: sugar in the blood should be reclaimed in the reabsorption process, but when there is too much it runs off through the tubules, causing kidney damage and excess urination. There are remedies for this. I had a case where we held kidney deterioration at bay for several years until the patient could get a pancreas and kidney transplant. The remedy used in that case was gravel root *(Eupatorium purpureum)*.

In my experience, the great remedy for diabetes mellitus or insipidus with profuse urination is *Rhus spp.* (an astringent). This remedy cured a case I saw where high blood pressure had damaged the kidneys; the patient had profuse urination as well as profuse sweating. *Rhus typhina* removed the high blood pressure, and the doctor cheerfully told her, "I will write down in your medical records, 'cured by an herb.'" Blueberry or huckleberry leaf *(Vaccinium myrtillus)* should have similar properties.

Another problem causing kidney distress is insomnia. If a person is unable to relax at night, the kidneys will not relax, and there may be excessive urination—only at night. Prostate problems present excess urination all the time.

The Six Tissue States and Renal Conditions

The tissue state model can be very helpful in analyzing renal disease. This is one area where I don't find the Chinese model helpful enough, although it is good for some indications, as we will see.

Heat/Excitation: The kidneys can be overstimulated by a number of causes. In hot weather, the skin sweats out water to keep the body cool, and the kidneys are left with less water to remove protein wastes. The herbal remedy for this is *Cucurbita citrullus* (watermelon seed). When Osama bin Laden was killed, one of his wives was asked why he wasn't on kidney dialysis, since it was known that he had kidney failure. "Oh," she said, "he cured that a long time ago with a home remedy—watermelon" (paraphrase).

If alkaline or electrolyte waste products are building up, the preferred remedy may be *Fragaria vesca* (strawberry) leaf. This is also a remedy for dental plaque, an indication of high alkalinity. A large amount of protein waste can cause an allergic reaction, resulting in urine retention and puffing-up of the lower back, sometimes with hives or lesions. I had a client like this, thirty-plus years ago; cortisone shots saved her life but were needed constantly. One dose of homeopathic honeybee (*Apis mellifica,* 30c) cured her permanently.

Cold/depression: Warmth in the kidneys can also be caused by kidney infection—bacteria comes up the ureters and lodges in the kidneys. This condition needs antibiotics immediately. However, if the infection is stubborn, or one gets the case at the same time as the doctors, give herbs. I find that this condition usually comes from overwork in school. The residual pain and low-level heat has often responded well to *Verbena.*

Cold or depression of kidney function is associated with either edema from low renal function or excess urination from poor reabsorption. Both of these conditions are called "kidney yang deficiency" in TCM, meaning that the heat or "yang of the kidneys is too low to transform the water." In addition to renal symptoms, other symptoms usually include: a sore, stiff lower back and knees; aggravation from cold, or getting the feet cold; cold coming up the legs to the kidneys; and cold in the lower back. Remedies are warming (yang) tonics and warming astringents. Warming kidney remedies are *Solidago* (tired feet, tired lower back), *Chimaphila* (lymphatic and kidney stagnation), and *Tsuga canadensis* (this is more of a warming remedy for the lower back and back pain than a kidney remedy *per se*).

Relaxation: Also classified under "kidney yang deficiency" are conditions where the kidney apparatus is "too relaxed" and does not hold onto the urine, resulting in excess urination. This condition responds to astringents—*Rhus spp., Citrus limonum*, and probably others. The urine is clear and frequent, and the tongue is damp or (paradoxically) dry due to fluid loss. Renal anemia occurs with relaxation of the kidneys, resulting in general anemia, damp tongue, and excess clear urination—use *Rhus typhina*, etc.

Tension: The kidneys are not strongly innervated, and should not be subject to tension, but in my now-getting-long career, I have a few times seen edema come and go suddenly—indicating wind or tension. I discuss this in *The Book of Herbal Wisdom*, under *Agrimonia* and *Potentilla*. *Agrimonia* was a kidney remedy well attested to by John Scudder and the eclectic medical movement. Also recommended: *Dioscorea* and *Piper methysticum*.

Dry/Atrophy: The late William LeSassier used to say in his classes, "don't rip off the kidneys"—meaning, don't use forceful diuretics. Medical diuretics force the kidneys to remove water, which weakens them over the long run. Instead, he recommended the use of nutritive diuretics that strengthened the renal function, such as nettles *(Urtica)*, bean pod *(Phaseolus)*, and self-heal *(Prunella)*. *The majority of herbal diuretics are not very forceful; those that are include* Apocynum *and* Juniperus. These very stimulating remedies are used only for the cold/depressed tissue state, and only in small doses. If a diuretic needs to be used continuously, and is not making the condition better, it will ultimate make it worse.

Lack of fluids in the kidneys is called "kidney yin deficiency" in TCM. The symptoms are dry tongue and skin, dry joints, and darker, concentrated urine in small amounts.

Drying out of the skin and fluids generally causes excessive excretion through the kidneys, which are forced to make up for the lack of excretion from the skin. This can ultimately cause kidney failure or Bright's disease. The kidneys seem to be too damp, but the overall condition is one of drying.

Damp/Stagnation: The kidneys can't break down toxins like the liver or the immune system, so a damp/stagnant tissue state can only affect the kidneys when bacteria, pus, or toxins from other regions reach them. The kidneys can then get inflamed and, although antibiotics may help, it is not until the locus of the infection is found that the insult to the kidneys will be addressed and the condition cured. For example, the infected root of a tooth can cause pus to circulate, which inflames the kidneys. This kind of infection causes what the old doctors called "congestive chills," which are a lot like the chills of influenza except that they feel really deep. The traditional remedy here is *Cnicus benedictus*, "holy thistle" or "St. Benedict's thistle." I don't have much experience with this condition, but I have seen this remedy work twice on congestive chills in the kidneys caused by tooth problems, and once in hepatitis. These are problems where a person would usually be on antibiotics.

Edema, Water Retention: • Agrimonia (changeable edema) • Allium sativa • Anagallis • Apium (debilitated and languid) • APOCYNUM CANNABINUM (puffiness; area under eyes swollen, or wrinkled from recent swelling; infiltration into ankles; uremia; small doses or homeopathic) • Arctium (osmotic diuretic relieving sodium retention; acidosis; seed) • Arctostaphylos (relaxed, toneless tissues with draggy, weighty feeling; feeble circulation, lack of innervation) • ARALIA HISPIDA ("most efficient"—Scudder) • Aristolochia serpentaria (suppression of urine; small dose) • Asparagus officinalis • Astragalus (edema, heavy feeling in limbs, urinary difficulty) • Barosma • BERBERIS ("the grand specific for various diseases of the kidneys and bladder"—Stacey Jones)

• Betonica • Betula (birch leaf) • Borago • Camellia (edema, swollen ankles) • Capsella • Centella (mild but nutritive diuretic) • CHIMAPHILA (the great diuretic; swelling in joints, scanty, suppressed urine, lymphatic stagnation) • Collinsonia • Cynara (nephrosclerosis) • CUCURBITA CITRULLUS (watermelon seed is a most effective cooling diuretic) • Daucus (stimulating; cold and chronic conditions) • Equisetum • Erigeron • Eryngium yuccifolium (swollen and hard tissue) • EUPATORIUM PUR-PUREUM (atonic; mucus discharge; albuminuria) • Filipendula (nervous, irritable) • Fragaria (cooling diuretic; leaf) • Fumaria • Galium • Genista tinctoria • Helonias • Hydrangea • Junipe-rus (depressed, cold conditions with harsh, dry skin, pitting in ankles, dragging in lumbar region) • Larix (tamarack) • Ledum (edema of feet) • Leonurus (albuminuria in pregnancy) • Levis-ticum • Liatris • Mentha spicata (spearmint tea) • Mitchella (edema during menses, pregnancy) • Onosmodium (edema, stones) • Oxydendrum (cooling) • Parietaria • Petroselinum • Piper methysticum (spasm) • Rosmarinus (cardiac edema) • Scoparium • Solidago (for exhausted kidneys, lower back pain, tired feet and back; internally—Treben; albuminuria—Weiss; externally for back pain) • Stellaria • TARAXACUM (leaf), • TRIBULUS • URTICA (kidney failure) • Vaccinium • Verbascum (dysuria; suppression) • Vitis • Zanthoxylum • Zea mays.

Excessive Urination (Copious, Light Urine): • Agrimonia • Citrus limonum (juice, daily) • Eupatorium purpureum • Geranium robertianum • Hypericum • Linum (older men; fresh ground seed) • RHUS SPP. (sweating and urinating in profusion; anxiety; diabetes insipidus and mellitus type II; brings down blood sugar and high blood pressure) • Solidago (exhausted kidneys, tired feet) • TARAXACUM (to replenish potassium; raw or roasted root) • Verbascum (keeps the feet warm; root).

Deficient Urination (Dark, Scanty Urine): • Achillea (darkish-red, scanty urine; removes proteins and fats; can make the urine cloudy and oily; decoction) • Agropyron (increases water output and dilution of solids) • Eupatorium purpureum • Galium • Solidago (muscular pain in back).

Kidney Infection, Nephritis (take antibiotics as well): • Achillea • Agrimonia (chronic irritability) • Agropyron (chronic renal weakness and inflammation; increases water output and dilution of solids) • Althaea (mucilaginous diuretic; pain, irritation) • Arctostaphylos uva-ursi (astringent antiseptic; acute, sub-acute; dysuria, pyelitis, lithuria, cystitis, mucus, moderate hematuria) • Barosma • BERBERIS (pains radiate from kidneys; urine thick with mucus, or sedimentous) • Chimaphila (with lymphatic stagnation, arthritis; glomerulonephritis, acute or chronic) • Chionanthus (with liver problems) • Cimicifuga (inflammation of kidneys and ureters) • Commiphora myrrha (chronic, non-inflammatory) • Cordyceps • Cnicus (chills and fever) • Dioscorea (kidney colic; pains shooting up the back and down the legs; passing of small stones) • Equisetum (edematous) • Eupatorium purpureum • Gaultheria (acute, mild; with fine hyaline casts) • Glechoma (acute and feverish) • Hydrangea (deep-seated pain) • Juniperus (chronic, non-inflammatory; infection from renal depression; never use during an active infection) • Leonurus • MONARDA FISTULOSA (cool, sweaty skin) • Parietaria (inflammation, infection of kidneys, bladder, nephritis; renal colic) • Petroselinum • Sambucus ebulus (with deficient excretion) • SOLIDAGO (acute, chronic; deep-seated pain; anuria) • Verbena hastata (kidney infection from straining and exhaustion) • Zea (stones; high in potassium; also see "Albuminuria," below).

Note: Because of the serious nature of kidney infection, always use antibiotics with herbs as a supplementation. Anyone suffering from severe pain in the region of the kidneys should be referred to the doctor first, to determine if there is an infection.

Kidney Infection (Pyelitis): • Agropyron (chronic; tensive) • Arctostaphylos uva-ursi (ascending cystitis; relaxed mucosa; mucus and blood cells in urine) • Barosma (acidic urine; mucopurulence) • Chimaphila (ascending cystitis; relaxed mucosa; alkaline urine; mucus and blood cells in urine) • Dioscorea (chronic; tensive) • Eupatorium purpureum (after passing a stone; painful urination) • Glycyrrhiza (with salt) • Monarda fistulosa • Parietaria • Piper methysticum (after passing a stone; painful urination; spasms) • Solidago (after passing a stone; painful urination, lower back) • Zea (acute, initial stages; with painful urination; alkaline urine).

Note: The information above is primarily from Michael Moore.

Kidney Pain: • Agrimonia (deep soreness or tenderness; sharp, cutting pains—Scudder) • Agropyron (heavy, dull ache; sacral-lumbar) • Berberis (stiffness, lameness in lower back) • Centaurium (chronic colic) • Dioscorea (renal and bladder colic, clonic spasm) • Eupatorium purpureum • Hydrangea (painful lumbar region) • Juniperus (lower back pain; exhausted kidneys resulting in extensive edema; nervous system weak, with heart symptoms) • Lycopodium (severe spasm with atrophy) • Melilotus • Nymphaea odorata • Pinus strobus (exhaustion; external) • Piper methysticum (constriction and spasm in urinary tract) • Solidago (pain over kidneys, exhaustion, tired feet) • Taraxacum • Tsuga (to warm kidneys and lower back; pain, cold, exhaustion; Canada hemlock oil, external).

Kidney Failure: • Ajuga reptans (albuminuria, with rapid pulse) • Agropyron (chronic renal weakness, with inflammation; frequent, scanty, burning, scalding urine; increases water output, dilutes solids) • Apium (languid, debilitated) • Chimaphila

(incipient and advanced albuminuria) • CORDYCEPS
("degenerative kidney disease"—D. Winston) • Echinacea
(toxic albuminuria) • Eupatorium purpureum • Gaultheria
• Juniperus (chronic structural change) • Solidago (weak lower
back and kidneys, exhaustion; does not deplete kidney energy)
• Taraxacum • URTICA (proteins in urine; has gotten dozens of
people off dialysis and prevented numerous others from starting;
seed or leaf).

Albuminuria: • Ajuga reptans (with rapid pulse) • Caulophyllum
(nervous weakness) • Echinacea (toxic albuminuria) • Leonurus (nervousness; tea, not tincture; small dose).

Kidneys, to protect during chemotherapy and other drugs:
• Cordyceps.

Kidney Stones: • AGRIMONIA (pains in the kidneys; pain
from passage, holding breath from pain, dribbling after passing
stones) • Agropyron (accumulation of "sand" in the pelvis; back
pain) • ALTHAEA (sharp, inflammatory pains; lubricates the
passages, increases amount of urine) • Ammi (to facilitate passage) • Armoracia (external on kidneys—needs confirmation)
• APHANES (dysuria, strangury, edema, stones) • Arctium
(with hyperuricemia) • Arctostaphylos (diuretic astringent)
• Asparagus officinalis (diuretic) • Apium (decalcifying
diuretic) • Barosma (acid, muddy, or brick-dust urine) • BER-
BERIS (chief remedy for prevention, lodgment of stone; excess
mucus, from calculi; gravelly urine, pain in back and loins; tincture) • Beta (dietary for chronic production) • Calluna
• Capsella (poor tone; sharp, inflammatory pain; hematuria)
• Centaurium (chronic colic from stone passage) • Chimaphila
(5–10-drop doses, every three hours) • COLLINSONIA (small
dose, when stone causes constriction in passage; large doses
consistently, to destroy the tendency) • DAUCUS (decalcifying diuretic) • Dioscorea (passage of stone, with clonic spasms,

writhing pains) • Equisetum • ERYNGIUM MARITIMUM (frequency, hematuria) • EUPATORIUM PURPUREUM (dissolves stones, increases capillary profusion of water into kidneys) • Fragaria (traditional antilithic) • GALIUM • Harpagophytum • Hernaria (reduces spasm) • HYDRANGEA (dissolves stones; sharp pain in the kidneys, sallow) • Levisticum • Linum • OCIMUM (passage of stone with "agonizing pain, twists about, screams and groans; red urine with brick-dust sediment"—Clarke) • Ononis • Onosmodium • PARIETARIA (dissolves stones) • Platanus (bark, twigs, or heartwood) • POLYGONUM HYDROPIPEROIDES (or other variety of smartweed) • Rhodiola • Rubia (reduces spasms) • Sabal (reduces spasms; lubricates) • Sambucus ebulus • Senecio aureus • Smilax (worn-down and wasted) • Taraxacum (leaf) • Tribulus • Ulmus (lubricates the passage) • Urtica • Verbena • Veronica • Zea (irritation and sharp, inflammatory pain).

Note: Many claims have been made by herbalists past and present about the ability of plant agents to reduce kidney-stone size and production. Although it has not been scientifically proven that herbs can remove stones, many practitioners can attest to this through their own experience.

Phosphaturia: • Agropyron (pain in kidneys) • Aristolochia serpentaria (aggravated by cold and winter) • Cannabis (irritable bladder) • Capsella (irritable bladder) • Erigeron (pain in kidneys) • Hydrangea (pain in kidneys, pain on urination) • Medicago • Zea (muco-purulent urine).

Prophylactic (needs confirmation): • Agropyron • Citrus limonum • Eupatorium purpureum • Hydrangea, Polygonum spp. • Taraxacum (root) • Zea.

"Weak Kidneys Impeding Recovery of Illness Elsewhere in the Body": • Agathosma ("hereditary weakness of the kidney or prior illness, specially chill of the kidney, or past STD causing difficulty with the menstrual cycle; delayed, spotting before, emotional lability, migraine, nausea"—Croft) • Arctostaphylos ("combine with *Urtica* when there is permanent catheterization in a para- or quadriplegic; kidneys become heavily taxed, resulting in hyperreflexia; this combination has a strong energetic effect through the kidneys and spinal cord"—Croft) • CAPSELLA ("strep throat or tonsillitis cycling from tonsils to kidneys; recurrent tonsillitis in child, usually at three-week intervals"—Croft) • SOLIDAGO (almost better from acute disease, then it comes back or another starts; recovering from acute disease, urine turns dark, healing stops) • URTICA (urine turns dark and smelly from large amount of proteins after burn, dietary change, or sickness).

Note: I had to make up the above category because it is not found, to my knowledge, in any system of medicine. It was developed in coordination with herbalist Glenda Croft of Wagga Wagga, Australia. The indication for Solidago *comes from J.G. Rademacher, as described in my* The Book of Herbal Wisdom, *and I have often confirmed it in practice.*

FORMULARY

Agropyron—with Levisticum, Parietaria, Apium (edema). BHP 1983, 131.

Althaea—with Aphanes arvensis (kidney stones). BHP 1983, 28.

Eupatorium purpureum—with Daucus, Parietaria, Galium, Hydrangea, Eryngium maritimum (kidney stones and kidney conditions). BHP 1983, 78, 85.

Hydrangea—with Eupatorium purpureum, Polygonum hydropiperoides or Verbascum (kidney stones).

Parietaria—with Aphanes, Arctostaphylos, Juniperus, Barosma (kidney stones). BHP 1983, 153.

Urtica—with Phaseolus (pod), Prunella (nutritive diuretic). William LeSassier's favorite "triune formula" for the kidneys.

KIDNEY STONE PROTOCOL

Rudolf Weiss gives an extensive protocol for the nonsurgical treatment of kidney stones. During the stage of colic: (1) A very hot bath will sometimes dislodge the stone; hot compresses to the kidney region may also be sufficient. (2) Encourage diuresis only when the acute stage has passed; it often flushes the stone. (3) Sip *Chamomilla* tea slowly, for a spasmolytic and anodyne effect during passage. *Aesculus hip.* can also reduce edema in the mucosa of the ureter, to help the stone move.

After the colic stage: (4) If the stone has not passed, drink large amounts of warm water, then *Taraxacum* leaf infusion (1–2 tablespoons per ½-liter), and more water. (5) As a preventive afterwards, take *Taraxacum*, *Agropyron*, and *Zea*, preferably as tea.

This does not exploit the herbal possibilities very thoroughly, so I would add: reduce pain and spasm with hot *Agrimonia* or *Potentilla* tea if available, or tincture if not; *Eupatorium purpureum* to increase profusion of water out of the capillaries into the kidneys; *Hydrangea* and *Citrus limonum* to mildly decalcify stones; *Althaea* root decoction for mucilaginous soothing and lubrication, with mild diuresis; and *Polygonum spp.*, traditional for stone removal. Afterwards, other remedies may be needed to repair lingering tissue damage and pain.

Bladder and Urethra

The urine arriving from the kidneys through the ureters is collected in the bladder, and builds up until the pressure demands release. The bladder is like a large, thick, plastic bag that fits into the space between the organs and muscles as it slowly fills up. When it is full, the muscles that surround the bladder get the signal—"I need to go"—and the search is on for a suitable place. When one is reached, the muscles relax and let go, and the pee comes along.

This process can be interfered with by any of the six tissue state imbalances. Excitation or irritability of the bladder walls, or even autoimmune allergic reactions in the mucosa, can cause inflammation and excessive urging—this is classified as idiopathic (self-induced) bladder inflammation. The bladder is overactive and over-responsive.

In tissue depression, the opposite state, the cells in the bladder walls have a low metabolism; bacteria live off the dying cells, or come up the urethra from outside to infect the cells, spreading exotoxins that shorten cell life. This results in the typical bacterial bladder infection, or cystitis. Women are unfortunately more prone to this because they have a shorter urethra, so the bladder is closer to the outside world and all those darn bacteria. Cystitis causes inflammation, with difficulty emptying the bladder.

The tense tissue state is related to spasm of the muscles around the bladder. It can be due to neuromuscular tensions that often arise elsewhere. Unproductive urges are a typical symptom of spastic bladder. The opposite tissue state, as we usually think of it, is relaxation. This means the bladder muscles and bag are too relaxed to hold the urine, so it runs off easily, dribbles, and/or the person can't hold it for long. This may be caused by kidney problems as well.

Cystitis: • ACHILLEA (spasm, infection, bleeding, febrile)
• Agrimonia (chronic irritation; strangury; burning, scalding)
• AGROPYRON (irritation; frequent, difficult urination; mucus in urine; cramps, pain; increases water output, dilutes solids)
• Allium sativa • ALTHAEA (inflamed, painful; palliative or curative) • Anemopsis • Apium (languid, debilitated) • ARCTO-STAPHYLOS (antiseptic astringent; relaxed, mucoid discharges; alkaline urine) • Arctium (weak supporting tissue, lower back, and pelvis) • Armoracia • Avena • BAROSMA (acid urine; frequency, mucus, profuse; cystitis, chronic irritability; urethritis, prostatitis) • Berberis (low-grade, chronic infection, ill-health, radiating pains) • Bidens • Calluna • Cannabis (scalding, burning, frequent urination; irritability more than pain) • Capsella
• Chimaphila (burning, scalding, urging; chronic irritability)
• Chondrus • Crataegus • Cucumis sativus (low back pain, turbid urine, irritable tract, sharp pain in loins) • Cucurbita citrullus (painful, scanty; in infants) • Curcuma (straining; bacterial

inflammation from depressed mucosa) • Daucus • Echinacea • Equisetum (acute and chronic; urethritis, cystitis; tissue weakness) • Erigeron (irritation of bladder, uneasy and painful urination) • Eriodictyon (mucus in urine) • Eryngium spp. (cystitis, urethritis, proctitis; frequent urge, burning, itching) • Eupatorium purpureum (chronic; full, uneasy feeling; incontinence; in pregnancy) • Filipendula (urinary weakness, atonicity; acute catarrhal cystitis) • Gaultheria • HYDRANGEA (frequent, painful urination from gravel and alkalinity, with phosphatic urine) • Hydrastis (irritability; tones mucosa, nerves) • HYPERICUM (chronic inflammation) • JUNIPERUS (cold, depressed tissue state, sepsis) • Lamium • Levisticum • MONARDA FISTULOSA (cold, clammy skin; burning pain, tension, straining; idiopathic) • PARIETARIA (infusion of the root is "unexcelled" in cystic "irritability"—Parton) • PETROSELINUM (cloudy urine, pain, frequent urging; fresh parsley, chopped and infused; use for two weeks; avoid in pregnancy) • Peumus • Pinus • Piper cubeba (chronic; burning and scalding; during menstruation) • PIPER METHYSTICUM (urethritis, tension, pain) • Plantago major • Polygonum bistorta (stimulating astringent) • Populus • Sabal (nervous bladder, painful urination, tenesmus) • Senecio aureus (painful urination) • SMILAX (rheumatic or skin problems with cystitis) • Solidago (tired, painful lower back, inflammation, irritability, exhaustion) • Turnera (urinary antiseptic; in women, from intercourse) • Tsuga (strong stimulant; tired lower back) • Urtica (mucoid flow; chronic irritability) • Vaccinium macrocarpon (antiseptic, protective; acute, chronic; urethritis, cystitis; large doses of juice, up to 500 ml/day;) • Viola tricolor • ZEA (difficult or scanty; for children; soothing to urethra; tea of good-quality corn silk).

Mucus Discharges: • Agropyron • Arctostaphylos • Barosma • Chimaphila • Eriodictyon • Petroselinum • Urtica.

Irritable Bladder (Frequent Urge): • Agrimonia • Agropyron
 • Apis (homeopathic; puffy, swollen, painful, difficult passing
urine) • Arctostaphylos • Avena • Barosma (chronic) • Berberis
(female especially; burning, cutting, sticking pain in urethra,
during and after urination; frequent urge; small doses)
 • Cannabis (irritability more than pain) • Chimaphila (chronic)
 • Erigeron • Eryngium • Eupatorium purpureum • Glycyrrhiza
 • Hydrastis • Lobelia • PARIETARIA (root infusion "unexcelled" in cystic "irritability"—Parton) • Urtica (chronic) • Zea.

Urethritis: • Agropyron (irritation, frequent, difficult urination;
increases water output, dilutes solids; mucus in urine; cramps,
pain) • Althaea (inflamed, painful) • Anemopsis • Apium
 • Arctostaphylos (antiseptic astringent; relaxed, inflamed urethral opening with mucoid discharges; highly acid urine)
 • BAROSMA (frequent mucusy, profuse, acid urine; cystitis,
urethritis, prostatitis) • Berberis (see "Irritable Bladder," above)
 • Cannabis (scalding, burning, irritable, frequent urination)
 • Curcuma (straining) • Dioscorea (urethral pain) • Echinacea
 • Equisetum (acute and chronic; tissue weakness) • Eryngium
spp. (cystitis, urethritis, proctitis; frequent desire, burning, itching) • Eupatorium purpureum (chronic; full, uneasy feeling;
incontinence; pregnancy) • Galium (acute or relapsing; burning,
pain, straining; of cystic outlet; in febrile states) • Hydrangea
(frequent, painful, from gravel and alkalinity, with phosphatic
urine) • Lamium • MONARDA FISTULOSA (cold, clammy
skin; burning pain, tension, straining; idiopathic) • Petroselinum (cloudy, painful, frequent urine; fresh parsley, chopped
and infused; use for two weeks; avoid in pregnancy) • PIPER
METHYSTICUM (tension, pain) • Sabal • Senecio aureus
(painful urination) • Solidago (cystitis, urethritis, pain, inflammation, irritability, exhaustion) • Turnera • Vaccinium macrocarpon (antiseptic, protective to mucosa; large doses of juice, up
to 500 ml/day; acute, chronic; urethritis, cystitis).

Dribbling of Urine: • Agrimonia (after passing a stone) • Allium sativa (atonic; poor flow) • Betonica (general weakness) • Equisetum (involuntary, in old people; desire without relief) • Eupatorium purpureum (incontinence due to kidneys, bladder, or prostate; in elderly, both sexes) • Lycopodium (general weakness) • Populus tremuloides (dribbling, irritating, reduced flow) • Rhus spp. • Thuja.

Bedwetting, Incontinence, Enuresis: • Achillea (insensitive nerve) • Agrimonia (children stressed about toilet training; after passage of stone; chronic nephritis; acute urinary tract infection) • Arctostaphylos (stress) • Aquilegia (insensitive nerve; flowers and leaves — Native American) • Asafoetida (not sure whether they need to go or not — needs confirmation) • Avena (nutritive) • Equisetum (poor bladder control) • Eryngium spp. (menstrual; menopausal; aggravated by movement; after recent sexual activity; in sedentary, previously sexually inactive males — M. Moore) • Eschscholzia (also probably for paralysis) • Eupatorium purpureum (children hold their urine too long; bedwetting in children with bad dreams) • Galium • Gentiana (20 drops, midday and evening — Weiss) • HYPERICUM (insensitive nerve; children afraid of the dark, spirit phenomena) • Lentinula • Polygala (involuntary urination in sleep) • Polygonum aviculare (knotgrass tea) • Polygonum bistorta (stimulating astringent) • Pulsatilla (chronic inflammation or catarrh of bladder "with incontinence in bed at night" — Clarke; homeopathic low potency) • RHUS SPP. (children, elderly, nervous people; light, clear urination) • Rubia • Schisandra (combines well with Agrimonia) • TARAXACUM (root) • Thuja (elderly males; with enlarged prostate, poor bladder control) • VERBASCUM (insensitive nerve signal; poor bladder tone and enervation; root — M. Moore) • Vinca major • Zea.

Dysuria (painful urination): • Achillea (great pain) • Agropyron (pain in back, difficult urination) • Althaea (strangury)

- Arctostaphylos (muco-purulent, scanty urine; strangury)
- Barosma (chronic acidic urine and pain) • Cannabis (great pain) • Erigeron • Eryngium spp. (in women during menses, after coitus, in menopause; worse from movement) • Eschscholzia (strangury) • Eupatorium purpureum (dark or milky urine)
- Fouquieria (congestive prostatic enlargement in sedentary men — M. Moore) • Hydrangea (alkaline urine; great pain)
- Mitchella (with painful menstruation; congestive prostatic enlargement in sedentary men — M. Moore) • Piper methysticum (spasmodic) • Serenoa (with partial impotence)
- Smilax (pain after) • Tribulus (partial impotence) • Verbascum (chronic acidic) • Zea (strangury).

Calculi: See "Kidney Stones," in previous section.

Paralysis: • Eschscholzia (needs confirmation).

FORMULARY

Agrimonia (neutral) with *Chimaphila umbellata* (eliminating) and *Zea* (nourishing); this is William LeSassier's basic triune formula for the bladder.

Barosma — with Achillea, Arctostaphylos, Foeniculum (bacterial cystitis) modified from BHP 1983, 93.

Barosma — with Althaea, Arctostaphylos, Agropyron, Zea (cystitis). BHP 1983, 30.

Barosma — with Capsella, Equisetum, Agropyron, Rosmarinus, in tea. This has been my basic general recommendation for cystitis for twenty-five years; it can be tweaked to fit the case.

Barosma — with Petroselinum, Agropyron, Hydrangea (acute cystitis). BHP 1983, 155.

Rhus aromatica, Rhus spp. — with Agrimonia, Equisetum, Gentiana, Verbascum (nocturnal enuresis). Modified from BHP 1983, 179.

Rhus aromatica — with Cucurbita pepo (oil), Piper methysticum, Sabal, Humulus (weak, nervous bladder).

Rhus aromatica—with Equisetum, Viburnum opulus (urinary incontinence). BHP 1983, 179.

Rhus aromatica—can substitute Rhus typhina or R. coriaria in these last two formulas.

HOMEOPATHIC STAPHYSAGRIA
(DELPHINIUM STAPHISAGRIA)

My cousin, the late Julian Winston, a well-known lecturer and author in the homeopathic field, told a story that perfectly illustrated the chagrin and feeling of violation that leads to the typical *Staphysagria* bladder infection. He needed a plumber, and called ahead in good time to get one. He was given a day when the plumber would come, and waited at home, missing work, for the fellow to arrive. At a quarter to six, the plumber finally showed up. By this time, Julian was seething in anger for being made to wait all day, but he knew he couldn't complain, because he didn't want the guy to leave. The plumbing was fixed, but that evening Julian came down with a bladder infection—quickly cleared with *Staphysagria*.

Urine

Appearance, Contents, Sensations: • Achillea (bloody; great pain on urination) • Agrimony (foul-smelling, cloudy urine from mucus, calcium, urates, or phosphates; bloody urine) • Agropyron (high solids, low water content; muco-purulence; great pain on urination) • Alnus serrulata • Arctium (strong, dark, gritty) • Arctostaphylos (mucoid discharge) • Barosma (acid and muco-purulent; profuse cystorrhea) • Bidens (essential hematuria) • Cannabis (great pain on urination) • Chamomilla • Chelidonium (loaded with bile; high specific gravity) • Cichorium (sand and gravel) • Chionanthus (presence of sugar; orange urine) • Chimaphila (thick and ropy in the aged; glycosuria) • Epigea (bloody pus in urine) • Equisetum (bloody urine; cystic irritation; vapor bath, compress, or internal use) • Eryngium

yuccifolium (sexual desire with urinary desire) • Eupatorium
purpureum (acidic, highly colored urine, with blood and solids, voided with pain; chronic, passive bleeding) • Filipendula
(asthenic; oily, red, sandy) • Fragaria • Galium aparine (retention) • Gaultheria (purulent, ammoniacal; oil) • Geranium
maculatum (bloody) • Geranium robertianum (excessive night
urination) • Hydrangea (alkaline; great pain on urination)
• Hypericum (blood from kidneys) • Iris (scanty; with clay-like
stools; liver and glandular involvement) • Lamium) • Leonurus
(blood protein) • Lycopus (bloody) • Mentha spicata (highly
colored) • Phytolacca (somewhat opaque) • Plantago (pale or
bloody urine; damp constitution) • Pulsatilla (pale urine, nervousness, difficult control of urination; flooding pulse) • Rhus
spp. (light, copious, frequent) • Salvia (low specific gravity)
• Senecio aureus (bloody) • Solidago (dark, heavy sediment; or
light, frequent; with tired feet) • Syzgium (glycosuria) • Thymus • Trillium • Urtica • Vaccinium macrocarpon (simple urinary tract infection) • Vaccinium myrtillus (glycosuria; leaf or
fruit) • Xanthium • Zea.

Lithuria: see "Kidney Stones" in the Kidneys section.

Female Sexual System

The modern conceit is that reproductive problems should be treated
with hormones, or herbs that contain hormone-like substances. This
is only a small part of the picture, however, because the female organs
are also subject to tissue imbalances. The uterus can be stretched,
atonic, or spastic, and these conditions may reflect the general constitution or simply the overall tone of the pelvic cavity. In fact, in my
experience, tissue imbalance is a more important factor than hormonal imbalance. And the hormones must be processed by the liver
to complete their journey in the body. If the liver is not up to the job,
hormones will linger in the bloodstream after they are supposed to
have departed, which will also cause "hormone imbalances."

Fortunately, the field of gynecology has been reasonably represented in herbal literature, despite the prejudice against female practitioners. In the middle ages, female physicians were an accepted part of the field, and Trota of Salerno was the author of a major text on the subject; her name was attached to several later volumes, together known as the *Trotula*. The humanist authors of the Renaissance, however, bitterly opposed female involvement in medicine, and reattributed the authorship of the *Trotula*. Women increasingly practiced only as "nurses" and "midwives."

Until the nineteenth century, the wives of British country squires were often placed in charge of the medical needs of the community, either undertaking the task themselves or ensuring that a competent practitioner was available (Griggs 1997). Many of these women left logs and journals, a few of which have been published. Many American women were also able herbalists and midwifes, but we lack a good review of their writings, such as Barbara Griggs's work. A male doctor who was especially able in the field of obstetrics, gynecology, and the sexual-urinary tract was Finley Ellingwood, author of *The American Materia Medica* (1919). Finally, an extensive treatment of all facets of this field has been rendered in an excellent fashion by Susun Weed; see her works in the bibliography.

Puberty, Menstruation, and Menopause

Puberty: • Achillea (increases circulation) • Agrimonia (difficulty establishing flow; relaxant) • Alchemilla (pelvic floor astringent; can use with Achillea) • Angelica sinensis (delayed menarche) • Caulophyllum (delayed menarche; increases pelvic circulation) • Celastrus (blue bands under eyes, general pallor, precarious appetite; nervous, feeble; adrenocortical deficiency, vaginal prolapse) • CIMICIFUGA (delayed menarche; never well since; spasm, brooding) • Cnicus (strengthen liver; female regulator; can use with Mitchella) • Helonias (anemia; delayed menarche) • Lactuca (acne, negative thinking) • Leonurus (menstrual irregularity and nervousness) • Medicago sativa (nutritive,

cleansing, blood-thinning; delayed menarche) • Mitchella (with
Cnicus) • Panax quinquefolius (delayed menarche after recent
growth spurt and increased pubic hair—M. Moore) • PULSA-
TILLA (delayed menarche; never well since; irregular menses,
emotional lability, dreamy, nervous) • Rumex crispus (fractious,
irritable sleep that does not refresh, especially at puberty and
in young women with menstrual irregularities; with anemia;
bleeding elsewhere during menstruation; nervous symptoms
predominant) • SENECIO AUREUS (functional amenorrhea
of adolescence; worse before, better after periods—Boericke;
minute or homeopathic dose) • Turnera (delayed menarche)
• Vitex (irregular menses; feeling unready, fear of transition,
"late bloomers"; small doses—Welliver).

Amenorrhea (Menses Absent or Scanty): • Achillea (lack of
peripheral blood flow) • Alchemilla (anemic, pale) • Aletris
(undernourished) • Aloe barb. (with constipation) • Angelica
(see Cook for an American use of Angelica as a female remedy)
• Angelica sinensis • Anthemis (tension, pain, weight, heaviness) • Aristolochia serpentaria (after recent viral infection,
exposure to cold; in chronic, debilitating conditions; minute or
homeopathic doses) • ARTEMISIA ABROTANUM (psychogenic amenorrhea) • Artemisia absinthium (suppressed by cold
or emotion) • ARTEMISIA VULGARIS (functional amenorrhea; cold; stiff hips, lower back; delayed, irregular menses)
• Asarum (suppressed by cold, after viral infection; crampy)
• Asclepias tuberosa (after recent viral infection) • Betonica
(weak and nervous; ungrounded, malnourished) • Calendula
• Carthamus • CAULOPHYLLUM (delayed menarche; after
cold weather; feet wet and cold; increases pelvic circulation and
tone) • Chamomilla (whining, peevish) • CIMICIFUGA (congestion, brooding, pelvic and back pain) • Commiphora myrrha
(uterine torpor) • Daucus (helps the membrane slough; regulates the period, but contraceptive while used; increases blood

to Fallopian tubes) • Dicentra • GOSSYPIUM (backache, fullness, aching pelvis; sensation as if the flow will start, but it does
not) • Hedeoma (from chill; crampy) • HELONIAS (anemia,
weak uterus; restorative of menses after using birth control)
• Hydrastis (pelvic heaviness; atonic) • Inula • LEONURUS
(debility, nervousness, irritation, bearing-down pains; pelvic and
lumbar pain) • Levisticum (delayed, absent, or painful menses)
• Mentha piperita (from sudden chill; longstanding, with pallor,
coldness, anemia, languor; dark circles around eyes; pain in back
and loins; full, prominent veins) • MENTHA PULEGIUM
(nervous shock or chill) • Mitchella (swollen feeling, congestion
of kidneys) • Monarda fistulosa, M. punctata (suppressed by
chill or emotion) • Nepeta (delayed or painful menses; agitated,
nervous, excitable) • Origanum (suppressed by chill or emotion) • Petroselinum (lacking or scanty; weak and anemic)
• Polygonum hydropiperoides, punctatum (hot infusion; amenorrhea from cold or emotional cause, pelvic heaviness; low
cardiac function with poor circulation to the surface) • PUL-
SATILLA (labile moods and cycles; nervous excitability; cold
extremities) • Ricinus • Rubia (anemia) • Rumex crispus (anemia; for girls at puberty; nervous, fractious, irritable) • RUTA
(Weiss) • Senecio aureus (minute or homeopathic dose; pallor,
blood loss, excessive secretions of blood, mucus, pus; uterine
prolapse, infertility, feeble appetite, backache; at adolescence;
fallopian congestion, debility) • Solidago (from chill) • Thymus
• Viburnum prunifolium (tense, bearing-down pains) • Viscum
• Vitex (pituitary dysregulation) • Zanthoxylum.

Note: Warm the feet if amenorrhea is from chill.

Dysmenorrhea (Menstrual Cramp and Pain): • Achillea (from
congestion of blood) • Acorus • Agrimonia (denies the pain;
dysuria) • Alchemilla (tea) • Aletris (painful, scanty, or excessive) • ANGELICA ARCHANGELICA (works as well as the
following; confirmed—Kress, Buhner, Wood) • ANGELICA

SINENSIS (blood stagnation causing dysmenorrhea; lengthy cycles) • Anthemis (pain) • Apium (languor, debility) • Artemisia vulgaris • Asarum canadense • Bidens • Calendula • Cannabis (painful, spasmodic) • Capsella bursa-pastoris (oozing blood, from weak uterine muscles) • Carum • CAULOPHYLLUM (congestion, with lengthy cycles) • Chamomilla (irritable, complaining of pain) • Cichorium (tea) • CIMICIFUGA (brooding, delayed, better from onset) • Collinsonia (menses aggravate rectal spasms and hemorrhoids) • Crocus sativus (warming and nourishing; painful, irregular periods; menopause, infertility, anemia) • DIOSCOREA (griping, twisting pain, worse bending down and lying down, better standing erect and bending back) • Erigeron • Gelsemium (apply cream over uterus; internal nonhomeopathic use is toxic) • Gossypium (menses tardy, with backache, clots; iatrogenic complications from antihistamines, anti-inflammatory medications) • Hedeoma • Helonias (pelvic fullness) • Hydrastis (congestive) • Lactuca (stiff and cold) • Lamium (tea) • Leonurus (irritability, unrest, lumbar and pelvic pain and cramping; better from onset of menses) • Levisticum • Lilium longiflorum (conflicting desires) • LIRIODENDRON (increases flow, decreases spasm) • Liatris • Lobelia (painful torsion) • Magnesium salts • Melilotus • Mitchella (pain in kidneys and lower back from mild edema) • Nepeta (delayed, painful menses) • Passiflora (neuralgic) • Petroselinum (weak and anemic; scanty periods or very severe dysmenorrhea) • Piper methysticum • Piscidia (cramp, tension, insomnia, pain) • Polygonum aviculare (tea) • Pulsatilla (progesterone deficiency; changeable—happy/sad, tearful, nervous, on-edge) • Rosa • Rubus canadensis (cramps towards the end of menses, with red blood) • SAMBUCUS (painful, heavy flow from endometrial excess—Wolff) • Senecio aureus (pallor, blood loss, backache; "its action on the female organism has been clinically verified"—Boericke) • Symplocarpus • Tanacetum parthenium • Thymus (compress, tea) • TRIFOLIUM (hot flashes, night sweats, mood changes, depression, menstrual cramps, vaginal dryness, low desire) • Valeriana • Verbena hastata (food cravings; feels driven) • VIBURNUM OPU-LUS (uterine spasm, before and during menses; with intestinal cramps referred to thighs and sacrum; PMS) • VIBURNUM PRUNIFOLIUM (tension; intense spasms before, during, after menses; colicky lumbar and pelvic pain; scanty flow) • Viscum • Vitex (progesterone deficiency; headache, migraine, menstrual pains, breast tenderness, acne) • Zanthoxylum (tortured, as if ovaries are being ripped out by wires) • Zingiberis (muscle spasm; warm tea or liniment).

Note: Warm the feet if dysmenorrhea is due to cold. Magnesium salts are always indicated during and after spasm.

Menorrhagia, Metrorrhagia (Excessive Bleeding): • ACHIL-LEA (profuse bleeding) • Alchemilla (astringent; passive hemorrhage, menorrhagia) • Aletris (too frequent, weak, pale, insufficient flow) • Angelica archangelica (with cramping) • Angelica sinensis (with cramping) • Bidens (metrorrhagia) • CAPSELLA (heavy, dark, oozing, clotted) • Capsicum • Cimicifuga (with diarrhea and colon cramp) • Cinnamomum spp. (early and profuse menses; polyps and fibroids) • Codonopsis (thin, weak, drying out) • Crocus sativus (dark, clotted) • Equisetum • Erigeron • Fraxinus (severe hemor-rhage) • Geranium • Geum (hemorrhage) • Gossypium • Hamamelis • Helonias • Hibiscus (excitation; hemorrhage) • Hydrastis (congestive, atonic menorrhagia) • Juniperus • Krameria (menorrhagia) • Leonurus (excess flow) • Lycopus (irregular pulse) • Mitchella (congestion) • Polygonum bistorta (excessive menses) • Pulsatilla (changeable cycles and moods) • Sanguisorba (metrorrhagia) • Scoparium • Senecio aureus (too soon, too long, painful; excess blood loss, prolapse, pal-lor, feeble appetite, backache) • TRILLIUM (pelvic weak-ness, fibroids, endometriosis, prolonged periods, uterine prolapse, menopausal bleeding) • Urtica (spotting) • Viburnum

(menopausal metrorrhagia) • VINCA MAJOR (menorrhagia)
• Vitex.

Menses Too Frequent: • Capsella (bleeding elsewhere during menstruation; poor uterine tone causes oozing, possibly
throughout the month) • Erigeron • Senecio aureus (blood loss)
• Trillium.

Menses Delayed: • Achillea (brings blood to the surface) • Aletris
• Capsella (poor expulsive power of womb) • Cimicifuga (dark
mood until arrival of menses) • GOSSYPIUM (backache, fullness, aching pelvis; sensation as if the flow will start, but does
not) • Mitchella (backache, mild edema) • Pulsatilla (irregular
or late periods due to pituitary dysregulation) • Senecio aureus
(blood loss, anemia, backache; when "women do not cycle well
or at all"—Sedlacek).

Restorative after Birth Control Pills Discontinued: • HELO-
NIAS • Hypericum (helps liver clear hormones) • Nuphar
• Vitex (after coming off the pill; can cause severe depression in women with high progesterone; other side effects
reported—Welliver).

Menses Irregular: • Achillea • Alchemilla • Aletris • Angelica
sinensis (cycles longer than 28 days) • Capsella bursa-pastoris
• Cinchona • DAUCUS (take once a month at full or new moon
until periods are regular, then discontinue) • Helonias • Hypericum (helps liver clear hormones) • Linum • Nuphar • PULSA-
TILLA (no two periods are alike) • RUBUS CANADENSIS
(menses "too much, too little, too seldom, too frequent, too painful," etc.—Kress) • SENECIO AUREUS (known as "female
regulator" in the nineteenth century; "women do not cycle well
or at all"—Sedlacek) • Vitex (after coming off the pill; can cause
severe depression in women with high progesterone—Welliver;
other side effects reported).

Mittelschmerz: (pain in the middle of the cycle, from ovulation): • Cimicifuga (with colon cramp or diarrhea) • Dioscorea • Paeonia • Viburnum.

Pre-Menstrual Syndrome (PMS): • ANGELICA SINENSIS (chronic; cramping and clotting menses, pain, headache, mood swings, insomnia, low energy) • Avena (easily startled, jumpy; adrenaline discharges) • Bupleurum (congested liver; drug and alcohol abuse; bloating, nausea, breast swelling, constipation, diarrhea, indigestion, overstimulation, tension, anger, irritability), Chamomilla (whining, regressing) • CIMICIFUGA (black state of mind, brooding; delayed menses; headache, water weight) • DIOSCOREA (neuromuscular relaxant; administer during last half of cycle) • Glycyrrhiza (anxiety, stress, headaches, exhaustion) • Leonurus (muscular rigidity, nervous tension, pain in chest) • Lepidium (normalizer; acne, infertility, low libido) • Mahonia ("catabolic-dominant" thin people with efficient detoxification abilities, but prone to drying out and malnutrition—M. Moore) • NEPETA (nervous agitation; light and tardy flow; in feeble, excitable women) • Ocimum • Passiflora (insomnia; restless in evening) • Populus tremuloides (chronic, every month, without insomnia; take for 3 days before onset—M. Moore) • PULSATILLA (emotional lability; gloomy, tearful, happy, nervous; irregular menses) • Scutellaria (nervous irritability, depression, sensitivity, mood swings, sleeplessness, anxiety) • Smilax • TARAXACUM (water weight, bloating) • VERBENA (food cravings, overactive mind, tension headache; driven) • Viburnum opulus (PMS cramps) • VITEX (menstrual and hormonal headaches; anxiety, irritability, insomnia, mood changes, tension, breast tenderness, water weight, bloating, sugar craving).

Menopause: • Achillea (hot flashes and night sweats; stuffy, hot feeling—Treben) • Alchemilla (night sweats) • Althaea (thin, dry, atrophic, infertile) • Amygdalus (hot and dry) • Angelica archangelica (poor circulation, pelvic congestion, cold hands and feet, hot flashes; with Glycyrrhiza for adrenocortical strength) • Angelica sinensis (naturally occurring and surgically induced; flushing, sweats, insomnia, bladder weakness, bloating, water retention, vaginal dryness and spasm, fatigue) • Arctium (leaf or root) • ASPARAGUS RACEMOSA ("she of a thousand husbands"; restores fluids) • Avena (insomnia; melancholia after hot flashes; "sense of pressure and pain in ovaries, uterus, sacrum, bladder, with nervousness and sense of confusion"—M. Moore) • Betonica (uncentered) • Borago (overworked; exhausted, nervous) • Calendula (fibroids) • Capsella bursa-pastoris • Caulophyllum (hot flashes; pressure and pain in pelvis, discomfort refers down legs from pelvis) • CIMICIFUGA (muscle pain, nervous irritability, depression, headache, dizziness, poor sleep; flustered feeling with hot flashes; osteoarthritis in wrists, hands, fingers; pain on movement; low estrogen) • Cnicus • Equisetum (early-onset osteoporosis) • Glycyrrhiza (pituitary balance; adjuvant) • Helonias (hot flashes; heavy, bloated abdomen; headache, depression; for surgically induced menopause) • Humulus • Hypericum (helps the liver process hormones; "menopausal neurosis," easily excited—BHP) • Juniperus (with recurring dysuria but no inflammation) • LEONURUS (lumbar and pelvic pain and cramping, vaginal dryness; palpitations, hot flashes, insomnia, nervousness; unrest, irritability, freaked-out appearance) • Lepidium (low hormones) • Medicago (osteoporosis) • Nuphar (pain refers down legs from pelvis) • Ocimum (brain fog) • Osmunda (osteoporosis) • Paeonia (hot flashes, night sweats) • Panax quinquefolius (dryness; "cloudy thinking"—Kuhn and Winston) • Passiflora (insomnia) • Polygonum multiflorum (increases libido and stamina) • Pulsatilla (night sweats, anxiety, heart palpitations) • Rheum • SALVIA (night sweats; drying out of skin, mucosa, vagina) • Selenicereus (anxiety; asthenia) • Senecio aureus (hot flashes, nervous instability, hemorrhage) • Scutellaria • Smilacina racemosa ("PMS psychobitch from hell"—Crow) • Taraxacum (hot flashes) • Tilia (anxiety) • Trigonella (hot flashes, vaginal dryness) • Valeriana (insomnia) • VERBENA (hot flashes, night sweats, tension, anxiety) • Viburnum prunifolium (nutritive tonic for debility) • Viscum • VITEX (perimenopausal menstrual irregularity, heavy bleeding, hot flashes, night sweats; "lack of spiciness and libido later in life"—Donahue) • Withania (hot flashes, night sweats).

Note: Also refer to Susun Weed's New Menopausal Years (2002).

Female Organs

Vagina: • Achillea (heat, fever) • Alchemilla (relaxed, atonic mucosa, vaginal prolapse; torn or stretched tissue from rape or obstetric medical injury) • Allium sativa (douche) • Althaea (dryness, vaginitis) • Anemopsis (relaxed, boggy mucosa; sub-acute vaginitis; sitz bath, internal) • Angelica sinensis (vaginal dryness) • Arctostaphylos (vaginitis, often bacterial; prolapse) • Asparagus racemosa (dryness; restores fluids) • Berberis (bacterial infection) • Calendula (abrasions; fungal, bacterial, or HPV infection; sitz bath, external) • Caulophyllum (vaginitis; internal) • Cimicifuga (large, dragging uterus causes vaginal pain, worse from movement; vaginal atrophy in menopause) • Collinsonia • Commiphora myrrha (vaginitis) • Coptis • Cornus florida (weakness) • Echinacea (vaginitis; douche) • Geranium (bleeding; prolapse—needs confirmation) • Gossypium (vaginitis; internal) • Helonias (relaxed tissue; vaginitis) • HYDRASTIS (mucosal tonic; discharge thick, yellow, due to staph, strep, etc.; douche) • Inula (vaginal catarrh) • Krameria (prolapse; douche) • Leonurus (restores elasticity, lubrication) • Lipedium (low hormones, vaginal dryness, libido) • Mitchella (relaxed tissue) • MAHONIA (dry, inflamed) • Monarda fistulosa (draws out heat; cf. Origanum) • Nymphaea (vaginitis) • Origanum (oil of wild oregano; douche, external wash) • Staphysagria (homeopathic; tearing, violation) • TRIGONELLA (dryness, soreness, inflammation; dry skin in general;

low hormones, menopause) • Ulmus (chronic inflamed mucosa, itching, irritation; douche).

Vaginal Secretion: • Aletris (dry, atrophic; infertility) • Leonurus • MONARDA FISTULOSA (vaginal dryness, burning sensations, with "lack of passionate steam"—Flint) • Panax quinquefolius (dryness, menopause) • Salvia (dryness, withering, menopause) • Ulmus (dryness).

Vulvitis: • Aconitum (homeopathic; acute, with fever) • Alchemilla (*pruritus vulvae;* douche) • Anemopsis (with or without Bartholin-gland cyst inflammation) • Berberis (itching) • Collinsonia (with chronic pelvic congestion) • Coptis • Gossypium (acute, with incontinence) • Myrica (sub-acute) • Piper cubeba (acute, with irritation and burning) • Tabebuia (sub-acute; internal) • Thuja (small dose, internally).

Yeast Infection, Vaginitis, Leucorrhea, Discharge, Candida: • Acacia (douche) • Acetum acidum (local spray; vehicle for other agents) • Achillea (sitz bath) • Agrimonia (trichomonas) • Alcea rosea (anti-inflammatory mucilage) • ALCHEMILLA (topical) • Aletris (asthenia) • Allium sativa • Althaea officinalis (anti-inflammatory mucilage) • Anemopsis (local, for itch) • Angelica sinensis (viscous, fetid) • Baptisia (antiseptic stimulant for putrid discharge) • Berberis (chronic, low-grade infection) • Bidens • Calendula • Chelidonium • Chimaphila (internal) • Collinsonia • Commiphora myrrha (infection) • Dicentra (viscous, but without smell, with pelvic atony and hemorrhoids) • Echinacea (fetid) • Equisetum (sitz bath) • Gentiana (with Hydrastis and Chelone) • Geranium • Geum urbanum • Grifola • Hamamelis (chronic leucorrhea; viscid, fetid) • HELONIAS (abdomen feels bloated, heavy, swollen; anemia and leucorrhea; viscid, fetid) • Hydrastis (hypersecretion; 1-drop doses as a mucosal tonic) • Inula (chronic bacterial infection) • Juglans nigra (leaf douche) • Larix (tamarack)

• Larrea (for unusual and difficult-to-treat microorganisms; sitz bath for local itching and pain) • Mahonia (dryness) • Mitchella • MONARDA FISTULOSA (specific when skin is clammy and cool) • Myrica (atonic) • NYMPHAEA (tongue pale, coated white) • Ocimum • OLEA (leaf) • ORIGANUM (oil of wild oregano) • Polygonum aviculare (knotgrass tea) • Polygonum bistorta (stimulating astringent) • Pulsatilla (free, thick, milky, yellow, bland discharge) • Quercus alba (Q. rubra may also be used) • Rosmarinus (warming and drying) • Rubus canadensis • RUMEX CRISPUS (specific when tongue is carmine-red, pointed, coated) • Senecio aureus (irregular periods with yeast infection; tenderness of inguinal glands; small dose) • Smilacina (berries in brandy) • Tabebuia (viscid, fetid) • Taraxacum • Trillium • TSUGA (cold, painful lower back) • Usnea • Vaccinium marcrocarpon • Vaccinium myrtillus • Viburnum spp. (poor mucosal tone) • Vinca major.

Note: Try to take a constitutional approach for vaginitis, rather than using "natural antibiotics." In my experience, Monarda fistulosa, *wild bergamot (or* Origanum, *oil of wild oregano),* Nymphaea odorata, *and* Rumex crispus *cover most cases.*

Cervix: • Aesculus hip. (engorgement) • Althaea (dysplasia) • Angelica sinensis (cervicitis with blood congestion in pelvis) • Baptisia (erosions, discharges) • Calendula (infection, erosion) • Caulophyllum (chronic inflammation and debility) • Cimicifuga (spasm) • Echinacea (dysplasia) • Fouquieria (cervicitis with hemorrhoids, varicose veins, pelvic stagnation) • Hamamelis (congested, flabby, atonic) • Hydrastis (inflammation, erosion, polyps) • Lilium longiflorum (dysplasia, neoplasia) • Lobelia (rigid spasm) • Mitchella (cervicitis) • Oenothera (oil on cervical opening) • Rubus canadensis (raspberry leaf; cervicitis, dysplasia) • Thuja (dysplasia).

Ovaries: • Apis (homeopathic or mother tincture) • Asparagus racemosa • Echinacea (salpingitis) • Hamamelis (dull pain) • Helonias (inflamed Fallopian tubes; ovarian neuralgia) • Lilium longiflorum, L. candidum (soft, moveable cysts; mucus in menses, brown and stringy discharge) • Lilium tigrinum (ovaritis) • Melilotus (ovarian neuralgia) • Paeonia (congestion, heat at midcycle) • Phytolacca (dragging pains in) • Salvia (atrophy) • Senecio aureus (atrophy, pain; Fallopian tubes) • Smilax • Stellaria (cysts) • Trifolium.

Cysts: • Achillea (blood-filled ovarian cysts) • Anthriscus (breast) • Arctium • Bupleurum (breast) • Ceanothus • Cimicifuga • Equisetum (external) • GALIUM (fibrous breast tissue, numerous cysts) • Glechoma (fibrocystic breasts) • Glycyrrhiza • Humulus • Iris • LILIUM LONGIFLORUM (breast, ovarian cysts; one or two at a time, swelling with the period) • Oenothera (evening primrose oil) • Phytolacca (breast; external) • Prunella • Scrophularia • STELLARIA (fatty tumor, lipoma) • Trifolium (breast, hard cysts; have the cysts checked) • Vitex (breast).

Note: Dietary recommendations for cysts include the juice of fresh beetroots and carrots, with a tablespoonful of blackstrap molasses (traditional/ confirmed—Patel).

Uterus (Fibroids, Polyps): • ACHILLEA (with bright-red blood, fibroids in wall of uterus; sitz bath—Treben; often confirmed—Wood) • CAPSELLA (dark, oozing bleeding; asthenia; myoma with oozing—Weiss; confirmed—Wood) • Calendula (menopausal) • Cimicifuga • Daucus (bleeding uterine polyps) • Fraxinus • GALIUM • Helonias • Hydrastis • Leonurus • Mitchella (polyps) • Myrica (polyps—needs confirmation) • Nymphaea • Oplopanax • Quercus • Rubus canadensis (polyps—Light) • Thuja • Trillium (with cyclic bleeding) • Viola • Vitex.

Note: Fibroids are often assumed when polyps are present; polyps are the number-one cause of bleeding in postmenopausal women.

Uterus (Congestion, Prolapse, Displacement): • Achillea (sitz bath) • Alchemilla (soggy muscles) • Aletris (weak or displaced uterus; infertility, anemia, poor nutrition; backache) • Agrimonia • Angelica sinensis (atonic) • Arctium (pain, congestion in pelvis, worse from standing; prolapse) • Artemisia vulgaris (scar tissue from abortion, miscarriage) • Astragalus • Capsella (weak muscles; dark, oozing, spotting) • Caulophyllum (chronic uterine inflammation with related arthritis in small joints) • Cimicifuga (prolapse) • Collinsonia (congestion, with hemorrhoids or dull, aching urination; portal stagnation) • Crocus (spotting; stimulant) • Erigeron (acute hemorrhage) • Eryngium maritimum (prolapse and irritability) • EUPATORIUM PURPUREUM (inflammation, displacement, during and after pregnancy) • Fouquieria (pelvic congestion) • Fraxinus (astringent; severe; with hemorrhaging) • Gossypium (congestion, prolapse) • Hamamelis (general pelvic engorgement and congestion, fullness and dragging, enlarged veins) • HELONIAS (uterine weakness, prolapse, atony; back pain) • Mitchella • Myrica • Petroselinum (parsley) • Polygonatum (weak uterine ligaments) • Senecio aureus (relaxed tissue; pallor, blood loss, prolapse, infertility, feeble appetite, backache; small or homeopathic dose) • Tsuga (stimulating astringent; cold lower back; prolapse—BHP).

Uterine Inflammation: • Calendula • Caulophyllum • Cimicifuga • Dioscorea (with cramps) • EUPATORIUM PURPUREUM (inflammation, displacement, during or after pregnancy) • Gossypium • Nuphar • Piper cubeba • Trillium • Viburnum opulus, V. trilobum.

Endometriosis: • Achillea • Angelica archangelica (pain) • Angelica sinensis • Caulophyllum • Daucus (with mucus) • Dipsacus

• Galium (cysts) • Helonias • Lilium longiflorum (with mucus—
Wood) • Phytolacca • SAMBUCUS (with Phytolacca—Wolff)
• Scrophularia (cysts) • TRILLIUM (often confirmed—Wood)
• Vitex.

Metritis: • Baptisia (septic tendency) • Collinsonia (relaxed tissue;
chronic recurrent endometritis with inflammatory episodes)
• Commiphora myrrha (septic tendency) • Echinacea (septic
tendency) • Myrica (needs confirmation).

Pelvic Floor: • ALCHEMILLA (relaxation) • CAPSELLA (atrophic muscles) • POLYGONUM PERSICARIA (pelvic relaxant) • SMILACINA (unequal tensions).

Fertility and Pregnancy

Infertility: • Achillea (fibroids, bleeding, congestion) • Alchemilla
(sensitive, weak, pale, anemic) • ALETRIS (thin, poorly nourished; "if you don't want to get pregnant, don't go anywhere
near this plant"—Christopher; may have to use homeopathic,
because now endangered and rare) • Angelica (blood congestion) • ANGELICA SINENSIS (blood congestion) • Aralia
racemosa (needs confirmation) • Arctium (lipid digestion and
metabolism, to build steroids; weak lower back, tired feet—
Hall) • ARTEMISIA VULGARIS (cold uterus; after abortion, miscarriage, setback; infertility from scar tissue has been
resolved by this; stiff lower back—Bernard) • ASPARAGUS
RACEMOSA (increase libido and fertility) • Caulophyllum (in
older women; increases pelvic circulation—Keewaydinoquay)
• Cichorium (anemia, atrophy, weakness) • CIMICIFUGA
(amenorrhea) • Cordyceps • Daucus (take until cycles are
regular, then discontinue to get pregnant) • Dioscorea (nutritive
tonic) • Eleutherococcus (adrenal exhaustion) • Glycyrrhiza
• HELONIAS (thickens endometrium, improves implantation)
• LACTUCA (tight lower back, cold uterus; has worked many
times—Wood) • LEPIDIUM (increases fertility, birth weight,

number of offspring) • Leonurus • LILIUM LONGIFLO-
RUM (polycystic ovarian syndrome; mucus in Fallopian tubes,
womb; has worked many times—Wood) • Marrubium (mucus
in tubes and womb) • Mitchella (amenorrhea, exhaustion,
edema) • Panax quinquefolius • Panax ginseng • Petroselinum
(corpus luteum) • POLYGONUM MULTIFLORUM (good
for older men and women) • POLYGONUM PERSICARIA
(infertility, tonic for uterine mucus—Turner; confirmed many
times by Wolff and her students; this is really an exceptional
remedy) • PULSATILLA (irregular cycles, pituitary dysregulation) • Rubus canadensis (nutritive, sweet, astringent
tonic) • Sabal (if *vata*) • Salvia (dose everyday in first half
of cycle) • Senecio aureus ("women do not cycle well or at
all"—Sedlacek) • Smilax (androgen normalizer) • Trifolium
• Veronica • Viscum (tincture) • VITEX (irregular periods;
wants to conceive but unready—Welliver; polycystic ovarian
syndrome—Chevallier).

Miscarriage, to Prevent: • ALETRIS (asthenia; habitual)
• Capsella (poor uterine muscle tone, displacement) • Dioscorea
(impending, with cramps as main symptom) • Helonias
• MITCHELLA (history of miscarriage; in first and second
trimesters) • RUBUS CANADENSIS • Viburnum • VIBUR-
NUM PRUNIFOLIUM (high blood pressure, history of
miscarriage).

*Note: William Cook recommends stimulants and astringents as the general
treatment plan.*

Miscarriage and Abortion, Side Effects: • Achillea (hemorrhage)
• Artemisia vulgaris (seems to lessen scar tissue, re-establish fertility) • Polygonum hydropiperoides (atonic hemorrhage). Also
see "Pregnancy, Postpartum," below.

Cesarean (following): • Achillea (pelvic blood stagnation) • Angelica sinensis (pelvic blood stagnation) • Dipsacus (scar tissue; tonic). Also see "Pregnancy, to Prevent Cesarean," below.

Varicosities, to Prevent or Reduce (for external use): • Achillea (fresh plant poultice is best) • Hamamelis (poultice) • Potentilla • QUERCUS (large, knobby, corrugated, blue/black and yellow varicosities of pregnancy). Also see "Varicose Veins" under "Heart/Vasculature."

Pregnancy: • Aesculus hip. (hemorrhoids) • ALETRIS (weakness; threatened miscarriage; low progesterone; undernourished) • Aralia racemosa (in last trimester for irritability, nervousness, stress) • Ballota (nausea) • Capsicum (poor muscle tone; flabby; heart murmurs; small dose) • Cimicifuga (traditionally used in small doses, in last month, for ease of delivery; now disqualified as an emmenagogue) • Dipsacus (restless fetus; muscular pain) • Eupatorium purpureum (supports kidneys during late pregnancy) • Helonias (nausea, vomiting) • Leonurus (nervousness; albuminuria; tea, not tincture; small dose) • MITCHELLA (in last 2–6 months of pregnancy) • Monarda fistulosa (nerve relaxant, nutritive) • Polygonatum (nutritive; tones tight or loose ligaments) • Quercus (varicose veins, loose teeth, decalcification of teeth—Christopher; often proven—Wood; this strong astringent should always be used in small doses) • RUBUS CANADENSIS (astringent, nutritive; tones uterus, mother and fetus; reduces nausea, tones bowels; tea, last 2 trimesters, several days a week) • Rumex crispus (anemia; thrush) • SCUTELLARIA (restless fetus; gestational diabetes) • URTICA (nutritive; anemia, strengthens muscles) • VACCINIUM MACROCARPON (prevents or reduces urinary tract infection in pregnancy) • Viburnum spp. • VIBURNUM PRUNIFOLIUM (to prevent abortion, lower blood pressure, nourish fetus and mother).

Note: Rubus canadensis *(raspberry) has been used for hundreds of years as a pregnancy tonic. Modern physicians have mistakenly assumed it is an emmenagogue and abortifacient, and tend to discourage even the consumption of raspberry fruit and tea during pregnancy. This has no basis in scientific research or fact;* Rubus *is not an emmenagogue but a nutritive astringent.*

Pregnancy, Labor: • Achillea (clumsiness before delivery due to hormonal changes loosening the tendons — Fogg; used afterwards to prevent excessive bleeding and pain) • Anthemis (cross, peevish, contradictory) • Agrimonia (unwraps the cord from around the baby; confirmed many times — Wood and several midwives) • Aristolochia serpentaria (homeopathic; depressed and septic tissue state; exhaustion, cold feet and general cold; ineffective labor, with great sense of coldness — this was often followed by childbed fever in the old days;) • Ballota (false and premature labor pains) • Betonica (anticipation, hysteria, weak contractions; during last three weeks of pregnancy) • Caulophyllum (used for delayed labor, low oxytocin; erratic and exhausted contractions; weak uterus; rigid os; history of inflammation; almost never fails, but large doses stress the baby, so it is only used in homeopathic or small doses) • Chamomilla (see Anthemis) • CIMICIFUGA (weak, irregular contractions; rigid os; Braxton Hicks pains; feeble, erratic contractions; in first stage of labor) • Commiphora myrrha (uterine inertia — 7Song) • Dioscorea • Dipsacus • Erigeron (postpartum bleeding) • GOSSYPIUM (poor oxytocin release, simple uterine exhaustion) • Helonias • Hydrastis (5 drops every twenty minutes) • Lactuca • Leonurus (encourages labor, relieves false contractions; tincture, not tea) • Lobelia (prolonged labor, severe spasms; rigid os) • Mitchella (to prevent hemorrhage) • Myrica (has moved the baby from breach position; eases labor; last few days of pregnancy) • Panax quinquefolius (reduces labor pains — Weiss) • Piscidia (erratic labor pains) • Potentilla • Ricinus (castor oil pack, to induce) • Sambucus (last three weeks of pregnancy when there is a blue complexion, inactive

fetus; 3 drops, 3 times a day) • Scutellaria (nervous fear, anticipation) • Smilacina (uneven loosening of pelvic floor; loosens
the symphysis pubis — Wolff) • Trillium (promotes labor, lessens
hemorrhage and prolapse) • Ustilago (uterine inertia)
• Valeriana • Verbena (tension, depression, exhaustion;
increases contractions, relaxes system generally) • Viburnum
opulus, V. trilobum (bearing-down and explosive labor, Braxton
Hicks contractions) • VIBURNUM PRUNIFOLIUM (premature contractions) • Ulmus (mucilage used to lubricate the birth
channel in the last few days) • Zingiberis (muscle relaxant; tea).

*Note: When clumsiness sets in, labor will follow within forty-eight hours,
according to Wendy Fogg. A round of ginger tea in the room, as labor starts,
relaxes everyone, according to my friend Margi Flint. Remember Dr. Bach's
Rescue Remedy for stress or panic in the mother or those attending.*

Pregnancy, to Prevent Cesarean: • Agrimonia (unwinds cord
from around the neck; confirmed in over ten years' practice —
a midwife, and Wood) • Artemisia vulgaris (moxibustion to
"warm the uterus") • Cayenne (exhausted labor, in women with
atonic muscles) • Cimicifuga (cervical spasm) • Lobelia (cervical spasm) • Myrica (breach presentation — moves the fetus;
uterine weakness, confirmed) • Ricinus (castor oil pack, to
induce labor) • Ustilago (uterine inertia) • Zingiberis (cup of
tea at beginning of labor as a relaxant).

Pregnancy, Postpartum: • ACHILLEA (hemorrhage, tissue
trauma; for immediate use; up to 1 ml in the mouth — Piorier),
• ALCHEMILLA (blood loss, anemia, weakness; torn, atonic
tissues; emotional depression) • APIUM (exhaustion, electrolyte loss, and pain; stalk, leaf, seed tea) • Arctostaphylos
(tearing or episiotomy; sitz bath) • Aristolochia serpentaria
(toxic — use homeopathic doses only; to expel placenta; low
febrile state from childbed fever) • Arnica (bruising; but see
Bellis) • Asparagus racemosa

• BELLIS (homeopathic, though herb can be used too; deep internal bruising, common to most births; "save your arnica" — Murphy) • CALENDULA (bleeding, tearing, irritated, or dry vaginal walls; episiotomy) • Cannabis (childbed fever with mania) • Capsella (subinvolution of the uterus; passive bleeding becoming chronic) • Caulophyllum (after pains) • Ceanothus (poor coagulation) • Cinnamomum (with oil of Erigeron — Ellingwood's famous formula for profuse bleeding) • Cimicifuga (puerperal mania) • Crocus sativum (suppressed lochia) • Dipsacus (torn muscles) • Erigeron (oil) • Geranium • Gossypium (lack of contraction; passive hemorrhage) • Hamamelis (soreness after delivery) • HEDEOMA (retained placenta, with pungent heat; "one of the best" — Scudder) • Helonias (postpartum hemorrhage) • HYDRASTIS (passive hemorrhage) • Hydrangea (back pain) • Hypericum (injured nerves; pain in coccyx) • Leonurus (suppressed lochia; depression after delivery; use tincture, not tea) • Mentha piperita (suppressed lochia) • Rehmannia (for rebuilding blood; cooked) • Ricinus (castor oil on stretch marks; use for 4–6 months) • Rubia (expels placenta) • Rubus canadensis (recuperative) • Senecio vulgaris (small dosage — Weiss) • Silybum ("milk thistle"; pelvic, venous congestion, stasis, prolapse after birth; initiates and promotes milk) • Staphysagria (homeopathic; after cesarean) • Tribulus • Ulmus (convalescent nutritive tonic) • URTICA (slows postpartum bleeding, reduces hemorrhoids, increases milk) • Ustilago (passive hemorrhage) • Veratrum viride (homeopathic only; strong pulse following overexertion, with nervousness, anguish, pelvic tension) • Verbena (exhaustion after hard labor) • VITEX (to reset postpartum pituitary regulation).

Uterine Subinvolution (prolapse following birth): • Asclepias asperula (with poor drainage) • CAPSELLA (muscular weakness, oozing blood) • Cimicifuga (dull ache, sense of heaviness) • Collinsonia (dull ache, rectal symptoms, aggravated by diet;

congested portal vein backing up to gall bladder) • Fraxinus
(with headache of crown, occiput; hemorrhagic bleeding).

Lactation and Breast Health

Note: Also see Susun Weed's Breast Cancer? Breast Health! The Wise
Woman Way (1996).

Lactation: • Acacia (sore nipples; external) • ALCHEMILLA
(restores tone after lactation) • Agnus • Selenicereus (to initiate;
depression after cessation of lactation) • ANETHUM (increases
milk) • Aralia racemosa (opens the ducts) • Baptisia (antiseptic;
sore nipples) • Borago (increases milk) • Calendula (engorgement; external) • Carum carvi (increases milk) • Centaurium
• CHAMOMILLA (mother angry or irritable; inflammation,
sore nipples; suppressed, cheesy milk) • Cimicifuga (excess
reflex pain) • Cetraria • Codonopsis (fatigue, weak digestion,
blood deficiency; increases milk) • CNICUS (blessed thistle; to
initiate) • Cynara (can reduce milk production) • FOENICU-
LUM (increases milk in mild sympathetic excess, nervousness,
causing suppression) • GALEGA (increases milk) • Gossypium
(poor letdown or oxytocin release) • Hydrastis (salve, when
the baby has sore mouth) • Medicago (increases milk quantity and quality) • Melissa • Ocimum • Pimpinella (increases
milk) • Pulsatilla (painful, swollen breasts) • Ricinus (to bring
in the milk, reduce inflammation and swelling, open ducts; oil,
external only) • Rosmarinus (to reduce excessive flow) • Rubus
canadensis (exhaustion of lactation) • Rheum (to "keep the milk
cool and healthy"—Tilke; small doses) • Salvia (to check galac-
torrhea; otherwise avoid during lactation) • Sambucus (deficient
flow with spoiling of milk; breast swelling) • SCROPHU-
LARIA (enlarged and indurated glands; very useful in dissipa-
tion of breast tumors, drowsiness; for women with large breasts;
specific affinity for the breast; tincture and first dilution) • Silybum (initiates, increases flow) • Tribulus • Trigonella (increases

milk; restores tone, cycle after lactation; assists infantile digestion) • Urtica (stimulates milk, provides iron; 5 drops in hot
water every 4 hours) • Verbena • VITEX (increases quantity).

*Note: Cabbage leaf may be placed around the breasts to prevent mastitis. Add
bananas to the diet to balance deficient potassium.*

Breast Infection, Mastitis, Abscess: • Acacia (fissured nipples;
external) • Aralia racemosa (opens the ducts) • Bellis (red
streaks radiating from a central point outwards)
• Bryonia (homeopathic; "with swollen lymphatics, marked
inflammation"—M. Moore; "as soon as the first symptoms"
appear—Clarke) • Calendula (congestion, pain deep in lymphatic ducts, sore nipples) • Capsella (hot compress)
• Chamomilla (pain, irritation, short-tempered mother or child)
• Cichorium (sore breasts from abundance of milk)
• Chimaphila (indurated glands) • Daucus (cracked nipples;
external) • Mentha piperita (mastitis; external) • Melilotus
(soothing poultice for congestion) • Mitchella (sore nipples)
• PHYTOLACCA (pain during breastfeeding; mastitis; indurated glands; abscess; painful nipples; external only—do not get
in baby's mouth) • Plantain (external) • Pulsatilla (nervous,
painful and swollen breasts) • Salvia (excess flow; weaning;
contraindicated if milk production is desired) • Sambucus (add
to breast remedies when there is fever) • Sinapis alba (cold compress) • Smilax (retracted nipples) • Trifolium (encysted gland)
• Symphytum (poultice on abscess) • Thymus serpyllum (mastitis; oil; do not use externally) • Ulmus (external) • VERBENA
(restorative, for postpartum exhaustion; increases milk secretion
and flow; increases absorption of nutrients from food).

Breast Health: • Achillea (removes congealed blood from bruise,
which is believed to cause cancer) • Aloe vera (external)
• Angelica sinensis (breast tenderness, stagnation, congestion)
• Aralia racemosa (opens ducts) • Astragalus (increases blood

flow to surface) • Baptisia (smelly discharge from nipple) • Bellis (bruising) • BUPLEURUM ("swollen and painful breasts or nodules"—Huang) • Calendula (swollen glands) • Ceanothus (fibrocystic breast disease) • Chimaphila (for large-breasted women; lymphatic stagnation with kidney deficiency causing damp stagnation; sexually inactive) • Cimicifuga (breast pain at menopause; breast lumps) • Equisetum (tones) • Fucus (source of iodine, required for breast health) • GALIUM (fibrocystic breast disease; extensive cystic tissue; discharge) • Helonias • LILIUM LONGIFLORUM (fibrocystic breast disease; soft, moveable cysts) • JUGLANS NIGRA (Native American women rub on breasts to prevent cancer—needs confirmation) • Medicago (nourishing) • Melissa (tenderness, pain) • Oenothera (oil) • Phytolacca (tenderness, pain; hard, dangerous lumps; large-breasted women; fibrocystic breast disease) • Rosmarinus (tenderness, pain) • Rubus canadensis (tones) • Sabal (nutritious for breast tissue; swollen, tender) • Scrophularia (congestion of lymph and blood; large-breasted women; specific affinity to the breast) • Smilax (sarsaparilla) • STELLARIA (hard breast tissue) • Stillingia (lymphatic stagnation) • Trigonella (paste on breasts for enlargement and tone—Chevallier) • TRIFOLIUM (hard, dangerous cysts) • Vitex (tenderness, pain; prolactin regulation).

Breast Cysts and Lumps: • Ceanothus (large, painful cysts; lymph stagnation) • Chimaphila (in large-breasted woman, lymphatic stagnation) • Cimicifuga • Fucus (internal, external) • GALIUM (fibrocystic disease; many small cysts) • LILIUM LONGIFLORUM (soft lumps, changing from cycle to cycle) • PHYTOLACCA (hard, suspicious cysts) • STELLARIA (external) • TRIFOLIUM (hard, suspicious cysts) • VITEX (hormonally responsive cysts; continue over several months).

Breast Cancer: • Achillea (from a bruise) • Calendula • CONIUM (homeopathic, originally used as an herb on the breast; from a bruise to the breast) • Phytolacca (oil, externally) • Quercus (lymphedema after removal of glands) • Trifolium (encysts the tumor but does not destroy it; excellent in combination with surgery) • Viola.

Note: In Traditional Chinese Medicine, Native American medicine, and homeopathy, it is believed that a blow causing a bruise can result in cancer formation on the bruise site. Our Native teacher, Tis Mal Crow, used to say, "always treat a bruise, because a bruise can turn to bad blood, and bad blood can turn to cancer." When I repeated this to a Kickapoo Indian from Mexico, she smiled and said, "Yes, that is always what they told us."

Another comment needs to be made about red clover: it very often grows an encysting membrane around the tumor, limiting its interaction with the environment and controlling but not eradicating the cancer. Therefore, it should be used in combination with surgery. This remedy is particularly good for younger women in their late thirties or early forties with aggressive breast cancer. Finally, many other cancer remedies listed as general cancer remedies in the "Cancer" section can be used for breast cancer.

Libido, Relationships, Emotions, Female Constitutions

Sexual and Romantic Desires and Issues: • Acorus ("lack of mental presence interfering with sexual presence"—Donahue) • Agrimonia (tension, stress, "bad-hair day"—Wood; "it's hard to feel sexy with bad hair"—Sedlacek) • Albizia (difficulty feeling glad) • Angelica sinensis (increases sex drive, especially for menopausal and postmenopausal women; dry skin and vagina) • Apium (increases flexibility, for sexual enjoyment) • Aristolochia serpentaria (depressed circulation and intestinal function; emotional distraction and cooling of the skin during lovemaking) • Artemisia vulgaris (lost romantic aspirations from hardship—LeSassier) • ASPARAGUS RACEMOSA ("she of a thousand husbands"; increases libido, fertility) • Chamomilla (for the partner that whines) • Cimicifuga (withdrawn, brooding, abusive relationship) • Codonopsis (weak, thin, dried-out, tired) • Crataegus (opens the heart and imagination) • Eleutherococcus (reduces stress—hard to want sex when feeling stressed) • Gossypium (arousal, but weak and vague uterine contractions—M. Moore) • Humulus (excessive nervousness, anxiety) • Lavandula (overly fastidious) • Leonurus (menopausal and hormonal nervousness, bossiness) • Lilium (conflicted desires, especially sexual) • Melissa (nervous, anxious) • MONARDA FISTULOSA (increases sensations, helps deal with passion; "lack of passionate steam" with vaginal dryness, burning sensations, speaking loudly here!—Flint) • Nuphar (trapped, dry pelvic heat causing irritable libido; seeks sex for release of tension but is unconnected and unfulfilled; corresponding creative blockages—Hale; confirmed—Donahue) • Nymphaea (lascivious thoughts; lovesickness) • Ocimum (calming, centering) • Oplopanax (increases sexual confidence, establishes healthy sexual boundaries, increases desire) • Origanum (lovesickness) • Panax quinquefolius (fatigue; vaginal dryness) • Passiflora (anxiety, mental chatter, inability to relax) • Piper methysticum (anxiety; pelvic tension) • Polygonum hydropiperoides (aversion) • Prunus serotina (misuse of heart by another; irregular pulse) • Pulsatilla (nervousness, performance anxiety, fear of no arousal, depression regarding sexuality, male-dependence, sensitive to criticism of her own sex; easily manipulated) • Rosmarinus (out of the mood from a headache) • Salix nigra (lascivious thoughts, excessive desire) • Salvia (excessive desire) • SCHISANDRA (lack of libido from exhaustion; "seldom fails"—Patel) • Scutellaria laterifolia (overstimulated, nervous) • Smilacina (pelvic discomfort) • Smilax (sexual debility) • Tribulus (low desire) • Turnera (depression with loss of libido; sexual performance anxiety; calming and energizing; heightens sense of touch) • Verbascum (increases sensations) • Verbena (stiff neck, nymphomania from hormonal imbalance; idealistic, neurotic) • WITHANIA (deficient energy and libido; hypothyroidism).

Relationships: • Agrimonia (sorts out legal issues fairly in a divorce) • Artemisia absinthium, A. vulgaris (cruel and unfeeling; repetitive-cycle relationships) • CHAMOMILLA (one party whines) • CIMICIFUGA (attracted to deep emotional ties that are later hard to break; withdrawn; magnetic women) • Geranium (helps separate energies quickly in a breakup) • Mitchella (can't understand what her partner wants—traditional Native American use) • PULSATILLA (mate-dependent, has difficulty thinking for herself, feels she needs directions; emotionally labile, outside herself) • Sepia (homeopathic; loves husband and children, but so exhausted she can't cope) • Solidago (exhausted from divorce, broken covenants; tired feet) • Trillium (helps relationships) • Verbena (thin, stiff-necked; perfectionist, idealist).

Sexual Exhaustion, Neurasthenia: • AVENA ("slow-acting, but unbeatable if used for a long time"—Sedlacek) • Eryngium spp. (nymphomania; overly sensitive urethra) • Nuphar (dryness) • Panax ginseng (depression associated with sexual inadequacy) • Panax quinquefolius (dry, atrophic, debilitated; loss of fluids; exhaustion of brain, nervous system; menopause) • Polygonatum multiflorum (profound sexual exhaustion) • Smilax (sexual debility) • Salvia (premature menopause; excessive or deficient desire) • Staphysagria (homeopathic; with violation issues) • Turnera (sexual debility) • Vitex (sexual exhaustion from abuse, exploitation, or overactivity).

Sexual Suppression (effects of long-term celibacy): • CONIUM (homeopathic).

Physical Constitution: • Achillea (sanguine, athletic, but clumsy before period) • Alchemilla (pale, anemic, sensitive women with vaginal disorders) • ALETRIS (thin, dry, atrophic, infertile; poor digestion) • Angelica (pale, asthenic; or full, sanguine) • Capsella (thin, dry) • Caulophyllum (large, full build with poorly toned tissues; with uterine pains and tenderness) • Cimicifuga (dark, introspective, magnetic) • Helonias ("backachy

females"—Boericke) • Lilium longiflorum (glowing skin) • Liriodendron (wiry, tough, dried-out, spastic) • Mitchella (thin, tall,
angular, dark-haired, athletic; too much on their minds) • Phytolacca (large-breasted, fatigued) • Pulsatilla (emotionally labile,
dependent, nervous, sometimes blonde) • Rosmarinus (pale,
weak, cold; amenorrhea) • Senecio aureus (relaxed, atonic conditions; pallor, anemia, blood loss, excessive fluid loss; uterine
prolapse, infertility, backache) • Scrophularia (large breasts)
• Verbena (thin, overly intense, neurotic; food cravings).

Rape, Abuse: • Alchemilla (vaginal tear) • Artemisia absinthium
(1-drop dose, once a week, to process memories of abuse—
Wood; "one week of therapy per drop"—Donahue; do not use a
larger dose) • Artemisia vulgaris (recovery from hardship, pov-
erty, abuse, obstetric injury, abortion; "female nature injured"—
LeSassier) • Cimicifuga (dark, brooding state of mind; after
abuse) • Nuphar (pelvic tension) • Oplopanax • Pulsatilla (sug-
gestible, uncertain of emotions) • Rosmarinus (poultice on genitals for rape trauma, even long afterward) • STAPHYSAGRIA
(homeopathic specific for feeling violated) • Vitex (small doses,
after rape or assault—Welliver).

Emotions: • Aralia racemosa (nervous, assumes fetal position)
• Cimicifuga (brooding before periods) • Geranium (difficulty
separating from children) • Juglans nigra (too much under the
influence of another, whether parent, spouse, or child) • Leonurus (history of bossy or fearful mother) • Nigella (PMS and
hormonal changes) • Pulsatilla (happy/sad, PMS) • Turnera
(performance anxiety) • Verbena (feels crazy before periods;
tall, thin, stiff-necked, perfectionist, idealist; hormonal food
cravings).

Hair: • AGRIMONIA ("bad-hair day"; "always doing something
with her hair" such as bleaches, dyes—Wood; great for alopecia)
• ARCTIUM (seed in oil on scalp) • Arnica (external)

- Artemisia vulgaris (wash to maintain—Native American)
- Betula (alopecia; oil or inner bark) • Cimicifuga (dark-haired women) • EQUISETUM (hair thin, breaks easily; nervous) • POLYGONUM MULTIFLORUM (darkens and thickens hair) • Prunus serotina (redheads) • Pulsatilla (blonde, fair-haired women) • URTICA (local application; returns color, thickens; confirmed).

FORMULARY

Alchemilla—with Trillium and Bidens (menorrhagia). BHP 1983, 19.

Angelica archangelica—with Equisetum, Medicago (early-onset osteoporosis).

Angelica sinensis—with Glycyrrhiza (after "surgical menopause"). Michael Moore.

Arctium—with Betula and Nettle (alopecia; local application). I would add Agrimonia.

Asparagus racemosa—with Vitex, cooked Rehmannia (postpartum tonic). "Practice changer," from a Canadian naturopath.

Ceanothus—with Gossypium (internal), Phytolacca (mastitis; external).

Geranium—with Trillium, Nymphaea (leucorrhea; douche). BHP 1983, 151.

Helonias—with Artemisia abrotanum (amenorrhea). BHP 1983, 32.

Helonias—with Trillium (female tonic). BHP 1983, 60.

Hydrastis—with Trillium (uterine hemorrhage). BHP 1983, 114.

Leonurus—with Ballota (false labor pains). BHP 1983, 38, 130.

Leonurus—with Passiflora (menopausal insomnia).

Mitchella—with Cnicus (menstrual regulation in teenage girls).

Mitchella—with Rubus idaeus, R. canadensis (pregnancy tonic).
Pinus spp.—with Prunus serotina. "Pitch Pine buds and small wild Cherry Tree, but two-thirds of the Latter boiled together—good for young Women whose Flowers are stopped by weakness of Nature"—Samson Occom, Mohegan medicine man, 1754.

Pulsatilla—with Petroselinum, Chamomilla, Viburnum prunifolium (dysmenorrhea). BHP 1983, 155).

Rubus—with Smilax (infertility).

Senecio aureus—with Avena, Hypericum, Viburnum prunifolium, Pulsatilla (menopausal disturbances).

Senecio aureus—with Chamomilla, Ruta (suppressed menses). BHP 1983, 184.

Senecio aureus—with Helonias, Leonurus, Salvia (delayed menses). BHP 1983, 195.

Trillium—with Krameria (menorrhagia from prolapse, atonicity). BHP 1983, 126.

Trillium—with Lycopus (menstrual bleeding), frequently used in the mid-nineteenth century.

Trillium—with Vinca major (metrorrhagia and menorrhagia). BHP 1983, 232.Tsuga—with Trillium and Hamamelis (leucorrhea; douche). BHP 1983, 219.

Viburnum spp.—with Cinchona, Dioscorea, Zanthoxylum (cramps). BHP 1983, 67, 230.

Viburnum prunifolium—with Gossypium, Pulsatilla (dysmenorrhea). BHP 1983, 106.

THE HERITAGE GIFT OF THE NATIVE AMERICAN FEMALE REMEDIES

Western herbalism possesses nearly a dozen medicinal plants that are specifics for the female reproductive tract and only used secondarily, if at all, for other purposes. This includes black cohosh *(Cimicifuga)*, blue cohosh *(Caulophyllum)*, true unicorn root *(Aletris)*, false unicorn root *(Helonias)*, cramp bark *(Viburnum opulus, V. trilobum)*, black haw *(Viburnum prunifolium)*, birth root *(Trillium)*, female regulator *(Senecio aureus)*, wild yam *(Dioscorea)*, raspberry leaf *(Rubus canadensis)*, and partridge berry *(Mitchella repens)*. These *all* grow in the Eastern woodlands of North America and were adopted from Native American practice. They comprise a precious "heritage gift" from the original inhabitants of this continent.

By comparison, European, Chinese, and Ayurvedic medicine each contain less than half a dozen such specifics. From Europe we have lady's mantle *(Alchemilla)*, pasqueflower *(Anemone pulsatilla)*, ergot *(Secale)*, and peony *(Paeonia);* from China tang kwei *(Angelica sinensis)*, peony root *(Paeonia)*, and cooked rehmannia root *(Rehmannia)*; from India shatavari *(Asparagus)* and probably others. Very few of these Old World remedies are used to make pregnancy or delivery more free of pain and stress, while fully six of the Native American remedies are used in this fashion. In China raspberry is a male remedy and is not used, as it is in Native American medicine, to render a safe and quick labor and a healthy mother and child.

We must ask, "What is the reason for this disparity?" Old World religious and social institutions sometimes diminished the importance and position of women in society, and organized medicine banned them from membership. However, the American Indian people imagined that such remedies existed, looked for them, and developed a *materia medica* for nearly every facet of female reproductive health, from puberty through the childbearing epoch to menopause. The modern Western herbalist is the bearer of this precious tradition and should be aware of the origin of these medicines and importance of maintaining knowledge about them in the face of racist supposition that the science of one culture is more sophisticated than that of others.

Male Sexual System

One of the few books to emphasize treatment of the male system is fortunately a very good one: James Green's *The Male Herbal: The Definitive Health Care Book for Men and Boys* (2007). There is a real shortage of both remedies and specific indications for male remedies in the literature. Many indications we owe to single individuals; their contributions have been noted.

Like the female's, the male sexual system is certainly influenced by hormonal imbalances. However, it too is composed of structures and tissues, and therefore responds to tissue state treatment. For example, new evidence indicates that prostate swelling may be caused by venous stagnation retaining androgens too long in the prostate. This could be treated by stimulants and astringents, which ease stagnation by improving blood flow and drainage. Impotence is influenced, not only by hormones, but also by fluid dynamics that influence erection—not to mention emotional issues.

Impotence, Sterility: • ACHILLEA (astringent and cooling; impotence, premature ejaculation—Bonaldo) • Aesculus hip. (pelvic venous congestion) • Alchemilla • Angelica sinensis (in men with depressed testosterone levels, low sperm count) • Arctium (improves lipid digestion and metabolism for hormone production) • Aristolochia serpentaria (depressed circulation and intestinal function; emotional distraction and cooling of the skin during lovemaking—M. Moore; small or homeopathic dose) • Astragalus (increases sperm count, muscle tone, sexual function) • AVENA (nervous, irritable men with seminal discharge too early, at stool, or with slightest excitement—Bartram; infertility—Rogers) • Betonica (weakness) • Capsella bursa-pastoris • Chimaphila (testicular atrophy) • CONIUM (homeopathic; side effects of long-term celibacy or sexual suppression) • Cordyceps (impotence; increases sperm activity) • CORNUS OFFICINALIS (asthenia, low sex drive) • Crocus sativus (impotence) • Gingko • Gossypium (arousal but weak ejaculation; low testosterone, low sperm counts—M. Moore) • Heracleum • Lactuca • Liriosma (aromatic astringent) • Lycopodium (homeopathic; weakness) • Nuphar (dry irritation; compulsively seeking sex for release of tension, but finding it unfulfilling—Hale, Donahue) • Nymphaea (lascivious thoughts interfering with sex, relationship) • Oplopanax • PANAX GINSENG (increases sex drive) • Panax quinquefolius (neurasthenia, loss of fluids; dry, atrophic, debilitated persons; exhaustion of brain, nervous system) • Polygonatum (said to increase semen production) • Polygonum multiflorum (low libido, sperm count, sperm motility; *cf.* following; use herb, not root) • POLYGONUM PERSICARIA (pelvic relaxant;

premature ejaculation or priapism; can cause or cure both states—Wolff) • Pulsatilla (constant anxiety and depression regarding sexuality; fear of no erection) • Salix nigra (excessive desire) • Salvia (excessive desire; premature andropause) • Smilax (sexual debility) • Quercus alba (varicose veins) • Rhus spp. (excessive urination, fluid loss, probably also impotence) • Sabal (malnutrition) • Schisandra • Silphium integrifolium ("make a new man out of an old one"—Howard; "renewed vision of life"—Schnell) • SMILAX (normalizes androgens) • TRIBULUS (impotence, infertility; with dysuria) • Trigonella • TURNERA (erectile dysfunction, premature ejaculation, testicular atrophy; performance anxiety) • Verbena (high ideals, neurosis) • WITHANIA (sexual debility, fatigue, anxiety; mix with ghee or honey).

Note: "Some say tequila works also...."—Michael Moore (1994).

Sexual Overexcitement: • Arnica (overexertion) • Avena (nervous exhaustion) • Betonica • Dioscorea (seminal emissions with lustful dreams; weak knees, cold genitals—Bartram) • Eryngium spp. (urethral irritation) • Humulus (excessive desire; priapism) • Lactuca (priapism) • Mentha piperita (chronic use of peppermint can decrease sex drive) • Nuphar (compulsive unfulfilling sex for relief of tension and irritation—Hale, Donahue) • Nymphaea (lascivious thoughts; lovesickness) • Panax ginseng • Piper methysticum (excessive sexual activity) • Polygonum multiflorum (herb) • Polygonum persicaria (premature ejaculation, priapism) • Salix nigra (lascivious thoughts, nocturnal emissions) • Turnera (intellect interferes with arousal—Donahue) • Verbena (neurosis).

Prostate: • Aesculus hip. • Agrimonia (bacterial prostatitis) • Agropyron (sub-acute and chronic enlargement, prostatitis, strangury, hematuria) • ANEMOPSIS (boggy prostate; discharge, inflammation) • Angelica sinensis (enlarged, with dull ache, in older men)

• ARCTIUM • Barosma (prostatitis) • Betonica (inflammation) • Arctostaphylos (bacterial infection; with muco-purulent or acidic urine) • Barosma (bacterial infection; with muco-purulent or acidic urine) • Bidens • CEANOTHUS • Chimaphila (swollen, indurated) • Cimicifuga (with pelvic and sacral pain) • Collinsonia (portal backup from liver, gall bladder) • Cucurbita pepo (male nutrition; oil) • Echinacea • EPILOBIUM • EQUISETUM (enlargement, acute inflammation) • ERYNGIUM MARITI-MUM (enlarged prostate; prostatitis with frequent urination, irritability) • Eupatorium purpureum (sub-acute, chronic, after inflammation; pelvic and sacral pain) • Fouquieria (congestive prostatic enlargement in sedentary men) • Gossypium (enlarged, with pelvic congestion; dull ache in older males; after protracted celibacy) • Hydrangea • Hydrastis (mucosal tonic, antimicrobial) • Juniperus (enlarged, with discharge but no inflammation) • Leonurus (BHP) • Mahonia • Mitchella (with urethritis; conges-tive prostatic enlargement, in sedentary men – M. Moore) • Monarda (inflamed) • Nuphar (acute) • Piper methysticum (from excessive sexual activity; with urethritis—M. Moore) • POPULUS TREMULOIDES • Pulsatilla (prostatitis; depressed, nervous) • PRUNUS PYGEUM (swelling, inflam-mation; perhaps this remedy can be used in small or homeopathic doses—unfortunately, it is being unsustainably harvested and faces environmental concerns) • RHUS SPP. • SABAL (for *vata* men; swollen, painful) • Salix nigra • SALVIA APIANA (enlarged, with dull ache in older males; tendency to congestion in general, phlegmatic; decreases sex drive while in use—LeSassier) • Seleni-cereus • Senecio aureus (prostatitis) • Silybum • Smilax • Thuja (enlarged, inflamed; incontinence) • Tribulus terrestris (enlarged, inflamed) • TRIFOLIUM (concentrate, for cancer; internal) • URTICA (enlargement, pain, urgent urination; root) • VAC-CINIUM MYRTILLUS • Verbascum (root) • Zea.

Testicles, Orchitis, Epididymitis: • Angelica sinensis (hydrocele; chronic, in elderly) • Bryonia (tender with pressure)

- Ceanothus (hydrocele) • Chimaphila (to prevent atrophy)
- Clematis (orchitis, inflammation) • Collinsonia (varicocele, hemorrhoids, portal backup from liver; gall-bladder congestion)
- Eryngium maritimum (hydrocele) • Fouquieria (pelvic congestion) • Galium • Hamamelis (varicocele) • Lactuca (blow to testicle; pain, inflammation) • Paeonia • Phytolacca (orchitis; hard nodes in groin) • Pulsatilla (congested, enlarged, sensitive; inflammation from mumps) • Rhus tox. (non-venereal skin eruption on scrotum from sex; homeopathic) • Sabal serrulata (atrophy) • Salvia apiana (chronic, in elderly) • Sambucus ebulus (hydrocele) • Serenoa (atrophy) • Thuja (hydrocele) • Trifolium (swollen, inflamed; mumps) • Turnera (atrophy) • Viola.

Note: Tonic foods for the testicles include pumpkin seed, tomatoes, and goji berries. An active sex life is also good for the prostate.

FORMULARY

Gossypium—with Cucurbita pepo (prostate tonic).

Humulus—with Scutellaria and Valeriana (reduces excess desire).

DEVIL'S WEED *(DATURA SPP.)*

"Put the seeds of Datura in the pockets of a man who abuses women; it will drive him crazy."

—TIS MAL CROW.

Anyone who is acquainted with the properties of this plant can see the logic of this application. On a more positive note—

PERIWINKLE *(VINCA SPP.)*

"Venus owns this herb, and saith that the leaves, eaten by man and wife together, cause love between them."

—NICHOLAS CULPEPER (1652, 196)

Endocrine System

The major hormone-secreting glands of the endocrine system form a "cascade" from top to bottom: from the hypothalamus (which "reads" the blood and sends out messages to correct imbalances), to the pituitary (undertakes command of the hypothalamus), then to the thyroid (regulates metabolic levels), the adrenal cortex (mediates stress response), and the gonads (regulate sexual function). These form a feedback loop and operate as a relative unit, returning signals to the hypothalamus. Other glands and organs also communicate by hormone but are not a part of this "cascade" and are therefore not listed here.

The anterior pituitary gland regulates the thyroid, adrenal cortex, gonads, and thus the production of human growth hormone (HGH) and prolactin (for milk production). The posterior pituitary regulates retention of water by the kidneys (and blood pressure) and oxytocin (uterine labor contractions).

The liver breaks down old hormones, and therefore functions in effect as part of the endocrine system; if the blood is not well cleansed of old hormones, the hypothalamus will not be able to accurately monitor hormone signals in the blood. Hormones also pass through the extracellular fluids, so the extracellular matrix surrounding all the cells must be kept clean. This is assisted by lymphatic drainage. So the liver, cellular matrix, and lymph must all be well maintained for proper endocrine function to occur.

My "stick-man" approach to the endocrine system, describing it as a "cascade" from the top down, is a standard model for learning the subject, and I think it is the best way to organize a repertory. However, Stephen Buhner correctly describes the endocrine system as a circle. He emphasizes that the heart, set like a gem in the midst of the circulatory system, also acts as an endocrine-secreting gland. The environment of the heart is controlled by hormones and neurotransmitters that are controlled by the hypothalamus and the heart; therefore, to maintain its "comfort" within this ever-fluctuating environment, the heart also sends signals back to the hypothalamus.

The thyroid controls the temperature of the interior of the body, the posterior pituitary controls the peripheral blood pressure (through vasopressin), adrenaline influences fluctuations in blood pressure, etc. The heart reacts to all of these changes and sends signals back to the hypothalamus, so the whole system is a circle (or even a sphere) emanating out from the hypothalamus and back again. For more detail, see *The Secret Teachings of Plants* by Stephen Harrod Buhner (2004).

My knowledge of the endocrine system and the majority of the remedies listed below is derived from discussions with Phyllis Light and her class handout "Dysfunctions of the Endocrine System" (2001). Many of our alternative medical ideas about the endocrine system are not recognized by mainstream medicine. However, a huge number of patients are unsatisfied by conventional treatment, suggesting that biomedicine may well have much to learn here.

Hypothalamus and Pituitary

The major symptoms of hypothalamo-pituitary imbalance are over-sensitivity to heat and cold; stress in general; emotional lability; and (in women) irregular menstrual cycles.

Anterior Pituitary: • ARALIA RACEMOSA (nervous, exhausted; "burned-out adrenals," dark circles under eyes—LeSassier; has a slight preference for women) • Arctium (strong but yet-to-be-defined action) • Caulophyllum • Cnicus • DAUCUS (irregular menses and other hormonal imbalances) • ELEUTHEROCOC-CUS ("adrenal burn-out;" dark circles under eyes—LeSassier; smaller doses may be more effective) • Foeniculum • Fucus • Inula • Hypericum (detoxifies, so that hypothalamus can more clearly assess/adjust blood) • Medicago • Mitchella • Panax ginseng • Panax quinquefolius • Passiflora • Piper methysticum (small-to-moderate dose relaxes, large dose stimulates) • Pulsatilla (emotional lability, menstrual irregularity) • Salvia • Sassafras • Smilax • Turnera • Trigonella • Urtica • Vitex (to reduce FSH [follicle stimulating hormone]).

Posterior Pituitary: • Citrus limonum (excess urination; fresh juice, essential oil, dried peel) • Ledum (needs confirmation) • Rhus spp. (excess urination and other fluid discharges).

Note: The posterior pituitary secretes antidiuretic hormone (ADH) or vasopressin, which increases the peripheral vascular tension, causing urine (and other fluids) to be retained in the body. It also secretes oxytocin, which stimulates uterine labor. The above remedies act on ADH; for those that act on oxytocin see "Labor" under "Female Sexual System."

Thyroid

The thyroid gland, situated over the windpipe just above where the latter plunges into the thorax, secrets calcitonin, a hormone that sends calcium to the bones, and thyroxine, which is metabolized in the liver into a more active form that is picked up on cellular receptor sites and raises the metabolic rate or temperature in the cells.

We do not usually consider calcitonin as involved in "thyroid problems" because it usually does its job in such a satisfactory fashion. It balances the action of the parathyroid gland, which releases a hormone (parathormone) that, when calcium levels are low, takes calcium out of the bones and sends it into the serum so it can be available to assist magnesium in sedating muscles.

If there is overbuilding of bone, we usually use the "anti-lithics" or stone-removers, which act on the kidneys, such as gravel root (*Eupatorium purpureum*), hydrangea (*H. arborescens*), and celery seed (*Apium graveolens*). If there is not enough calcium, the person is thin, long-boned, and twitchy, and the parathyroid kicks in. This was called the "consumptive" or "tubercular" type in nineteenth-century herbals and medical books, since the body needs calcium to control the tuberculosis bacteria. The remedies are the "rabbit medicines" of Native herbalism, which are for thin, delicate, twitchy persons. These are listed under "Stages of Life" in the "Chronic Conditions" section.

Most troubles included in "thyroid problems" in popular speech revolve around thyroxine and its unusual component, iodine. Lack of iodine, goiter, hyperthyroidism, Hashimoto's disease (autoimmune attack on the thyroid), and hypothyroidism constitute these common "problems."

There are raging debates inside and outside medicine about the causes of hypothyroidism in particular, so this is something we really must address. The following perspectives and approaches I have gathered through experience, and the occasional conversation with Phyllis Light, an herbalist who knows her thyroid!

Lack of iodine produces the simplest form of hypothyroidism, and may also cause goiter (neck swelling from thyroid enlargement), as the thyroid expands to pick up any iodine it can. However, goiter may also be caused by overactivity of the thyroid. Iodine is also needed elsewhere in the body, and acts as a general antiseptic when it is in the bloodstream; so there are other reasons beyond the thyroid to make sure we have enough. Seaweed is the usual source and, as long as it is clean, is one of the most nutritious foods available to us.

Assuming there is enough iodine in the body, we must assume there is enough signaling from the anterior pituitary, which sends thyroid-stimulating hormone (TSH) to tell the thyroid (based on feedback received by the hypothalamus) how much thyroxine it needs to produce. Low TSH levels may respond to wild carrot *(Daucus carota)*. High levels of TSH production are taken as a sign that the thyroid is not producing enough thyroxine, and is the usual measure for beginning medical supplementation. This does not, however, address the cause of the hypothyroidism, which is what we want to do in holistic herbal medicine.

The most common cause of hypothyroidism is Hashimoto's disease, where the body's own immune system attacks the thyroid. The causes of autoimmune disease are not well understood; often it involves an overreaction to a toxin. However, several times I have seen hypothyroidism or Hashimoto's disease caused by improper use of the voice (a teacher straining the voice to control kids) or tension in the shoulders, neck, and upper chest. The inflammatory and tension levels in the neck need not be very high for the thyroid to be mildly suppressed; chronic inflammation can cause the hypothalamus to lower thyroid action—why overheat the body? Yet supplementary heat from pharmaceutical stimulation is not the same thing as proper heat from a healthy thyroid. It's best to eliminate the chronic inflammation.

We do not know all the causes of Hashimoto's, but this I do know—it will often respond to black walnut hull *(Juglans nigra)*, which may work on several kinds of hypothyroidism. This gem of clinical herbalism I learned from Phyllis Light, and have confirmed again and again. It is probable that ashwaganda *(Withania somniferia)* also acts on autoimmune thyroid problems, since it is such a fine adaptogen, and it too may act on other kinds of hypothyroid.

"Wilson's Temperature Syndrome" refers to a kind of hypothyroidism believed to occur when the thyroxine released by the thyroid (T4) is not metabolized in the liver into T3, which is much more active on the cell binding sites. Hershoff and Rotelli (2000, 244) recommend bitter herbs *(Gentiana* and *Taraxacum)* as general remedies to stimulate metabolism. Such herbs may help alleviate this condition in particular.

Another kind of hypothyroidism is caused by "leaky gut" syndrome (food particles diffuse through the gut wall), or by oversensitivity to proteins in the gut wall. Either may set off an immune storm, increasing the metabolism in the liver (it has to deal with the large input of food/toxins) and cells. The thyroid then has to turn up the metabolism, but later crashes. Widely fluctuating thyroid and blood-sugar patterns indicate this problem. Blue flag *(Iris versicolor)* will usually treat this kind of hypothyroidism.

As Michael Moore stresses, it is the job of the adrenals to deal with stress, but when the adrenals are weak or worn out, "the thyroid takes the hit" (paraphrased). Therefore, the adrenal medulla and cortex need to be "firmed up" to support the thyroid. This effect is probably why remedies like *Eleutherococcus* and *Borago* end up with a thyroid reputation. And it may be another avenue upon which *Withania* operates. This would explain the experiences of several herbalists (Nancy Welliver, Lise Wolff) who claim that hyperthyroid remedies *(Leonorus, Melissa)* also work on hypothyroidism.

The only foolproof test for hypothyroidism is the underarm-thermometer method introduced by Dr. Broda Barnes—see his book

Hypothyroidism (1976). Visible symptoms include two creases across the neck, above and below the thyroid (Margi Flint) and ragged-to-missing outer halves of the eyebrows (medically attested).

Hyperthyroidism: • Borago • Equisetum • Filipendula (nervousness, irritability, restlessness, palpitations) • Fucus • Iris (fluctuating high and low levels) • LEONURUS (heart palpitations; menopausal) • LYCOPUS (looks like a hunted animal; tachycardia, dyspnea) • MELISSA (worse in heat) • Populus (asthmatic panting, worse in heat) • Prunella • Scutellaria (thyroid-supportive) • SELENICEREUS (heart palpitations) • Sinapis spp. (raw seed) • Veratrum viride (homeopathic; hyperthyroid goiter) • Zea.

Hypothyroidism: • Avena • Centella (Hashimoto's; "emotional depression, dry skin, cold extremities, poor digestion, weight gain, little endurance"—Gagnon) • Cetraria • COLEUS • Commiphora myrrha • Daucus ("flabby, flaccid, pale, water weight"—Piorier) • Echinacea (Hashimoto's) • FUCUS (iodine deficiency; listless, general debility) • Galium • Gentiana (promotes metabolism; Wilson's Temperature Syndrome) • IRIS ("leaky gut"; levels go up and down) • JUGLANS NIGRA (specific for hypothyroidism) • Phytolacca (2 drops a day for 10 days) • Polymnia (friction-application of ointment) • Sabal • STELLARIA (perhaps acts on receptor sites, increasing uptake of iodine or thyroxine) • Taraxacum (general metabolism; Wilson's Temperature Syndrome) • Urtica • WITHANIA.

Thyroid Nodules: • FUCUS • STELLARIA (externally and internally).

Goiter: • FUCUS (iodine deficiency; lymphadenoid) • Galium (tea) • Iris • Juglans nigra • Passiflora • Plantago (poultice) • Scrophularia (tea) • Trifolium • Urtica.

Adrenals

Adrenal Medulla (Hyperadrenalism): • Aconitum (homeopathic only; shock or exhaustion; animal fear) • AVENA (nutritive tonic) • BORAGO (long-term nervous exhaustion, persecuted feeling) • Cimicifuga • ELEUTHEROCOCCUS • GLYCYRRHIZA • LEONURUS • LYCOPUS • MELISSA • Rhus spp. (frequent urination with nervousness) • Rumex crispus • SCUTELLARIA • VERBENA (self-critical, perfectionist).

Adrenal Cortex: • ANGELICA (similar to Arctium, but warming) • ARALIA RACEMOSA (dark circles under eyes) • ARCTIUM (excellent for rebuilding lipid digestion, metabolism, and adrenals) • AVENA (nervous exhaustion from work, study, drugs, alcohol, sexual excess) • BORAGO (adrenal glands worn out by use of steroids, long-term nervous anxiety, feeling of persecution) • ELEUTHEROCOCCUS (dark circles under eyes) • GLYCYRRHIZA (adrenocortical deficiency, Addison's disease; or with immune deficiency) • GNAPHALIUM (normalizes; good for adrenocortical-excess types) • Helianthus (tissue under eyes sunken; tonic to adrenals — Wood) • Helichrysum (essential oil; use if Gnaphalium not available) • Juglans nigra (strengthens the thyroid, which supports the adrenals) • Ledum (for energy; minute doses — Powell) • Ligusticum porteri • Lomatium • Nigella sativa (seed or oil) • Oplopanax • Panax ginseng (uncured) • Panax quinquefolius • Passiflora (improves sleep) • RIBES NIGRUM (leaf, berry, buds; oil) • Rumex crispus (large, adrenocortical-dominant constitutions with hot, overactive digestion) • Salvia • SCHISANDRA • Smilax • Vitex.

Note: Adrenal burnout is due to hyperfunction of the adrenal medulla with suppression of the adrenal cortex. The former supports stress response, while the latter supports the rest-rebuild-and-digest pathways. The two are competitive: we cannot respond to stress and eat at the same time. To treat this condition, it is necessary to simultaneously (1) sedate the adrenal medulla and (2) fortify the adrenal cortex. To sedate the adrenal medulla, adrenaline excess, and nervousness, we need the standard nervines and sedatives mentioned throughout this repertory. For the adrenal cortex, a diet high in good-quality fats and oils is necessary because this gland is composed of lipids; even good ice cream or rich, indulgent foods are helpful if the person is thin and exhausted.

Note on Eleutherococcus senticosus *vs.* Aralia racemosa: *William LeSassier taught us to look for "dark circles under the eyes," his indication for adrenal exhaustion. Two remedies he recommended for this were* Eleutherococcus *and* Aralia racemosa.

David Winston writes, "In my clinical practice I use Eleuthero for stressed-out, type-A people who work long hours, don't get adequate sleep or nutrition, and have a motto of 'word hard, play hard, and hardly sleep'" (Winston and Maimes 2007, 160).

I found this interesting because I too use Eleutherococcus *for exhaustion in the more "yang" types — while I use its more warming cousin,* Aralia racemosa, *for adrenal exhaustion in people with lower stamina (a more "yin" type of person) — something I learned from Kate Gilday. So* Eleuthero *comes up more often for men and* Aralia racemosa *more often for women.*

Gonads

Also see "Female Sexual System" and "Male Sexual System" sections, above.

Gonads: • Angelica archangelica (lipid deficiencies) • Angelica sinensis (lipid deficiencies) • Arctium (lipid deficiencies) • Cimicifuga (low estrogen) • Cornus officinalis • SALVIA (decline, in aging; drying-out) • Verbena (progesterone excess; sexual neurosis) • Vitex (prolactin or progesterone deficiency).

General Endocrine System

Adaptogens: • ARALIA RACEMOSA (similar to Eleutherococcus, but warmer) • Avena (complementary) • CENTELLA (weak connective tissue; "emotional depression, dry skin, cold extremities, poor digestion, weight gain, little endurance"—Gagnon) • CODONOPSIS (weak, thin, dried-out, tired; shortness of breath, bloating) • Cordyceps (fatigue, exhaustion, low immunity, sex drive) • ELEUTHEROCOC-CUS (acts on hypothalamic-pituitary-adrenal axis; stress intolerance) • GANODERMA (fatigue, insomnia, anxiety; restores heart/mind connection) • Glycyrrhiza (adrenal cortex deficiency) • Grifola • Ocimum (clears fat-soluble toxins—Davis) • PANAX GINSENG (long-term stress, unbalanced sleep, fatigue, debility) • Panax quinquefolius ("yin deficiency"; loss of fluids in senescence) • Pfaffia paniculata (inflammation, fatigue, stress) • Polygonum multiflorum • RHODIOLA • SCHISANDRA • WITHANIA (nervine; calming, yet stimulating; extensive adaptogenic action).

Essential Fatty Acids: • Borago • Nigella sativa • Oenothera • Ribes nigrum.

Note: Essential fatty acids (EFAs) adjust the "thermostat" between over- and under-reaction of the adrenal cortex, immune system, and fever mechanisms. This can influence neuroendocrine balance. Each EFA has a specific affinity. An herb that may act in this way is Gnaphalium obtusifolium and its cousins. The aromatherapy equivalent—another cousin—is Helichrysum spp.

FORMULARY

Eleutherococcus—with Cordyceps, Rhodiola, Schisandra (tonic, for severely stressful work, night shifts).

BLACK CURRANT *(RIBES NIGRUM)*

This plant medicine has a long history of use in France, but is little utilized in the New World except in a general way as a source of EFAs. This old French folk remedy is one of the darlings of gemmotherapy, which uses buds to make medicine, and is widely used in professional French medicine today.

"If you had to choose only one gemmotherapy extract to take with you to a desert island, it would have to be black currant. It is as powerful as cortisone, without any of the adverse side effects."

—ROGER HALFON, FROM *GEMMOTHERAPY: THE SCIENCE OF HEALING WITH PLANT STEM CELLS* (ROCHESTER, VT: HEALING ARTS PRESS, 2005)

Nervous System

Nerve Injuries: See "Injuries, First Aid."

Nervousness: See "Mind, Emotions, Will."

Debility: See "Exhaustion, Low Energy, Fatigue."

Neuralgia: • Anthemis (poultice on painful area) • Asclepias tuberosa (intercostal and pericardial) • Apocynum cannabinum (lumbar, sciatic, crural) • Cannabis • Cimicifuga (cranium, spine, eyes) • Dicentra • Dioscorea (liver, abdomen, stomach) • Eschscholzia (nerve damage, sharp, shooting pain) • Heracleum (trigeminal neuralgia; Bell's palsy; fresh seed or root) • Hypericum (sharp, shooting pain; muscular twitching) • Melilotus (with cold extremities and chronic headache; "sharp stabbing pain"—D. Winston) • Monotropa (pain that overwhelms the senses) • Passiflora (large doses) • Plantago (toothache) • Scutellaria (with fear, agitation; CNS sensitivity) • Tussilago (small of back and loins) • Zanthoxylum (severe, agonizing pains).

Facial Neuralgia: • Achillea • ACONITUM (homeopathic) • Anthemis nobilis • Chamomilla • Chelidonium (right side of head and face; migraine) • Cimicifuga (muscle tension) • Eugenia (oil) • Heracleum • Humulus • Melilotus (from cold) • Mentha piperita • Passiflora • Plantago • Thymus • Verbascum.

Neuritis: • Cannabis sativa (extreme sensitivity) • Hypericum (traumatic, inflamed nerves; shooting pain) • Leonurus • Melilotus (asthenic persons, with sense of cold) • Scutellaria.

Nerve Disease: • GALIUM (nerve endings; Morton's neuroma, DuPuytren's contracture, neurofibromatosis; external or internal) • Passiflora (increases serotonin levels) • Verbascum (holds moisture around the nerve endings) • Zanthoxylum.

Neurasthenia (Nerve Weakness): • Apium (cerebral debility from overwork) • ARALIA RACEMOSA (enfeebled state of nervous system, anemia, general debility) • AVENA (debility, depression, melancholy) • Betonica (ungrounded; weak digestion and cognition) • BORAGO • Caulophyllum ("nervous feebleness with irritability," with cramps, twitching—Cook) • CENTELLA • Citrus aurantium (slow digestion, large quantities of gas; neurasthenia) • Echinacea (when due to toxins) • ELEUTHEROCOCCUS • Hypericum • Ilex paraguariensis (increases oxygen to heart, brain; stimulates without causing nervousness) • Iris (sympathetic nervous excess, alternating with exhaustion; hypoglycemia, thyroid ups and downs) • Humulus (hops pillow) • Lycopodium • Melissa • Panax ginseng • Panax quinquefolius (neurasthenia, loss of fluids, dryness, atrophy, debility, exhaustion of brain, nervous system) • Polygonum multiflorum (deep exhaustion) • SELENICEREUS (cardiac; hyperthyroid) • TURNERA • Veratrum viride (homeopathic; strong pulse, exhaustion, nervousness, tension; after fever, overexertion) • WITHANIA ("stressed, burnt out, wired, jittery"—Green).

Note: Also see "Exhaustion, Low Energy, Fatigue," "Brain and Head," and "Adrenal Cortex." The note under the latter entry explains the common folk medical term "adrenal burnout" and its treatment.

Peripheral Neuropathy: • Aesculus hip. • Cinnamomum • Hypericum • OSMORHIZA LONGISTYLIS (especially diabetic) • Plantago • Rhus spp. (especially diabetic) • Vaccinium (especially diabetic) • Zanthoxylum.

Restless Leg Syndrome: • Bupleurum • Humulus • Paeonia • Piper methysticum • Scutellaria • Viburnum spp. (crampbark and black haw) • Withania.

Epilepsy, Convulsions, Chorea: • Acorus • Allium sativa (cerebrospinal disorders of children, with convulsions) • AMMI • Apium (nervous debility) • Artemisia absinthium (night terrors) • Artemisia vulgaris • Cimicifuga (menstrual) • Convallaria • Crocus sativa • Galium verum • Hypericum (spasm from nerve inflammation; traditionally used for tetanus; said to be preventive and curative) • Hyssopus (petit-mal seizures) • PAEONIA (epilepsy — Galen) • Passiflora (convulsions; traditionally used for tetanus) • POLYGONUM PERSICARIA (with menstrual pain, spasms) • Sambucus nigra • Scutellaria • Tilia ("reputation for reducing severity of epileptic attacks" — Bartram) • Verbascum • VERBENA (seizures start in the nape of the neck; convulsions after fever; epilepsy and other kinds of seizures) • Viscum.

DuPuytren's contracture and Morton's neuroma: see "Hands, Wrists, Fingers" section of "Muscular and Skeletal Systems," below.

Intermittent Claudication: • Allium sativa • Gingko.

Parkinson's: • Amygdalus • Avena (severe pain; nightly dose) • Capsicum • Galium • Scutellaria • Verbena hastata (palliative) • Zanthoxylum.

Multiple Sclerosis: • Angelica sinensis (young women) • Eleutherococcus • Eupatorium perfoliatum • Oplopanax (if aggravated by blood-sugar shifts) • Panax quinquefolius • Populus gileadensis • Scutellaria.

Narcolepsy: • Avena • Cola.

Shock: See "Injuries, First Aid."

Stroke, Paralysis: • Achillea (external) • Arnica (external) • Eupatorium purpureum (external, on paralyzed part) • Heracleum (fresh root tincture, externally) • Pedicularis • SASSAFRAS (thick blood, pulse like oatmeal) • Urtica (affinity to weakness of inner thighs; paralysis after anesthesia—needs confirmation; internal or external) • Zanthoxylum (external).

Note: For stroke/paralysis, both the brain and the affected part need attention.

Rebuilding Nervous System After any Severe Addiction:
• AVENA (decoct for at least forty minutes) • Borago (needs confirmation) • Passiflora (quieting effect on nervous system; heroine addition).

Sensorium: • Monarda (sensory nerves weak or too intense) • Monotropa (sensory overload) • Psilocybe (reawakens senses) • Turnera (loss of pleasure in).

FORMULARY

Hypericum, Melissa, and Rosemary comprise William LeSassier's basic "triune formula" for the nervous system.

Medicago—with Chondrus, Ulmus (convalescence tonic). BHP 1983, 140.

Muscular and Skeletal Systems

Myalgia, "Rheumatism" (Muscles Injured, Painful, Inflamed, Bruised): • ACHILLEA (bruising; poultice, fomentation) • Acorus • Aesculus hip. (dull, throbbing pain) • Agrimonia (pinched nerve, muscle) • Agropyron (renal) • Aletris (undernourished) • Allium cepa (rheumatic pain in the tendons; tincture, external) • Anemopsis • Anagallis (acute rheumatism) • Angelica • Anthemis (poultice on pain) • APIUM (stiffness, pain, mental depression) • Aralia racemosa (rheumatism) • Aralia spinosa (rheumatism, spasm) • Arctium (lower back, pelvis) • ARNICA (bruising, stiffness, strain, overexertion; external) • ARTEMISIA VULGARIS (external, in moxibustion) • Betonica (chronic rheumatism) • BUPLEURUM (intercostal, chest, shoulder, neck fullness and pain, the "must-see" sign—Huang) • Calendula (pulled muscle) • Calluna • Cannabis (severe pain) • Carthamus (reduces soreness if taken before exercise; removes lactic acid) • Castanea (generalized fibrositis) • Caulophyllum ("neuralgic forms of rheumatism," with cramping, twitching—Cook) • CENTELLA (dull, throbbing pain) • Chamomilla (complains about pain) • Chelidonium (dull muscular ache) • Chimaphila (muscle pain from edema; kidneys) • CIMICIFUGA (pain, tightness, dull ache; whiplash, fibromyalgia, rheumatism, rheumatoid arthritis, intercostal myalgia, sciatica; from change of weather) • Cinchona (shoulders, wrists, fingers) • Cinnamomum (external, on cold, sore muscles) • CURCUMA (combine with pepper) • DIOSCOREA (tincture) • DIPSACUS (myalgia; adhesions and scar tissue; torn, wrenched—LeSassier) • Echinacea (dull, heavy pain) • Echium vulgare (inflammatory pain) • Eschscholzia • Equisetum • Eupatorium purpureum • Filipendula (tea) • Fucus (internal and/or external) • Gaultheria (oil, external) • Genista tinctoria • Guaiacum (rheumatism, feeble circulation, cold hands and feet, vital depression) • Hamamelis (strain, soreness, injury) • HARPAGOPHYTUM • Heracleum (temporomandibular joint syndrome, Bell's palsy, whiplash; 20–40 drops) • Hydrangea • Hypericum (oil, external) • Hyssopus • Iris (pains in pectorals, under scapula) • Jeffersonia (acute, non-inflammatory, with mild auto-toxicity) • Juniperus • Lactuca (tightness, tight lower back) • Lavandula • Ledum (rheumatic feet) • Leonurus • Lobelia (torsion, spasm, "rheumatic nodules"— BHP) • Lycopodium • Majorana • Melilotus (cold extremities, lameness, soreness; "sharp stabbing pain"—D. Winston) • MENYANTHES • Myristica (pain) • Nicotiana (external poultice) • Oplopanax • Opuntia (flowers) • Paeonia (spasm) • Panax quinquefolius (during recuperation from debilitating, protracted illness) • Pedicularis (sprains, pain; sharp muscle spasms; removes lactic acid) • Peumus • Petroselinum (internal, external) • PHYTOLACCA • Pilocarpus jaborandi (profuse or lack of sweat; fever, hard pulse; small doses) • Piper methysticum • Populus gileadensis (ointment of the bud) • Primula vera (acute rheumatism) • Quercus • Rhamnus frangula (external) • RHODIOLA (increases stamina) • Ruta • Salix alba ("muscular and arthrodial rheumatism with inflammation and pain"—BHP) • Salvia • Sassafras • SENECIO JACOBAEA (external) • Smilax • Solanum dulcamara (toxic for internal use; external for pain from cold and damp) • Stellaria • Symphytum (swollen) • Taraxacum (affinity to sternocleidomastoid muscle, neck; inflamed, swollen muscles) • Thuja • Thymus serpyllum (dilute oil) • Urtica (bath) • Vaccinium (solid extract) • Valeriana • Verbascum • Verbena (tight nape of neck) • Veronica (tincture, external, internal) • WITHANIA • ZANTHOXYLUM (weakness with pain; poor circulation, debility, agony) • YUCCA • Zea (tea) • ZINGIBERIS (fresh rhizome for spasm; dried rhizome for pain).

Muscles (Weakness, Asthenia): • Abies nigra (poor digestion, vascular weakness, pale mucosa) • Alchemilla (hernia; weak muscles and membranes) • Betonica (weakness) • Capsella • Capsicum (senility) • Cichorium (rub on atrophic limbs) • Cola ("depressive states associated with general muscular weakness"—BHP; senescence) • Ganoderma • Glechoma (lead poisoning) • Hydrastis (weakness, debilitated muscles) • Lycopodium (weakness, sometimes with severe spasms) • Melilotus • Myrica • Panax quinquefolius (weak) • Pinus • Polygonatum (convalescence) • Rhodiola • Rubus canadensis (tones and nourishes) • Ulmus (convalescence) • Withania • Zanthoxylum (weakness, pain).

Muscles (Spasms, Cramps, Myalgia): • Betonica • Cannabis sativa (spasmodic pain of nervous origin, with depression) • Caulophyllum ("neuralgic forms of rheumatism," with cramping, twitching—Cook) • Chamomilla • Cimicifuga • DIOSCOREA (cramps and intermittent claudication) • Epilobium (with diarrhea and dysentery) • Filipendula • GELSEMIUM (herbal cream; external only) • Heracleum • Lavandula (external) • Leonurus (spine, mental; muscles, especially when felt around the heart; tension from cold) • Lobelia (sthenic; torsion) • Lycopodium (asthenic cramping) • Majorana (relaxes, loosens) • Mentha piperita • Paeonia • Passiflora • Pedicularis • Piper methysticum • Rosmarinus (essential oil, in olive oil—rub on calf spasm) • Salvia (tea) • Scutellaria (tremors, tics, fits, nervousness) • Thymus (compress, tea) • UMBELLULARIA (muscle spasm; leaf or roasted nut) • Valeriana (uterine, lower back, with nervousness) • VERBASCUM (root; "effective remedy esteemed by countryfolk"—Parton; lacking modern verification) • Viburnum opulus (uterine, lower back, leg at night) • Viscum (tea) • Withania • ZINGIBERIS (fresh rhizome; external).

Note: Always use Magnesium salts during or after muscle spasm to replenish their loss. Magnesium sedates muscles, and without this element muscles are twitchy and spastic. It is assisted by calcium; see discussion of parathyroid, under "Thyroid."

Muscles (Strain, Sprain, Overexertion, Hyperextension): • Acorus • ARNICA (overexertion) • ARTEMISIA VULGARIS (external, in moxibustion) • Hypericum (sharp pain, pulled muscle) • Pedicularis (sharp pain) • Petasites (leaf compress) • Ruta • SYMPHYTUM (sprain, overexertion; leaf, external) • Thymus • TSUGA CANADENSIS (oil, external) • VERBENA (hyperextension) • Veronica (overexertion).

Tendons, Ligaments: • Arctium (withered tendons; leaf poultice) • Cimicifuga (deep, aching pain with muscle involvement)

• Cinchona (relaxed ligaments; aching pain after movement) • DIPSACUS (pulled, torn, wrenched, incapacitated) • Echinacea (chronic) • Equisetum (cartilage damage) • Eupatorium purpureum (dried-out muscles and tendons around joint; frozen) • Hedeoma (Achilles-tendon strain; oil) • Iris (tight tendons) • Linum (rub linseed oil; not for internal consumption – Hall) • Monarda fistulosa (burning pain) • POLYGONATUM (tendons tight or loose) • Symphytum • Thuja (Achilles tendon strain).

Convulsions: See "Nervous System."

Joints (Arthritis): • Acorus (cold, achy) • Agrimonia (out of joint; inflammation, pain) • Alchemilla arvensis • Anemopsis (inflammatory; bath) • Angelica (warming) • Apocynum cannabinum (arthritic pain with edema) • Arctium • Arnica (chronic; external) • ASARUM CANADENSE (chronic; external) • Asclepias tuberosa (acute inflammation, bursitis, intercostal, lack of lubrication, clicking in joints) • Betonica • BOSWELLIA (rheumatoid and osteoarthritis; fatigue, weakness; with digestive, metabolic disorder) • Capsella • Caulophyllum (fingers) • Centella (red, not inflamed) • Chimaphila (arthritic pain with edema) • CIMICIFUGA (trapezius, scapula; rheumatism in the depth of the muscle) • CURCUMA (inflammation from tissue depression; external, internal) • DAUCUS (in elderly) • DIOSCOREA (arthritis; cook until suds appear) • DIPSACUS (muscle spasm, joint pain, inflammation, Lyme disease) • Equisetum • Eryngium maritimum • Eupatorium purpureum (removes calcification) • Filipendula (tea) • Fucus • Galium • Gaultheria (oil, external) • Glycyrrhiza • GUAIACUM ("takes the heat out of any rheumatic or arthritic flare-up"—Bartram; atrophy, contraction, shortening of tendons; joint stiffness, deformities; affinities to the wrists, knee, limbs, spine) • Harpagophytum (rheumatoid arthritis, osteoarthritis) • Hydrangea • HYPERICUM (tight, painful, swollen hands; external; if it doesn't work within 15 minutes, it

won't work at all) • Inula • Iris (aching in the shafts of the long
bones) • Juniperus • Larrea (bath; pain, swelling, redness)
• Lavender (external) • Leonurus (stiff, cold joints; osteoporosis)
• Lycopodium • Medicago sativa • Menispermum canadense
(chronic arthritis with lymphatic swelling and weak digestion)
• MENYANTHES (rheumatoid arthritis and osteoporosis;
with liver, digestive disorder) • Oplopanax • PARIETARIA
• Petroselinum • Phaseolus • Phytolacca (apathetic, with lazy
habits; external, or small doses) • Pinus • POLYGONATUM
(pain relief in all kinds of arthritis, lack of lubrication) • Populus
• Prunus serotina • Prunus spinosa • Pulsatilla (shoulder joints)
• Rosmarinus (external) • Ruscus • Salix (external) • Sassafras (tonic, preventive; warms the joints, increases circulation to
extremities; external) • Senecio • Smilacina • Smilax • Stellaria
• Symphytum (arthritis, swelling) • Tanacetum parthenium
(swelling, tenderness; thins blood) • Taraxacum • Thuja • Thymus (chronic; warming) • Tsuga canadensis (especially for lower
back; oil, external) • URTICA (arthritis) • Verbascum (lubricating; bath) • WITHANIA • YUCCA (breaks up mineral deposits
in inflamed tissues) • Zanthoxylum (in weak-nerved older people
with painful joints; adjuvant to stimulate nerves and capillaries)
• ZINGIBERIS (muscular cramp and pain with arthritis).

Joints (Inflammation, Synovitis): • AESCLEPIAS TUBEROSA
(swollen, inflamed, hot; old adhesions) • BRYONIA (homeopathic; acute) • CENTELLA (acts on cellular matrix and
connective tissue) • CURCUMA (inflammation from tissue
depression) • Hypericum • Smilax.

Joints (Injured, Frozen): • Agrimonia (pinched tissues, dislocations) • Ajuga (dislocations) • Angelica (hot compress on
painful joint) • Asclepias tuberosa (dried-out synovial fluids;
adhesions; frozen) • Cinchona (relaxed ligaments; aching
pain after movement) • DIPSACUS (pulled, torn, wrenched,
incapacitated) • Equisetum (cartilage damage) • Eupatorium

purpureum (dried-out muscles and tendons around joint; frozen) • Hydrastis (torn bursa, meniscus, disc) • Hypericum (shoulder) • Hyssopus (oil, rubbed into dry, painful joints) • Lycopodium (compress) • Menispermum (chronic arthritis with lymphatic congestion and weak digestion) • POLYGONATUM (tendons tight or loose) • Smilacina • Symphytum • Tsuga canadensis (oil, external) • Urtica • Zanthoxylum (painful).

Joints (Rheumatoid Arthritis): • Agrimonia • APIUM (with mental depression, debility) • Boswellia • Caulophyllum • Centella • Chelone • CIMICIFUGA • Citrus limonum (excessively red, inflamed surfaces; elongated red tongue) • DIOSCOREA • Dipsacus (with Smilacina) • Echinacea (acute phase) • Equisetum • Fucus • Ganoderma lucidum • Gaultheria • Glycyrrhiza • GUAIACUM ("gouty nodes on fingers and knees, etc."—Bartram) • HARPAGOPHYTUM (specific; small doses relieve pain; large doses cause inflammation and reduce deposits) • Menyanthes • Piper Methysticum • POPULUS • Salix • SENECIO JACOBAEA (lotion) • Scrophularia • SMILACINA • Smilax • Symphytum (external) • Tabebuia • Tanacetum parthenium • Taraxacum • Teucrium • Withania • YUCCA.

Hands, Wrists, Fingers: • Arctium (DuPuytren's contracture; leaf) • Boswellia (DuPuytren's) • Caulophyllum (arthritic fingers) • Cimicifuga (cramps in wrists from gardening; external) • Crataegus (dryness, back of wrists) • Cimicifuga (wrist, joints swollen, inflamed, red) • GALIUM (almost a specific for DuPuytren's and Morton's neuroma) • GUAIACUM (DuPuytren's; shrunken tendons of hands) • Ledum (wrists, ankles) • MELISSA (sweaty palms) • *Polygonum hydropiperoides, P. punctatum* (arthritis) • Senecio aureus (chapped hands; cream) • Smilacina (rheumatoid fingers; combines well with Dipsacus) • Thuja (chapped) • THYMUS (for some reason, specific for when the fingers are dry).

Palms (plump parts) Red: • CRATAEGUS • PRUNUS SERO-
TINA (red and yellow) • ROSA (mottling with carmine- and
dark-red).

*Note: Redness of the plump parts of the palms indicates slowing-down of eryth-
rocytes as they pass through the capillaries. This is due to inflammation of
the capillaries (with or without cholesterol deposition), low or high blood pressure, or inflammatory processes. With mottling of dark-red and carmine-red,
it indicates heat burning into the tissues, which needs to be stopped to prevent
chronic illness.*

Raynaud's Phenomenon (White and Cold Fingers): • Achillea
• Artemisia vulgaris • CARTHAMUS (a true specific; oil,
external; tincture, internal) • HELICHRYSUM (oil, external)
• Hypericum (external) • Melilotus • Oplopanax (needs confirmation) • Zanthoxylum.

Repetitive-use Injury: • Hypericum • POLYGONATUM (external) • RHUS TOX. (homeopathic) • RUTA (swollen, very
painful, complicated) • SYMPHYTUM (external)
• VERBENA.

Nails: • Althaea • Arnica (infection; tincture externally) • Avena
(ingrown) • Calendula • EQUISETUM (fungus under nail;
hangnails; weak nails) • Juglans nigra (suppurating infection;
leaf tea externally).

*Note: Henna on the nails will slowly kill fungus and strengthen the nails. This
"beauty tip" is well-known in India and was passed on to Jim MacDonald at
a Hindu wedding. Frank Parton (1931) gives general directions: "Look to the
general health; take at least a pint of milk daily; soak the nails in almond oil
nightly."*

Hip Joints: • Allium cepa (rheumatism) • Cannabis (palliative in
hip-joint disease) • Cimicifuga (dull pain; sciatica) • Dioscorea

(hip-joint disease) • Helianthemum (hip-joint disease) • Hypericum (sciatica) • Polygonatum (ligamentous tension) • Melilotus (sciatica) • Pulsatilla (pain in hip joint) • Smilacina (ligamentous tension).

Legs: • Aesculus hip. (phlebitis) • Mahonia (night pains in shin-bones) • Melilotus (rheumatic and neuralgic lameness) • Mentha piperita (flower essence; directs to lower limbs) • Nymphaea (sores) • Paeonia (shaky leg) • Plantago (ulceration) • Pulsatilla (phlebitis) • Rosmarinus (essential oil, in olive oil—rub on calf spasm) • Ruta (shin splints; acute, chronic) • Solidago (skin irritation) • Stellaria (ulceration; ointment) • TARAXACUM (flower, in oil). Also see "Restless Leg Syndrome," above.

Knees: • Althaea • Chamomilla • Chelidonium (right knee pain, drawing of muscles up to liver) • Cinchona (relaxed ligaments, with ache) • Helianthemum (swollen) • Nymphaea (weakness) • Polygonatum • Sambucus • Symphytum.

Ankles and Feet: • Acorus (tired feet; apply locally) • Althaea (swollen; footbath) • Arctium (tired, sore, painful hips, legs, feet) • Avena (tired feet; oatstraw bath) • Cinchona (ankle ligaments relaxed, achy from use) • Equisetum (sweaty; fallen arches; footbath) • Guaiacum (foot pain) • Juglans nigra (sweaty; leaf) • Juniperus (edemic pitting of ankles) • Larrea (foot pain) • Ledum (ankle joints swollen, soles of feet worse from warmth of bed) • Lycopodium (cramps in feet; homeopathic or herb) • Medicago (foot pain) • Petasites (on sore, chafed feet; leaf dressing) • Plantago (sore) • Polygonatum (bone spurs from unequal tensions on ligaments) • Polygonum hydropiperoides (to tone and relieve arthritis; footbath) • Rosmarinus (dark rings around ankles in the elderly; bad circulation to the head; "low blood") • Rumex crispus (sore feet) • Smilacina (arthritis) • Solidago (tired feet and kidneys) • SYMPHYTUM (footbath with bath salts) • Thuja (ingrown toenail) • Thymus (foot pain) • Tussilago (tired, swollen feet) • WITHANIA • Zanthoxylum (foot pain) • Zingiberis (chilled, cold, tight; decoction of the rhizome as a footbath).

Spinal Injury: • ACHILLEA (to prevent pressure of congealed blood on nerves, administer as soon as possible after a serious head or spine injury) • Aesculus hip. (swollen disks) • Agrimonia (pinched tissues) • Artemisia vulgaris (moxibustion) • ASARUM CANADENSE (old and very old injuries; stiff, sore, cold; external) • CIMICIFUGA (accumulation of cerebrospinal fluid; whiplash with tightness in trapezius; painful lower back, thighs, loins) • Dipsacus (torn, wrenched, pulled muscles) • Equisetum • Eupatorium perfoliatum (compression fracture) • Hydrangea (postpartum) • HYDRASTIS (herniated or ruptured discs) • HYPERICUM (nerve pain and inflammation, shooting pain, coccygeal pain; pain from torn disc) • Lobelia (whiplash with torsional spasm) • Petasites (inflamed, herniated, ruptured discs) • SOLIDAGO (bruised, tired; external, internal) • Verbascum (helps set spine straight) • Verbena (tension in nape of neck) • Zanthoxylum (writhing in agony from pain of torn disc).

Spine (Spasm): • Aesculus glabra (contraction, rigidity) • Aesculus hip. (lower back, sacrum, and sacroiliac pain; stiff, weak back that "gives out"; heaviness, swelling) • Agrimonia (pinched tissues; lumbar) • Angelica sinensis (back, pelvis, menstrual cramp) • Artemisia vulgaris (moxibustion) • Bupleurum • Cannabis (pain "between the shoulders"—Jones) • CIMICIFUGA (accumulation of cerebrospinal fluid; whiplash with tightness in trapezius; painful lower back, thighs, loins) • Cinnamomum (lower back pain, cold) • Dioscorea • HYPERICUM (nerve pain and inflammation, shooting pain, coccygeal pain) • Lactuca (lower back tight; cold constitution) • Lobelia (torsional spasm)• Piper methysticum • Piscidia (sedative, anodyne, antispasmodic; often palliative, not curative, but valuable for the pain) • Polygonatum (adjusts tensions on vertebrae; TMJ [temporomandibular joint syndrome]) • Sambucus (back pain, colic) • TSUGA (oil, on lower back) • VALERIAN (see Viburnum) • VERBENA (tension in nape of neck; TMJ) • VIBURNUM OPULUS (spasms, neuralgia, lower back, neck, pelvis, digestion, legs; back pain during menses) • Zingiberis (for spasm; fresh).

Spine (Dryness, Atrophy, Malnutrition): • Agrimonia • Aletris (uterine prolapse) • Althaea (dried-out) • APIUM (lumbago, debility) • ARCTIUM (lower back pain, worry, weakness, atrophy of tendons and ligaments) • Artemisia vulgaris (moxibustion) • Boswellia • CALCIUM PHOSPHATE (homeopathic; osteoporosis) • Castanea (compress) • CIMICIFUGA (bunching up of cerebrospinal fluid; of postmenopausal and reproductive origin) • Dioscorea (hip-joint deterioration) • Equisetum • Hydrangea • Hypericum (drying, but useful for nerve pain) • OSMUNDA (specific for lumbago, rickets; osteoporosis) • Parietaria • POLYGONATUM (adjusts tensions on vertebrae; TMJ [temporomandibular joint syndrome]; adjuvant) • Rosmarinus (external) • VERBASCUM (helps straighten spine).

Spine (Reproductive): • Aletris (uterine prolapse) • Angelica sinensis (back, pelvis, menstrual cramp, spasm) • Arctium • Artemisia vulgaris (infertility with cold, stiff, sore lower back; external, as moxibustion) • Caulophyllum (congested uterus and back muscles) • CIMICIFUGA (accumulation of cerebrospinal fluid; tightness in trapezius; painful lower back, thighs, loins) • Dioscorea (perimenopausal hip-joint deterioration) • Dipsacus • Hydrangea (postpartum) • Lactuca (tight lower back; cold constitution; infertility) • Smilacina (with Dipsacus, for pelvic instability; postpartum) • Symphytum (lumbar-sacral instability) • Valerian (see Viburnum) • Verbena (menopause) • VIBURNUM OPULUS (spasms, neuralgia in lower back, neck, pelvis, legs; digestion; back pain during menses).

Spine (Related to Kidney and Urinary-Tract Problems): • Agrimonia (lumbar) • Agropyron • Althaea (dried-out) • APIUM (lumbago) • Berberis (lumbago related to kidney congestion; weakness, weak muscles) • Chimaphila (urinary-tract origin) • Cucumis sativus (low back pain, turbid urine, irritable tract, sharp pain in loins) • Equisetum (needs confirmation) • Hydrangea • Hypericum • Juniperus • Parietaria • Piper methysticum • Rosmarinus (external) • Salix alba ("ankylosing spondylitis"—BHP) • Sambucus (back pain and colic) • Smilacina (with Dipsacus, for pelvic instability) • SOLIDAGO (cold kidneys; external) • TSUGA (cold kidneys; oil, on lower back;).

Spine (Aging and Deterioration): • Aesculus glabra (contraction, rigidity) • Aesculus hip. (low back, sacrum, and sacroiliac pain; stiff, weak back that "gives out;" heaviness, swelling) • Agrimonia (pinched tissues; lumbar region) • APIUM (lumbago) • ASARUM CANADENSE (cold; old injury, aging; external) • BOSWELLIA (stiffness, pain, inflammation, acute; improves circulation joints, sinews; *cf. Tsuga;* 2–4 weeks optimum use, even if acute) • CALCIUM PHOSPHATE (homeopathic; osteoporosis) • CIMICIFUGA (postmenopausal) • Cinnamomum (low back pain, cold) • DIOSCOREA (hip-joint deterioration) • Equisetum • Harpagophytum (pain, inflammation; rapid results or none at all) • HYPERICUM (nerve pain and inflammation, shooting pain, coccygeal pain) • Lactuca (tight lower back, cold constitution) • Leonurus (rounded spine, osteoporosis) • OSMUNDA (specific for lumbago; possible for osteoporosis) • POLYGONATUM (adjusts tensions on vertebrae; TMJ [temporomandibular joint syndrome]) • Rhodiola • Rosmarinus (external) • Salix alba ("ankylosing spondylitis"—BHP; probably just palliative) • Smilacina (with Dipsacus, for pelvic instability) • Symphytum (lumbar-sacral instability) • TSUGA (on lower back; oil) • VEBASCUM (dry, aging spine) • Zingiberis (pain; dried).

Spine (Cold): • Aesculus hip. • Angelica sinensis • ASARUM CANADENSE (cold, sore, old injuries, aging; external) • ARTEMISIA VULGARIS (moxibustion) • BOSWELLIA (stiffness, pain, inflammation, acute; improves circulation of joints, sinews; *cf. Tsuga;* 2–4 weeks' use is optimum even if acute) • Chimaphila (urinary-tract origin) • Cinnamomum (lower back pain) • Juniperus (urinary-tract origin) • LACTUCA (tight lower back; slow, hard pulse) • Rosmarinus (external) • SOLIDAGO (external) • TSUGA (on lower back; oil) • Zingiberis (pain; dried).

Spine (Lumbar): • Aesculus hip. (low back, sacrum, and sacroiliac pain; stiff, weak back that "gives out"; heaviness, swelling; with hemorrhoids) • Agrimonia • Agropyron (urinary-tract origin) • Aletris (uterine prolapse) • APIUM (lumbago) • ARCTIUM (lower back pain, worry; weakness, atrophy of tendons and ligaments) • Arnica (external) • Artemisia vulgaris • Asarum canadense (external) • Berberis (lumbago related to kidney congestion, weakness; weak muscles) • Boswellia • Castanea • Chimaphila (urinary-tract origin) • Cimicifuga (tightness in trapezius; lower back) • Cinnamomum (lower back pain, cold) • Dioscorea (hip-joint deterioration) • Dipsacus (torn, wrenched, pulled muscles) • Filipendula • Hedeoma • Hydrangea (postpartum) • HUMULUS (external) • Hypericum • Juniperus (urinary-tract origin) • Lactuca (tight lower back, cold constitution) • OSMUNDA (the great specific for lumbago) • Phytolacca • Smilacina (with Dipsacus, for pelvic instability) • Symphytum (lumbar-sacral instability) • TARAXACUM (flowers, in oil; "takes the aging out of the lower back"—Anonymous) • TSUGA (on lower back; oil) • Urtica • Valerian • VIBURNUM OPULUS (neuralgia; back, lower back, neck, pelvis, leg, menstrual spasm).

Spine (Intervertebral Discs): • Achillea (injury) • Agrimonia (pinched tissues) • Aesculus hip. (swelling) • Equisetum (needs confirmation) • HYDRASTIS (herniated or ruptured disc) • HYPERICUM (nerve pain and inflammation, shooting pain, coccygeal pain, pain from torn disc) • Petasites (inflamed, herniated, ruptured disc) • Verbascum (adjuvant; moistening to spine) • Zanthoxylum (writhing in agony from pain of torn disc).

Sacral and Coccygeal Pain: • Aesculus hip. ("aching worse by walking or standing, with constipation and blind [internal] piles; sacroiliac articulation"—Clarke) • Aloe (drawing and heaviness, worse in the evening, "with bleeding piles and diarrhea"— Clarke) • Berberis ("violent pain in, aching, bruised, dragging, or pressing; worse from lying, sitting, or stooping; with rectal troubles"—Clarke) • Collinsonia (pelvic pain from hemorrhoids; cf. Aesculus) • Fouquieria (tension in the pelvis, sacrum) • HYPERICUM (injury to coccyx).

Neck and Shoulders: • BUPLEURUM (tender, achy neck, shoulders, chest; tension; pulse wiry and thin; medium to thin, yellow constitution—Huang) • CHELIDONIUM (pain below occiput, sometimes down to shoulder blade, up to temporal region) • CIMICIFUGA (pain, stiffness; whiplash) • Glechoma • Lactuca (tension down sides of neck to shoulders, to chest) • Symphytum (stiffness) • TARAXACUM (SCM [sternocleidomastoid] muscle swollen, sore, reddish) • VERBENA HASTATA (tension down back of neck; stiff, atrophied, weak).

Bell's Palsy (Hemiplegia): • Asarum canadense (external) • Cimicifuga • Heracleum • Hypericum • Zanthoxylum.

Sciatica: • Arnica (better from warmth; external) • Cimicifuga • Filipendula • Gaultheria • Hypericum • Melilotus • Thymus serpyllum (oil) • Zanthoxylum.

Broken Bones: See "Injuries, First Aid."

Disc (Intervertebral Pain): • Aesculus (swelling) • EQUISE-
TUM • HYDRASTIS (herniated, ruptured, weak; deterioration; external) • HYPERICUM (pain of pinched nerves;
external) • Paeonia • Petasites (herniated, ruptured)
• Symphytum.

*Note: In order to repair herniated, worn-down, or ruptured discs, it is necessary
to reduce the inflammation so that tissue healing can take place.*

Infection in Bones: • Capsicum (mastoid) • QUERCUS (recalci-
fication afterward) • TARAXACUM (marrow, bones, mastoid;
recalcifies).

Sciatica: • Achillea • Amanita muscaria (specific from Finland)
• Arctostaphylos • Berberis • CIMICIFUGA • Gnaphalium
• Helichrysum (essential oil—analog to Gnaphalium)
• HYDRASTIS (for slipped disc) • HYPERICUM • Lobelia
• Menyanthes • Thymus • Valeriana • ZANTHOXYLUM.

Temporomandibular Joint Syndrome (TMJ): • Hypericum
• Polygonatum • Verbascum (root) • VERBENA.

Paralysis: • Avena • Collinsonia (infantile) • Eupatorium purpureum (impaired circulation) • Heracleum • Zanthoxylum (nerve
damage).

Bone, Congenital Weakness: • Centella • Cetraria • Equisetum
• Gnaphalium • Urtica.

Bone Spurs: • Polygonatum • Smilacina.

Bone Inflammation, Decay: • Helianthemum (decay) • Taraxacum (inflammation).

Corns (often caused by muscular and skeletal imbalance):
• Carica papaya (external) • Chelidonium (juice) • Symphytum (root; ointment) • Urtica (leaf and root; footbath, tea).

Osteoporosis: • CALCIUM PHOSPHATE (homeopathic, or supplement, or bone broth) • EQUISETUM • Eupatorium perfoliatum • Medicago • Osmunda • Quercus (confirmation needed) • Ulmus • Urtica.

Gout (Uric Acid Build-up): • Acorus (cold infusion; small dose) • APIUM (languid, debilitated) • Arctium (root; hyperuricemia) • ARNICA (very tender) • Asparagus • Barosma • Bidens • Calluna • Capsella (hyperuricema) • Chamomilla • Cimicifuga (with chronic muscular pain) • Daucus (hyperuricema) • Eupatorium purpureum • Filipendula (tea) • Ganoderma (footbath) • Guaiacum • Harpagophytum (hyperuricema) • Hypericum • Juniperus (chronic) • LARIX LARICINA (tamarack) • Ledum • Lilium longiflorum (inflames and removes; external) • Lycopodium • Mentha pulegium • Petasites (root; tea) • Plantago • Populus gileadensis (ointment) • Primula veris (tea) • PRUNUS (poor circulation to the periphery; irregular pulse) • Salix • Sassafras • Symphytum (bath) • Taraxacum (hyperuricemia; stems, eaten; roots, decocted) • Teucrium • Tribulus (hyperuricemia) • Trigonella • Tsuga canadensis (oil, external) • Veronica (internal, external) • URTICA (poor removal of uric acid by the kidneys) • Cercospora zeae-maydis.

Fatigue of Muscles from Exertion: • Arnica (prophylactically, gives excellent results) • Carthamus (soreness after exercise, in hypoglycemic and others) • Echinacea (exhaustion from overwork; with boils, carbuncles and abscesses) • Eleutherococcus (with nervousness) • HYDRASTIS (weakness of nerves and muscles in general, heart in particular) • Nepeta.

Note: Lactic acid as a food supplement can help remove lactic acid build-up in the muscles.

Dystonia: • SALVIA • Withania (needs confirmation).

FORMULARY

Apium—with Menyathes and/or Guaiacum (myalgia). BHP 1983, 29.

Apium—"therapeutic action appears to be potentiated by Taraxacum"—BHP 1983, 29.

Cimicifuga—with Apium (arthritis). BHP 1983, 66.

Cimicifuga—with Apium, Menyanthes, Filipendula, Castanea (myalgia, fibrositis). BHP 1983, 53, 144.

Cimicifuga—with a small amount of Lobelia (whiplash with torsion).

Cimicifuga—with Menyanthes and Populus (rheumatoid arthritis). BHP 1983, 169.

Cimicifuga—with Phytolacca, Zanthoxylum (myalgia, arthritis).

Cimicifuga—with Piper methysticum and Withania (fibromyalgia).

Cimicifuga—with Viburnum spp. and Dioscorea (rheumatoid arthritis). BHP 1983, 79.

Cinchona—incompatible with salicylates. BHP 1983, 67.

Eupatorium perfoliatum—with Leonurus, and a small amount of Lobelia (osteoporosis).

Gaultheria—with Fucus, Senecio jacobaea, "in a paraffin base for application as a plaster to affected joints in rheumatoid arthritis"—BHP 1983, 95.

Guaiacum—with Cimicifuga, Apium, Salix alba (rheumatoid arthritis). BHP 1983, 185.

Guaiacum—with Phytolacca, Zanthoxylum (muscular/skeletal). BHP 1983, 157.

Guaiacum—with Zingiberis, Menyanthes, Filipendula, Apium (arthritis, myalgia), varied by indications. BHP 1983, 108.

Lavandula oil—with Gaultheria oil, topically (myalgia). BHP 1983, 129.

Lycopodium—with Menyanthes and Rumex crispus (gout). "Ground pine … as an ointment melted with lard, buck-bean, and water-dock of any kind"—Samuel Westcott Tilke (1844, 333). We so seldom find an herbal formula for Lycopodium that I decided to include this one.

Polygonatum—with Chickweed in salve (connective tissue, tendons).

Populus—with Cimicifuga and Menyanthes (rheumatoid arthritis). BHP 1983, 169.

Rosmarinus—"Both the flower and leaves of this plant … made into oils or ointments, it will recover cold or benumbed joints and sinews"—Samuel Westcott Tilke (1844, 321).

Tsuga—salve, with Arnica or Solidago, and Artemisia vulgaris, in oil (warms the kidneys and lumbar region).

Zingiberis (fresh rhizome)—the great liniment for spastic muscles.

Zingiberis—with Echinacea, Phytolacca (rheumatic bone pain).

Skin

The cutaneous surface is very important for both diagnosis and health. Before the immune system is engaged, the surface adjusts for environmental stresses. Cold closes the pores and raises gooseflesh and hairs on end to keep in warmth (air is trapped and warmed by the raised hairs). Damp cold releases oily sweat, which protects us like the oil-infused wool clothing of fisherman and sailors. Our sweat pores open to cool the surface with perspiration. Arterioles clamp up to retain the warm blood in the surface when we are chilled and open to release it when we are overheated. That is why lighter-skinned people are usually pale or pink according to the weather. Ambient temperature change is the most common stressor for the living organism, except for our own thoughts and feelings. And actually, our deepest emotions use the same pathways to express themselves—sweating, blushing, turning pale, hair standing on end, etc. Therefore, the skin shows the dragon tracks of trauma, *both physical and psychological.* For this reason, doctors and grannies in traditional medicine always looked to the condition of the skin and treated that condition. This is true in Western, Ayurvedic, Chinese, and American Indian medicine. For further discussion of these principles see the discussion of *agni* under fever.

"Remedies act on the skin: (1) generally, through nerves, blood and lymph; (2) specifically, on structures of the skin; (3) indirectly, on the kidneys, stomach, bowels, and liver" (George M. Dash, *The Eclectic Gleaner* 4:35 [1908]); and to this must be added: (4) through the extracellular matrix (ECM), which supports, waters, and feeds the skin.

This section is divided into two parts: "Appearance," where the symptoms are useful for evaluation as well as treatment of conditions; and "Conditions," where we are looking to treat a specific problem. The latter can also be used for evaluation. For instance, identifying the different kinds of acne can point to remedies for constitutional treatment of the whole system.

Appearance (Diagnostic Indications)

General Appearance of Skin: • Achillea (red and blue) • Ajuga (for glossy sheen of health) • Althaea officinalis (very dry, hardened, inflamed, or pale) • Angelica (blue, green, grey, yellow) • Apocynum cannabinum (blanched, smooth, pitting, swollen) • Arnica (red and blue) • Asclepias tuberosa (dry and hot) • Calendula (chafed or abraded; swollen, tender, red) • Carthamus (red and blue) • CENTELLA (indolent, slow-healing wounds and cutaneous conditions; skin "red, hot, and inflamed"—D. Winston) • Ceanothus (doughy and sallow, expressionless) • Celastrus (chafy skin) • Chelidonium (sallow, greenish, with hepatic congestion) • Chionanthus (sallow, dirty-looking, with hepatic tenderness and expressionless eyes) • Echinacea (dirty) • Oenothera (dirty, sallow, full, and expressionless skin and tongue, with dyspepsia, vomiting of food, frequent desire to urinate) • Salvia sclarea (wrinkled, dehydrated) • Salvia (wrinkled, dehydrated; soft and relaxed; extremities cold, circulation weak) • Sambucus (red and dry skin, or blue and pale, moist) • Sassafras (blue and black, sooty appearance; cutaneous eruptions; head lice; external) • Veronicastrum (yellow, with pain in liver region).

Palms, Red: • CRATAEGUS (plump parts of palms red; slow capillary reflux; high or low blood pressure) • PRUNUS SEROTINA (plump parts red, the rest yellow) • ROSA (plump parts mottled carmine-red and deep-red, revealing penetration of heat into the tissues).

Note: This is a very useful indication, showing congestion in the capillaries, or poor peripheral circulation; associated with irritation of the capillaries, high or low blood pressure, and the heat/excitation tissue state.

Palms, Sweaty: • Calendula • Crataegus • Lavendula • MELISSA • Rosmarinus • Salvia • Taraxacum • Viola (if dry elsewhere).

Note: Sweaty palms are usually a symptom of sympathetic excess, or nervousness. Most of the above remedies are from my own practice picked up in discussions with Francis Bonaldo Begnoche and from Lise Wolff.

Ankles, Dark, in the Elderly ("Low Blood"): • Acorus • Capsicum • ROSMARINUS • Sambucus.

Note: See "Low Blood" in "Blood" section.

Conditions

Abscesses, Boils, Carbuncles: • Achillea (external) • Allium sativa (external) • Alnus (recurrent) • Althaea (poultice) • Anemopsis (external) • Amygdalus (leaf poultice) • ARCTIUM (external) • Aristolochia (small or homeopathic dose, or external) • Artemisia vulgaris (for skin and hair—Native American; wash with leaves)

• Astragalus (strengthens periphery) • Baptisia (indolent conditions; antiseptic ointment) • Calendula (lessens scar tissue; external) • Chamomilla (very tender) • Chelone • Commiphora myrrha • Crataegus • ECHINACEA (tendency to produce boils; skin looks dirty; external, internal) • Equisetum (external) • Trigonella (oil poultice) • Galium • Glechoma • Heracleum (external) • Humulus (hops poultice) • Iris (external) • Linum (fresh-ground seed poultice) • Phytolacca (after fevers; external) • PLANTAGO (abscess of tooth or skin; external) • Propolis (external) • Prunella (external) • Rumex crispus • Sambucus (external) • Stellaria (external) • Symphytum (external) • Thuja • Trifolium (internal) • Trigonella (external) • Ulmus (non-open; external) • Zingiberis.

Acne: • Achillea (sebaceous cysts; red, irritated acne; lukewarm tea or facial ointment) • Allium ursinum • ARALIA NUDICAULIS (androgen normalizer) • ARCTIUM (big, single pimples) • Baptisia (chronic) • Berberis • BETULA (inner birch bark compress) • CALENDULA (sebaceous cysts) • CENTELLA (scar tissue) • Chelidonium • Cichorium (tea) • Citrus limonum (juice, in mask with vitamin E and mayonnaise) • Daucus (domesticated carrot poultice) • Echinacea (associated with boils; with GI imbalance) • Eleutherococcus • Fragaria • Galium (blackheads; juice) • Guaiacum • Humulus (androgen excess) • Iris • Juglans (leaf; tea) • LACTUCA (androgen normalizer; chronic, pitting, scarring; juvenile acne) • LILIUM LONGIFLORUM (androgen normalizer; cyst-like acne; zygomatic arch) • Juglans nigra (back, neck, buttocks) • Mahonia (skin dry, rough) • Mentha piperita (hot packs alternated with cold packs) • PAEONIA OFFICINALIS (androgen normalizer; sore-like pimples on chin near outer lip crease, related to ovulation or PMS) • Panax quinquefolius • Phytolacca • Rumex crispus (back, neck, buttocks) • Sambucus (opens pores on cheeks) • Scrophularia (acne red and bluish) • SMILAX (androgen normalizer) • SOLIDAGO (sheets of small pimples on checks) • Taraxacum (root tea) • Thuja (external) • Urtica (tea) • Vitex (male and female).

Note: Acne is frequently due to androgens stressing the liver, and therefore is more common during puberty or menopause, under stress, or at different times in the female cycle.

Acne Rosacea: ("This is a tough disease and takes a longer period to cure"—Bhattacharya) • Achillea (Susun Weed) • Crataegus • Malus (feels unclean; bark or flower essence) • Rosa.

Note: Coconut oil is a good medium for external application.

Age Spots (Senile Keratosis): • Calendula (external) • Galium (external) • Rosa mosqueta (seed oil) • Thuja (external).

Allergies (Skin Rash, Hives, Heat Rash): • Althaea (external) • Apis (homeopathic) • Chamomilla (wash) • Equisetum (wash) • Juglans nigra (leaf wash) • Lamium (tea) • Plantago • Stellaria (external) • Taraxacum (stems, internal) • Tribulus • Urtica (tea, external) • Veronica.

Athlete's Foot: • Calendula (external) • Symphytum (leaf; external).

Birthmarks: • Calendula (external) • Galium (external) • Thuja (external).

Blisters on the Feet: • Calendula • Plantain.

Bruises: See "Injuries, First Aid" or "Face and Complexion."

Burns: See "Injuries, First Aid."

Cellulite: • Aesculus hip. • Fucus • Glechoma • Lycopodium (spore powder, externally, absorbs water out of skin) • Petroselinum.

Chilblains (unbroken): See "Injuries, First Aid."

Cradle Cap *(crusta lactea):* • Arctium • CHAMOMILLA (tea) • Iris (external) • Juglans nigra (leaf wash) • Quercus (oak bark wash) • Viola tricolor.

Dandruff: • ARCTIUM (external) • Arnica (external) • Rosmarinus (in water; hair rinse) • Valeriana (external).

Decubitus Ulcers (Bedsores): • Calendula • Commiphora myrrha • Echinacea • Quercus • Thuja.

Diaper Rash: • Calendula (do not use Symphytum, as it can seal the vaginal lips of very young baby girls).

Dry, Scaly: • Achillea (dry; incomplete, oily sweat) • Alnus rubra • Arctium • BORAGO • Crataegus (dry on backs of wrists) • Hypericum • Hyssopus • Iris (dry, thick, rough; rash, ulcerative) • MAHONIA • Pilocarpus jaborandi • Rosmarinus (dry cheeks) • Salvia ("lichenification," fine, dry wrinkling, usually in menopause) • Sambucus (red and dry) • Solidago (dry, scaly; red spots) • Trigonella.

Erysipelas: • Echinacea (external—Bergner) • Centella (needs confirmation) • Galium • Passiflora • Rhus tox. (homeopathic) • Sambucus (infusion of leaves; with Galium) • Veratrum viride (homeopathic).

Exudative Skin Eruptions: • Juglans cinerea • Juglans nigra • Quercus (skin cracking open) • Rumex (yellow serum discharges) • Stillingia (irritation, lymphatic involvement)

• VIOLA TRICOLOR ("eczema and skin eruptions with serous exudate, particularly when associated with rheumatic symptoms"—BHP).

Flesh-Eating Infection: • Aristolochia serpentaria (low-grade, septic fever; small or homeopathic dose) • Plantago (will digest corrupt flesh and "incarnate" new flesh—Gerard).

Formication: • Mentha pulegium.

Oily: • AJUGA (regulates sebum production; for glossy sheen of health) • Allium sativa • ARCTIUM (excess or deficient of oily sweat) • Helianthus (seed) • Hydrastis • Iris versicolor • Stillingia.

Note: excessive oil on the skin gives a "tacky" sensation, while excessive watery perspiration gives a moist, cool, or clammy sensation.

Cool, Clammy, Moist (Excessive, Spontaneous Perspiration): • ASTRAGALUS (this is not an astringent but a slightly warming nutritive for the periphery; spontaneous perspiration from weakness of the periphery; poor muscular tone) • CINNAMOMUM CASSIA (warming astringent; skin fair, firm, moist, easily sweats) • Citrus limonum (fresh juice in water) • Lavandula • Ledum (needs confirmation) • MELISSA (nervousness; damp palms) • MONARDA FISTULOSA (sympathetic excess; cool, clammy sweat over whole body) • Rhus spp. (profuse fluid loss from skin, kidneys, colon, lungs, menses) • Rosmarinus • Salvia • Senecio aureus • Taraxacum.

Eczema: • ALNUS RUBRA (pustular) • ALNUS SERRALATA • Ampelopsis (vesicular rash like poison ivy) • Angelica (with chronic poor fat digestion, dry, pale skin) • ARCTIUM (dry, red skin near joints; stubborn; seeds or roots; for long-term use) • Aristolochia (dry, hot skin; tissue depression) • Asclepias

tuberosa (obstinate) • BETULA (birch; compress of the inner
bark) • Chamomilla (bath) • Echinacea (sticky exudate, from
dirty system) • Fouquieria • Fumaria (chronic) • Galium
• Grindelia (itching rash like poison ivy; external) • Hydrastis
(eczema of external auditory canal) • Iris (chronic itch; psoriasis) • Juglans nigra (with constipation, flatulence) • Larix
• Larrea (chronic dry skin) • MAHONIA (dry; combines well
with Arctium) • Oplopanax (specific for eczema after emotional
crisis, drama) • Phytolacca (scaly; fissures, corners of mouth)
• Rumex crispus (dry, irritable, rusty patches turning to running
eczema) • Quercus (running eczema; external) • Sambucus
(dry, red skin over meaty areas) • Scrophularia (chronic)
• Smilax (eczema and psoriasis) • Solidago (scalp, lower
extremities) • STELLARIA (causes and cures itching of
eczema; external) • Stillingia • Thymus serpyllum (exudative)
• TRIFOLIUM • Veronica officinalis • VIOLA TRICOLOR
(exudative).

*Note: Echinacea "is of great service in skin diseases, locally as well as inter-
nally. It seems to act in any form of eczematous conditions, but especially in
the moist forms, with glutinous exudation associated with asthenic condition
of the system" (Massinger).*

Eruptive Fever, Exanthema: • Agrimony (erysipelas) • Arctium
• Asclepias tuberosa • ATROPA BELLADONNA (homeopathic; scarlet fever) • Calendula (measles; tea) • CAR-
THAMUS (low, septic fever with rash) • CHAMOMILLA
(external) • Cimicifuga (chickenpox; to bring out the rash)
• CROCUS SATIVA (formerly the main remedy for exanthema) • DROSERA (measles) • ECHINACEA (erysipelas;
scarlet fever; putrefaction; prevents side effects of putridity)
• Eupatorium perfoliatum (chickenpox) • GALIUM (measles)
• Inula (warm decoction) • Iris versicolor (chronic eruptive
and ulcerative conditions, lupus, tuberculosis) • Juglans nigra
(impetigo; hull) • Juglans nigra (pus-filled eruptions, stubborn

rashes; leaf) • Lithospermum (brings out the rash) • Lycopus
(scarlet fever) • Malus (feels unclean; flower essence) • Nepeta
(brings out rash) • Phytolacca (putrefaction) • Plantago
• Platanus (scarlet fever, with slow, tardy, or receding eruptions; heartwood for fever; twigs and bark for measles) • Potentilla • Pulsatilla (chickenpox) • Rhodiola • Sambucus (toxic
heat) • Sassafras (slow, tardy, receded eruptions) • Scutellaria
(chickenpox) • Taraxacum • Teucrium • Trifolium (measles)
• Viola tricolor (in children) • Zanthoxylum (capillary engorgement) • Zingiberis.

Fissures: • Alchemilla (rectal; external) • Anemopsis (rectal; sitz
bath) • Borago • Calendula (external) • Coptis (rectal; sitz
bath—only if not infected) • Hydrastis (*cf.* Coptis) • Hypericum
(pain) • Phytolacca (corners of mouth, vagina) • Symphytum
(external).

Freckles: • Calendula (external) • Citrus limonum (juice)
• Galium (external) • Thuja (external) • Urtica (tea).

Frostbite: See "Injuries, First Aid."

Ganglions (External): • Galium (ganglions, lipomas) • RUTA
(ganglions).

Hair, Unwanted: • Calendula (external) • Equisetum (sitz bath)
• Hypericum (oil) • Primula (juice) • Urtica.

*Note: Also recommended are medications that reduce androgens, or help the
liver break them down.*

Herpes, Shingles: • Anemopsis (external) • Commiphora myrrha
(external) • Coptis (external) • Glycyrrhiza (deglycyrrhized lic-
orice; external) • Echinacea (topical) • Helianthemum canadensis (shingles) • Hydrastis (external) • Hyssopus • Iris (shingles)

• Krameria (external) • Larrea • Lavandula (internal) • Leonurus (nerve irritation before the outbreak appears)
• Lithospermum (external) • Lysine (external) • MELISSA
(oil, external) • Monarda fistulosa • Olea (external) • Osmorhiza longistylis (herpes, shingles; external) • Plantago (herpes,
shingles; external) • Prunella • PRUNUS SEROTINA (specific when pustules do not point up in watery vesicles but are
red) • RANUNCULUS BULBOSUS (homeopathic; nearly
specific for red, water-filled vesicles) • Rhus glabra • Scutellaria
(nerve irritation, anticipation, before the outbreak) • STAPHY-
SAGRIA (homeopathic; eye) • Tilia.

Ichthyosis: • Oenothera *(pruritus)*.

Inflammation of Skin: • Calendula • Cucurbita pepo (stewed
flesh—applied hot to skin) • Plantago • Polygonum
hydropiperoides.

Insect Bite: See "Injuries, First Aid."

Insect Repellent (on the skin or as noted): • Achillea • Allium
sativa • Chrysanthemum • Citronella • Eugenia (oil, external)
• Eupatorium cannabinum (smudge) • Hedeoma (for mosqui-
toes, ants; external) • JUGLANS NIGRA (simmer a thick
decoction on a stove or campfire, to fill the air; hull) • Lavandula • LEDUM (flowers; external) • Mentha piperita (flies)
• NEPETA (external) • STAPHYSAGRIA (homeopathic; mos-
quitoes) • Tanacetum parthenium • Thuja • Thymus.

Itching (Pruritus): • Achillea *(pruritus senilis)* • Alnus (bark)
• Calendula • Chelidonium • Juniperus • Lithospermum (genital itching, herpes) • Marrubium (continual irritation) • Oenothera (ichthyosis) • Scrophularia • STELLARIA (external)
• Taraxacum • Urtica • Veronica *(pruritus senilis)*.

Leprosy: • CENTELLA (indolent ulcers; traditional).

Lichenification: • SALVIA.

Lipoma (nonmalignant fatty tumor): • Polymnia • Salvia • STELLARIA (external).

Lupus: • Centella (microorganisms, lupus, scleroderma, dermal tuberculosis, leprosy, psoriasis; acts on the matrix) • Codonopsis • Helianthemum (corrosive and dirty conditions of the skin) • Iris • Rumex acetosa • Stillingia • Tilia.

Poison Ivy/Oak: See "Injuries, First Aid."

Pregnancy Mask: • Potentilla • ROSA MOSQUETA (seed oil, external).

Proud Flesh: • INULA (hence the common name "scabwort") • Thuja.

Note: Another old remedy is to dice a raw potato and cover a wound with it.

Psoriasis (often difficult to treat): • Achillea • Alnus • ARCTIUM (root; alternate with Galium; "few cases can resist" — Parton) • Astragalus (strengthens the periphery) • Berberis • Calendula • Centella • Chelidonium • Cinnamomum spp. • Curcuma • Fouquieria • Galium • Iris • MAHONIA • Polygonatum • Quercus • RUMEX CRISPUS • Salix alba • Scrophularia • SMILAX (irritated, with heavy desquamation [flaking]) • Stellaria • Taraxacum • Thuja • TRIFOLIUM • Veronica • Urtica.

Ringworm: • *Azadirachta* (external) • Berberis • Chelidonium • HYDRASTIS (powder mixed with Calendula cream) • Juglans nigra (leaf; wash).

Scabies (external): • Calendula • Fumaria • Juglans nigra (leaf; wash) • Melaleuca (oil) • Phytolacca • Pimpinella • Polygonum aviculare (wash) • Tanacetum parthenium.

Scars: • Achillea (post-operative) • Artemisia absinthium (wash) • Calendula (post-operative) • CENTELLA • Dipsacus (wash, and internally) • Equisetum (keloids) • Galium (fibrous tissue) • Ichthammol (black ointment) • LACTUCA (acne) • Monarda fistulosa (burns) • Ricinus (oil; rub in; use for 4–6 months) • Rosa (seed oil, with castor oil; rub in, use for 4–6 months) • Withania.

Note: Vitamin E oil lessens the scar temporarily.

Scleroderma: • Artemisia vulgaris • Caulophyllum • Centella • CIMICIFUGA • Fucus • Glycyrrhiza • Iris • Scolopendrium • Symphytum • Zanthoxylum.

Scorpion Sting: • See "Injuries, First Aid."

Sebaceous Cyst: • ACHILLEA • ARCTIUM • CALENDULA.

Snakebite: See "Injuries, First Aid."

Suppuration, Purulent Discharge (external): • Arctium (with pyogenic membrane) • Baptisia • Calendula (external) • Commiphora myrrha • Echinacea (with necrosis) • Eupatorium purpureum • Plantago • Scrophularia • Thuja.

Tinea: • Phytolacca • Thuja (*tinea versicolor;* fresh leaf tincture).

Ulcers, Sores (External): • Agrimony (thighs, legs, colon, tongue, mouth; internal and external) • Ajuga • Alchemilla ("incurable ulcers"—Cech) • Alpinia • Aloe vera (internal and external)

• Anemopsis • Arctium • Astragalus (weakness of the periphery; chronic ulcers, watery, clear discharge, nonsuppurative)
• Baptisia (ointment on indolent ulcers) • Calendula • Centella (indolent) • Commiphora myrrha • Coptis (goldenseal's little brother) • Cornus florida • Daucus (advanced, deteriorative)
• Echinacea (bedsores) • Eucalyptus (fetid) • Grindelia (old, indolent; feeble circulation) • HYDRASTIS • Lamium (dressing) • Liatris (indolent) • Myrica (aphthae; indolent; poor peripheral circulation) • Phytolacca • Potentilla (root) • Ricinus (burns and wounds; oil, external) • Rubus canadensis (sweet, nutritive astringent) • Rumex crispus (running sores, yellow discharge) • Scrophularia (if scrofulous, hence the name)
• Stellaria (cooling; fresh plant; poultice or salve) • Symphytum (external, but be careful—this can seal foul matter inside)
• Thuja (bedsores) • Trifolium (skin cancer) • Trillium (indolent) • Tussilago (dressing) • Ulmus (dressing) • Usnea
• Vaccinium myrtillus.

Underarm Odor: • Arctium • Calendula.

Note: This condition is usually associated with lymphatic congestion.

Veins, Prominent (Face, Forearms): • ACHILLEA (blue veins showing through red skin) • ANGELICA (yellow/gray/blue/green around veins) • QUERCUS (veins blue and black, with yellow around them; swollen, like grapes).

Note: Also see "Varicose Veins" in "Heart/Vasculature" section.

Warts (External): • Allium sativa (with Zingiberis) • ALOE VERA (yellow sap to dissolve warts; clear gel to tone skin)
• Asclepias syriaca (milkweed sap) • Betula (inner bark)
• Calendula (fresh juice) • Chelidonium (fresh juice or tincture)
• Citrus limonum (fresh peel, externally, at night) • Juniperus (itching and burning warts; anal, genital) • Sanguinaria (very

irritating, but effective) • Taraxacum (apply fresh sap to wart) • THUJA (plantar warts; in moist places; constitutional tendency) • Zingiberis.

FORMULARY

Althaea—leaf, with Ulmus, in fomentation, poultice, or ointment (wounds, ulcers, boils, eczema). BHP 1983, 22.

Arctium leaf—with Plantago leaf (boils). This is an ancient Roman formula from Pliny. Sambucus leaf makes a good addition.

Arctium root—with Mahonia, Sassafras, Fumaria, Mahonia, Smilax, Scrophularia, and/or Trifolium (dry eczema).

Arctium root—with Stillingia, Iris, Rumex crispus, Fumaria (strong alterative cleansing formula). BHP 1983, 200.

Echinacea—with Arctium, Iris (boils). BHP 1983, 81.

Hydrastis—with Passiflora, Hamamelis leaf (pruritus). BHP 1983, 114.

Larrea—with Curcuma (stimulating salve for chronic skin lesions).

Mahonia—with Arctium (moistening, cleansing internal or external combination for eczema).

Rumex crispus—with Scrophularia (chronic skin disease). BHP 1983, 193.

Viola tricolor—with Rumex crispus (exudative skin disorders).

LAMIUM GALEOBDOLON *(YELLOW ARCHANGEL)*

"Most commended, for old, filthy and corrupt sores or corrupt Ulcers, yea, although they grow to be fistulous or hollow, and to dissolve tumors."

—JOHN PARKINSON (QUOTED IN BRUTON-SEAL AND SEAL)

Mucosa

The mucous membranes of the body have to handle some pretty harsh materials (hydrochloric acid, enzymes, bile, feces, urine, etc.), as well as extremely delicate ones (sperm, eggs), and although they are very tough they can suffer some awful insults. Fortunately for them, many herbs act strongly on the mucosa to cleanse, cool, stimulate, astringe, or moisten it. The herbalist needs to learn to think of the mucosa as a membrane that needs attention, even in babies (so prone to poor mucosal tone). He or she needs to learn to imagine what the mucosa may look like, even if it is not visible. I don't know how many times I heard some of the late, great teachers of herbal medicine, like William LeSassier or Michael Moore, use the term "mucosa" in their lectures. I would like younger students, who never heard them, to know that. In the previous section we learned how important it is to observe the condition of the skin or periphery of the body. The surface shows the evidence of disease hidden further within; it also needs to be restored to healthy functioning in order to maintain internal health. The mucous membranes are analogous to the dermis, and we must learn to think about them in the same way and to visualize their conditions, even if we cannot see them directly. The Chinese physicians, ever-so-wise, understood this relationship. The "Triple Heater" maintains both the health of the surface *(wei qi)* and the health of the linings of the internal cavities. This is paired with the "Heart Protector," which guards the heart against the shock of stressors external and internal. As we learned in our discussion of the autonomic nervous system and the regulation of the surface, powerful emotions use the same pathways in the periphery (blush, sweat, shiver) as environmental stressors—the heart is susceptible to both.

We can easily observe the mucosa in the mouth and tongue, and when we do we frequently find one or more of the tissue state imbalances. The mucosa are prone to all six of them (except tension), and thus we speak of refrigerants for heat, stimulants for cold, mucilages to moisten dryness, bitters to cleanse and purge dampness, and contractants or astringents for toning tissue that is too relaxed.

General: • Acacia (inflamed and irritable) • Achillea (inflamed; see peeled or feathered tongue) • ALTHAEA (inflamed and dry) • Arctostaphylos (damp, phlegmatic, atonic; bacteria) • Capsicum (atonic, inactive) • Collinsonia (congested, relaxed, irritable) • Commiphora myrrha (pale and relaxed) • Cornus florida (chronic, debilitated, relaxed) • Epilobium (gastrointestinal mucosa; profuse discharges, bacterial) • Erigeron (profuse discharges; bacterial) • Geranium (damp, atonic) • HYDRASTIS (stimulating bitter; feeble circulation, irritation, catarrh) • Linum (irritable hot mucosa; flaxseed oil) • Mahonia (dry; tumid with profuse secretion) • Monarda fistulosa (cool clammy skin, yeasty mucosa) • Myrica cerifera (laxity, catarrh, feeble venous flow, poor peripheral circulation) • NYMPHAEA (yeasty) • Phytolacca (atonic, congested) • Rheum (hot, inflamed, dry; poor persistalsis) • Rubus canadensis (atonic) • Rubus fructicosus (damp, atonic) • Rumex crispus (hot, inflamed, damp, atonic, yeasty) • Stillingia (red, glistening, and swollen; scanty secretions) • TABEBUIA (candida, mucosal problems) • Taraxacum (inflamed; see geographical tongue and dark red tongue body) • Tilia (inner bark is extensively used as a mucilage in France; flowers for autoimmune heat) • ULMUS (inflamed and irritable).

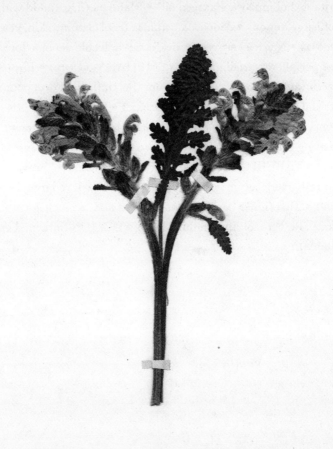

4. Chronic Conditions

Stages of Life

The first category below is offered somewhat tentatively, though I have personally seen *Gnaphalium* succeed in congenital cases. Traditional Chinese Medicine has remedies to offer here. Congenital weakness is called *jing* deficiency; *jing* is used to describe the life-essence or primal configuration. Another approach is found in some traditions of American Indian medicine; "Rabbit Medicine" is associated with congenital deficiency because of the weakness and vulnerability of this animal.

An important theory in modern TCM attributes the ill effects of aging largely to blood stagnation and increasing imbalances between blood and *qi*. The latter is considered the "commander of blood," meaning that blood circulation depends on *qi*. If circulation is not sufficient, blood will "congeal." This is considered the source of the joint and muscle pains of aging. Therefore, treating blood stagnation and circulation is of utmost importance in gerontology. Attention to circulation, of course, is appropriate in every stage of life.

Congenital Weakness: • Amygdalus (sensitive constitution; brain, spine, marrow tonic) • Aralia nudicaulis (Cree "rabbit root" — Rogers) • GNAPHALIUM (Cherokee "rabbit tobacco"; congenital problems or immune weakness from birth or first year of life) • Osmunda (bone weakness) • Rubus canadensis (used in pregnancy for hundreds of years to strengthen the mother and baby; often confirmed) • Urtica (used in pregnancy to strengthen mother and baby).

Infants and Children: • Aquilegia canadensis, A. vulgaris (bedwetting; flower essence or leaf tincture) • Agrimonia (acting out) • Allium cepa (baby fretful, nervous, sleepless, colicky; tea, for the lactating mother) • Aloe vera (diaper rash; apply locally) • Amygdalus (delicate, sensitive; insomnia) • Anagallis (rage) • Anethum (colic in babies; seed) • Betonica (fear) • Calendula (fear of the dark) • CHAMOMILLA (teething; constitutional, humoral, temperamental upset of babies; convulsions; in olive oil for cradle cap; "for babies of all ages"—Wood) • Cetraria (congenital weakness) • Chelidonium (scared by cartoons and images; 1-drop dose, as needed) • CICHORIUM (selfish, childish) • Chondrus (congenital weakness) • CRATAEGUS (attention deficient, loss of focus) • Eschscholzia (sleeplessness) • Dioscorea (teething spasms) • Epilobium (balances and helps to master will; wild, angry, overactive children are sedated, and shy children are strengthened; flower essence) • Filipendula (diarrhea; nervous, irritable, hyperactive children) • Foeniculum (infantile colic; seed) • Gentiana (fear) • GNAPHALIUM (congenital weakness; childhood asthma) • Humulus (delicate, sensitive children; bedwetting) • HYDRASTIS (1-drop doses to stimulate the ANS; diluted doses for sore mouth in baby; constipation in infants; skin rash, chafing, rawness—brilliant cures) • HYPERICUM (fear of the dark, night terrors; "Here Nature gives the St. John's Wort"—Parton) • JUGLANS spp. (children constipated, worrying about parental separation; black walnut, royal walnut, or butternut flower essence or herb; several successful cases) • Linaria (headstrong, willful children) • Mahonia (malnutrition due to poor anabolism, digestion; constipation, poor elimination, catabolism; dry constitution) • Nepeta (infants with colic, constipation and fever; bullying in children) • Nigella (hyperactivity) • Paeonia spp. (convulsions) • Panax quinquefolius (too nervous to play) • Papaver somnifera (fear from bad images, cartoons; constipation; seed tea) • Passiflora (atonic conditions; restlessness and insomnia in infants and the elderly) • Populus gileadensis (respiratory infection) • Rhamnus cathártica (syrup of berries with ginger, allspice, and honey or sugar; "considered one of the finest laxative remedies for children"—Tierra) • RICINIS ("for infants it is the safest"—Jones) • Rubus canadensis (childhood diarrhea) • Rubus fruticosus (childhood diarrhea) • Rosa (delicate constitution, low immunity; born by cesarean) • SAMBUCUS (pale, with blue swelling across nose; red, dry irritated cheeks—"the great infant remedy"—Wood) • Scrophularia (external; cradle cap) • Solidago ("for late development—brings them up to par"—Wolff) • Tilia (hyperactivity) • VERBASCUM (bedwetting) • Verbena (convulsions after fever) • Viburnum opulus (infantile enuresis) • Viola (dry skin, swollen glands, damp palms; flabby children) • WITHANIA (low weight gain, anemia, dark circles under the eyes).

Teenagers/Puberty/Young Adults: • Agrimonia (oppositional) • Amygdalus (thin, delicate, low immunity, pale skin, sensitivity) • Cimicifuga (girls brooding, never well since puberty) • Humulus (flat affect) • LACTUCA (cystic acne of teens and others; apathetic, indifferent, with negative thoughts) • LILIUM (cystic acne, in girls) • Nepeta (bullying, bullied) • Oplopanax (increases sexual confidence, establishes healthy sexual boundaries, increases desire) • PHYTOLACCA (in puberty, during glandular growth; apathetic, lazy, unclean; purple spot on tongue) • PULSATILLA (girls never well since puberty; young women with lack of confidence, male dependence, dependence on friends' opinions) • Quercus (sees skeletons, skulls in mind—one case only) • Vitex (calms down boys who are preoccupied by sex; regulates girls' cycles; inappropriate sexual acting-out).

Middle Age: • Capsicum (poorly exercised, flabby) • Chimaphila (weight gain, water retention) • Crataegus (loss of imagination in middle age) • Juglans cinerea (constipation) • Monarda fistulosa (loss of passion) • Rhus tox. (homeopathic; boredom with work, relationship, life) • Silphium integrifolium ("make a new man out of an old one" — Howard; renewed vision of life — Schnell) • Vitex (perimenopausal irregularity, heavy bleeding, hot flashes, night sweats; lack of spiciness and libido later in life).

Senescence (Physical and Mental): • Acorus (clarity of thought, articulation; digestion, arthritis) • Amygdalus (sensitive constitution) • Artemisia absinthium (a dose of absinth once in a while helps muscular soreness) • Artemisia vulgaris (moxibustion on cold, arthritic joints and muscles; or external application of herb) • BETONICA (mental, physical, digestive; tremendous for the elderly) • CALCIUM PHOSPHATE (homeopathic; osteoporosis) • Camellia sinensis (tea) • CAPSICUM (atonic debility of the digestive organs in senescence; weak peripheral circulation) • CENTELLA (circulation, memory, connective tissue) • Cetraria (weakness) • Chondrus • Cnicus (reduced circulation, memory) • Crataegus (heart, circulation) • Eleutherococcus (adrenal exhaustion, circles under the eyes) • Ganoderma • Gingko (cerebral circulation) • Hypericum (discouraged, depressed, and in pain) • Juglans cinerea (constipation, bowels; sluggish gall bladder; bark, if available, but the tree has lately been decimated by disease) • Juniperus (constipation from weakness of muscles) • Leonurus (rounded spine, osteoporosis; stiff joints; blood-mover in older women) • Lepidium • Lycopodium (homeopathic; "withered, dry, full of gas" — Boericke) • Nigella (oil or fresh-crushed seeds; forgetfulness, senility; combine with myrrh) • Panax quinquefolius (drying of skin, mucosa, joints) • PANAX GINSENG • Polygonum multiflorum • Rhodiola • Rheum (constipation in the elderly) • RIBES NIGRUM (many parts of this plant are used in several traditions) • ROSMARINUS ("low blood," dark around ankles; improves cerebral and peripheral circulation) • Rubia (blood stagnation; blue/gray tongue) • SALVIA (decreased hormones; withering, drying, wrinkling; weak tendons; blood stagnation;

blue/grey tongue, complexion) • Sinapis alba, S. nigra (delicate,
sensitive, frail, elderly; easily catches cold and comes down with
chronic respiratory problems; indigestion in old alcoholics)
• Turnera (loss of spirits, libido; depression in elders — Donahue) • WITHANIA (adaptogen).

Concentration, Memory (Lack of, due to senescence): See
"Mind, Emotions, Will."

Exhaustion, Low Energy, Fatigue

Requests for help with "low energy" are extremely common. These
problems can arise from chronic infection, endocrine imbalances,
malnutrition, nervous exhaustion, blood deficiency, excessive menstrual bleeding, sleeplessness, and many other causes. In energetic
terms, people may be suffering from tissue depression, stagnation,
atrophy, or lack of tone (relaxation).

According to the E-C-R cycle, a person is first overstimulated
(E — excitation), then tensed up (C — constriction), then overly
relaxed (R — relaxation). If this happens in excess the latter becomes
the chronic, and we get exhaustion, debility, fatigue, and weakness.
Or, by another route, constriction does not allow circulation into the
tissues, impeding nutrition and resulting in atrophy.

So the tissue states associated with this section are relaxation,
atropy, depression, and probably also stagnation. The tissue states
that first occur in excess — excitation and tension (constriction) —
should be treated before the exhaustion phase sets in, and sometimes
still need to be treated even after it has arrived. These people have
too much energy at first, but then they have too little. A small section
on these remedies has been included below.

Debility, Exhaustion, Weakness: • ALETRIS (in women; poor
digestion, atrophy, infertility) • Alnus serrulata (wasting)
• Apocynum cannabinum (watery infiltration of the tissues with
weak circulation and general dropsy) • ARALIA RACEMOSA

(adrenal exhaustion; dark circles under eyes; exhaustion in women) • ARCTIUM (adrenal burnout) • Arnica (from over-activity) • AVENA (exhaustion after fever; brain fog; sex and drug addiction; easily stimulated) • BAPTISIA (chronic fatigue syndrome; never well since glandular fever) • Berberis • Borago • Calendula (bone-weary feeling) • Cannabis (restlessness of nervous exhaustion) • Capsicum (feeble pulse and suppressed sweat) • Centaurium (lack of appetite and "digestive fire") • Centella (fatigue of mind and body) • Chamomilla (sitz bath, oil) • Chelidonium (with irregular bowels; beat-up feeling) • Chelone glabra (post-febrile liver problems) • Chimaphila (debility with glandular swelling) • Chondrus (nutritive) • CINNAMOMUM SPP. (weak, cold, with low immunity, hypoglycemia) • Cola (debilitated, atonic, asthenic, dyspneic; CNS depression) • Commiphora myrrha • Crataegus (lassitude and fatigue from overwork, overexcitement) • ELEUTHERO-COCCUS (adrenal exhaustion; dark circles under eyes; jet lag) • Equisetum (general weakness) • Euonymus (prostration with nerve irritation) • Ganoderma (sympathetic excess and adrenal burnout) • GENTIANA (malnutrition, discouragement, debil-ity) • Gingko • LAVANDULA (nervous exhaustion; in bath, to increase resistance to stress) • Leonurus (nervous debility; in elderly; irritation and unrest; lumbar pain and uneasiness) • Lycopus (post-febrile exhaustion with rapid pulse) • Medicago • Melissa (nervous exhaustion) • Menispermum canadensis • Olea • Oplopanax (asthenia; frequent sense of chill in warm room; fingers cold, appetite poor—M. Moore) • Osmunda (convalescence after exhausting diseases) • Panax ginseng (shortness of breath, after illness; collapse after severe fluid loss) • Panax quinquefolius (with loss of appetite, dryness) • Polygonum multiflorum (deep exhaustion and indifference; overworked, jaded) • Populus tremuloides (emaciation) • Pulsa-tilla (menstrual irregularity; emotional lability) • Rhodiola • Rumex crispus (feeble recuperative power) • Sabal serrulata (nutritive) • Scutellaria (nervous prostration) • Solidago (tired feet) • Trigonella (convalescent nutritive) • Tsuga canadensis (Canadian hemlock oil; apply externally over cold kidneys and back) • Tussilago (tired feet) • Ulmus (nutritive) • Urtica (tea) • Zanthoxylum (low nerve force; low dose) • ZINGIBERIS.

Sluggishness, Heavy Feeling: • Arctium (tired feet; internal abscess) • Armoracia • Carbo vegetabilis (homeopathic; sluggish, lazy, fat, with tendency to chronicity of complaints) • Capsicum (out of shape, needs exercise; pulse loose, unequal) • Gentiana • Phytolacca • Plantago (internal abscess) • Prunus serotina (weight on the heart, literally or metaphorically) • Sinapis • Solidago (tired feet) • Tussilago (tired feet).

Internal Abscess, Abscessed Tooth Causing Chronic Fatigue (patient should be on antibiotics): • Arctium • Aristolochia (small or homeopathic dosage) • Ceanothus • Cnicus (fever, chills, exhaustion) • Plantago (put next to the tooth) • Solidago • Taraxacum.

Relaxation (Lack of Tone): • Achillea (with free discharge) • Aesculus hip. • Astragalus (lax muscular tone) • Cinchona (weakness from loss of fluids, atonic muscles) • Erigeron (with profuse discharges) • Euphrasia (with profuse, watery discharges and acute inflammation) • Geranium maculatum (profuse, debilitating discharges) • Hypericum • Myrica (flabby, hypersecretion, catarrh) • Rhus spp. (free secretions, kidney anemia) • Rumex crispus (debility, from easily disordered homeostasis of fluids; ulceration, chronic skin disorders).

Irritability (Easily Overstimulated): • Amygdalus • Avena • Chamomilla • Crataegus • Lycopus • Melissa • Passiflora • Primula • Rosa • Scutellaria (mentally overstimulated).

Kundalini, Acute Crisis: • Peanut butter (or heavy, fatty meat; liberally and regularly, until condition subsides—Ryan).

Kundalini, Chronic Crisis: The homeopathic nightshades (Atropa belladonna, Hyoscyamus, Stramonium) and some venomous remedies (Lachesis, Tarantula, etc.).

FORMULARY

Rosa (hips, 5 parts) with Fragaria (2 parts), Tilia (2 parts), Thymus vulgaris (1 part). This "Breakfast Tea" tonic is a "prophylactic for healthy people." Les Moore 2002, 59. A cooling remedy with a circulatory stimulant (thyme).

Environmental and Dietary Toxins

In cases of acute poisoning, call the poison control center. An effective method for immediate removal of toxins or poisons is oil-pulling. This method used in Ayurvedic medicine places a dietary oil under the tongue, and the oil picks up toxins from the bloodstream. It is to be spit out after 15–20 minutes, or when it starts to taste bad. This can be done for either immediate poisoning or long-term toxicity. I have seen it stop anaphylaxis within minutes.

Poisoning: • Carthamus (oil-pulling to remove toxins) • ECHINACEA ("all diseases of blood poisoning, whether showing a great or small amount of cell destruction"; "powerful antidote to snakebites and poisonous insects"—Massinger) • Eupatorium purpureum (inhalation of poisonous vapors) • Fomes officinalis (an ancient and historical poison antidote) • Helianthus (oil, for oil-pulling) • LARREA (toxic headache, mucus congestion, sinus/respiratory troubles) • Veratrum (upper and lower respiratory).

Damp, Hot Weather: • Calendula (rash between legs, diaper rash) • GELSEMIUM (lethargy of mind and body due to damp, hot weather; this homeopathic remedy is the only well-attested remedy I know for this) • Lonicera (traditional, for exhaustion from damp, hot weather in the South—needs confirmation).

Drug Detox: • Ambrosia (ragweed; swelling of nasal turbinates from coke-sniffing) • AVENA (drug addiction—opiates, cocaine, cannabis, tranquilizers, sedatives, alcohol, coffee, tobacco, anti-depressants) • CENTELLA (cocaine) • Chamomilla (antidote to coffee) • ELEUTHEROCOCCUS • Eschscholzia (anxiety, tension, during withdrawal) • GERANIUM (restores lost part of self) • Hydrastis (cannabis; masks detection in tests) • Larrea (cocaine, speed, amphetamines) • OCIMUM (detoxification from cannabis; very effective; masks detection in tests) • Passiflora • Schisandra • Scutellaria (withdrawal) • SILYBUM (liver damage from alcohol and other drugs) • Zingiberis (craving and withdrawal from benzodiazepines).

Note: The above information is based on Hershoff/Rotelli and Brent Davis.

Electric Shock: • Juglans nigra.

Radiation: • Achillea • Althea • Chrysanthemum • Fagopyrum • Helianthus (used extensively and successfully after Chernobyl to remove radiation from the soil) • Larrea (a traditional Ute Indian medicine for prevention of cancer from exposure to radiation; confirmed) • TRAMETES VERSICOLOR (used in Japan for cancer associated with radiation).

Heavy Metals: • Coriandrum (leaf) • Eugenia (combine with Coriandrum) • GLECHOMA (lead, mercury, and other metals are removed efficiently; in fact, there is a concern that this plant may also remove nutritional iron and other required metals) • LARREA • OCIMUM (lipophilic toxins—Davis) • Stillingia (mercury).

Food Sensitivities, Gluten Intolerance: • PLANTAGO (leaky gut) • POLYGONUM PERSICARIA.

Rabies-Shot Side Effects: • Scutellaria.

FORMULARY

Glechoma—with Plantago, Prunella, Coriandrum (internally, to draw out heavy metals).

The Theory of Toxicity and Detoxification

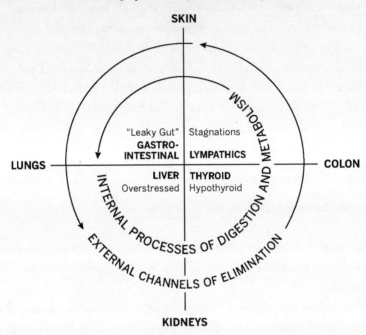

"Toxins" are incompletely metabolized substances which build up through lack of elimination, "leaky gut" or gut absorption issues, poor metabolism in the liver or the cells, low thyroid (causing low metabolism), exotoxin production by bacteria, and poor removal of waste from the extracellular matrix. Although frequently called "bad blood," "toxins in the blood," "impure blood," or "liver toxicity," these waste products build up in the extracellular matrix, between the cells. Originally called "humors" or "humors in the blood" in Hippocratic and English medicine, the terms "bad" and "impure blood" became popular in the nineteenth century. The idea is still popular in folk medicine and account for the popularity of "cleansing" diets and herbal protocols, not all of which are needed, but most of which are safe. The herbs used to "detoxify" the blood are called "alteratives" or "blood purifiers." They are assisted by laxatives.

Weight

Obesity, Overweight: • Alchemilla • Astragalus (loose tissue) • Camellia sinensis (tea) • Cichorium • Crataegus • Daucus (abdominal weight, beer belly) • Phytolacca (berries, not seeds) • STELLARIA • Trigonella • Zea mays (corn silk tea).

Thin, Underweight: • Acorus (bath, cold decoction) • Agnus castus • Chondrus (malnutrition) • Codonopsis (thin, weak, tired, dried-out) • Cornus (thin, low stamina and sexual energy) • Dioscorea • Glycyrrhiza • Gentiana • Trigonella ("general debility and anorexia of convalescence"—BHP) • Ulmus (convalescence).

Cancer

Cancer arises from many different causes and therefore requires many potential treatments. This is a very tough and formidable adversary, and *conventional therapies should not be shunned*. However, it should be remembered that many cancer patients die from biomedical treatments rather than the disease itself. It often seems that cancer therapy is geared towards helping the patient accept their eventual death by delaying the inevitable, or making the last months or years into a heroic battle. Making a person believe they are fighting an heroic battle for their life is, in my opinion, a worthy therapy, even if the cancer ultimately wins.

Alternative methods can be used alongside conventional methods. The following approaches should be considered, bearing in mind that other approaches are also possible:

- Treatments to strengthen the constitution.
- Organ and tissue treatments to strengthen regions affected by the cancer.
- Organ and tissue-directed treatment to strengthen body structures weakened by surgery or drugs—the extracellular matrix, lymph, and liver.

- Clearing stagnant blood (indicated by blue color in face, tongue, wrists, legs, etc.) Cancer often develops on old bruises, and thrives where blood is poorly oxygenated.
- Removing the cancer directly, through the use of escarotics that burn it away.
- Strengthening the immune system to reduce cancer-cell division; immune cells devour cancer cells.
- Strengthening the system by combating cachexia (wasting).
- Repairing the ECM (extracellular matrix) after surgery (pioneered by Alfred Pischinger).

Many of the following indications need confirmation, but some have proved surprisingly effective in clinical and anecdotal experience.

One final note: Always encourage the cancer patient or family to read the literature about their kind of cancer thoroughly. Doctors often don't have time to explain all the facts, or (understandably) can't deal with the emotions of their clients. Never allow intimidation to enter the medical relationship. Always bring an advocate, if possible. From hearing about numerous truly terrible experiences, I have to say that this is particularly true for women and minorities; but even a big, imposing man, faced with cancer, needs an advocate, friend, or family member present.

Cancer: • Achillea (breast cancer, from a blow) • Acorus (supportive in upper GI neoplasia; anorexia from therapy—Moore) • ALLIUM SATIVA (one ounce of garlic a week is believed to be preventative or suppressive to GI, breast, prostate, liver, lung, and brain cancers) • Apocynum cannabinum (Weiss) • Aristolochia (adenocarcinoma—Sherman) • Arctium (supportive, nutritive) • Astragalus (exhaustion, cachexia; increases cancer-fighting immune cells, supports recovery from radiation and chemotherapy) • Bellis (cancer resulting from a blow; to prevent or treat; homeopathic or herbal) • Beta (nausea and vomiting from chemotherapy; cachexia—Weiss) • Calendula (lymphatic cleansing; perhaps anti-tumor) • CAMELLIA (preventive; inhibits spread; for colon and rectal cancers; use decaffeinated tea) • CANNABIS (pain, glioma; nausea, anorexia from therapy) • CETRARIA (vomiting from chemotherapy; cachexia) • CHELIDONIUM (escharotic; liver support) • Commiphora myrrha (white blood cell deficiency) • CONIUM MACULATUM (sexual glands, breast, testicles; poultice on breast in old-time herbalism, now homeopathic remedy used internally—many confirmations in homeopathic literature) • Crataegus (skin, larynx, Burkitt's lymphoma—Rogers) • CURCUMA (cancer of mucosa, breast, lymphatics; preventive) • DAUCUS (skin cancer; seed oil externally) • ECHINACEA (supports the system stressed by chemotherapy and cancer; do not give in leukemia) • Epilobium (prostate) • Euonymus (anorexia from therapy) • Fouquieria (supportive in lymph dysplasias—Moore) • GALIUM (traditional) • GANODERMA (immune tonic; stomach, breast, lung) • Gentiana (supportive in upper GI neoplasias) • Glechoma ("beefsteak tongue" of advanced cases; palliative) • GRIFOLA (breast, colorectal, lung, bladder, liver, blood, lymph; inhibits spread, growth) • HYDRASTIS (worn, jaded look, yellow or sallow complexion, "hide-bound state of skin, low spirits, loss of appetite, chronic constipation"; 1-drop dose—Clarke) • INONOTUS (traditional on two continents for cancer; pharmacological mechanism is established; "more miracles from this than any other"—Wood) • LARREA (traditional and sometimes proven; "essential in neoplasia"—Davis) • Lentinula (to increase immunity, shrink existing tumors) • Lilium longiflorum (cervical dysplasia and neoplasia; confirmed—Wood) • Lithospermum (skin cancer; wash) • Monotropa (for pain of advanced cancer; lessens need for opiates and maintains conscious awareness; helps people deal with their regrets as they are dying—D. Winston; often confirmed) • Nigella (immune normalizer; traditional remedy for cancer; research shows action on cancer and tumor cells) • Panax ginseng • Panax quinquefolius (anorexia from therapy; to prevent metastases, strengthen the extracellular matrix)

• PHYTOLACCA (external, on breast cancer; traditional and sometimes confirmed; "tendency to fatness, sluggish circulation, lazy disposition, glandular enlargements"—Clarke) • Podophyllum (ovarian cancer—Weiss) • Potentilla ("drink tormentil tea"—Tilke) • Prunus serotina (liver) • Rhodiola (bladder, recurring) • Rheum • RUMEX ACETOSA (the most "active ingredient" in Essiac and also traditional; internal, external) • Rumex crispus (supportive) • SANGUINARIA (very corrosive escharotic; use with caution) • SCROPHULARIA (Hodgkin's lymphoma; specific affinity for the breast, and breast cancer, in women with large breasts—Boericke) • Silybum • Taraxacum (supports cleansing when tongue is dark-red, to bring heat to the surface and out of the body—Wood) • Thuja (skin, rectum, bladder) • TRAMETES VERSICOLOR (breast, colorectal; for radiation exposure) • TRIFOLIUM (skin, glandular, breast, lung, general; to prevent regrowth; internal or external; large dose or highly concentrated; traditional) • Vinca (acute leukemia in children; Hodgkin's lymphoma; solid tumors—Weiss) • VIOLA ("neoplasm in breast or alimentary canal" or lymphatic nodes; "after tumor extirpation, to protect from metastases"—BHP; often confirmed—Weed) • VISCUM (injectable form, for cancer) • Vitis (old saying: "when all hope is lost, resort to the grape cure"—or before hope is lost; fasting while eating only organic grapes) • WITHANIA (immune and general support).

Cancer from Congealed Blood, Bruise, Blow: • Achillea • Bellis perennis (usually homeopathic) • CONIUM (homeopathic) • Phytolacca (blue-purple complexion) • Symphytum (homeopathic).

Chemotherapy and Radiation Side Effects: • ACHILLEA (for radiation; flower essence) • ALTHAEA (dry, red tongue; burnt tissues from radiation—Fischer) • Arctium • Astragalus • Beta (nutritive) • Calendula • Cetraria (vomiting) • ECHINACEA

(low WBC count after chemotherapy) • Galium • Grifolia
• Hypericum • Lentinula • Mahonia • Rheum • Rumex crispus
• Taraxacum • Trametes • Trifolium • Uncaria • Withania.

Note: Give lymphatics, hepatics, and laxatives after chemo and radiation, to cleanse the system of toxins. Statistically, people who receive traditional therapy are expected to get cancer from the radiation within twenty years.

Cachexia (wasting): • Acorus • CETRARIA • Chondrus • Cola
• Sabal.

Pain: • Acorus (palliative for stomach pain in inoperable cases)
• CANNABIS • MONOTROPA (introduced by David Winston to lessen the pain of dying from cancer without diminishing consciousness; has often been confirmed; helps deal with regrets when dying) • Petasites (tumor pain).

Escharotic: • Calendula (not destructive to dermis) • Chelidonium
• Sanguinaria (very destructive to dermis) • Thuja • Trifolium.

Note: Escharotics are used externally on skin cancer to overheat the cancer cells (which already have a high metabolism) and destroy them. They are a form of chemotherapy because they particularly act on cancer cells. Although an "alternative" treatment, some escharotics are quite destructive; though not harmless, they can be skillfully used, as can conventional cancer treatments.

"For an excellent overview of Essiac, Hoxsey, and other historical and current herbal cancer formulas, consult Ralph Moss's *Herbs Against Cancer*."
—HERSHOFF AND ROTELLI

FORMULARY

Arctium (52 parts) —with *Rumex acetosella* (16 parts), *Ulmus* (4 parts), *Rheum* (1 part). This is the famous "Essaic Formula" for cancer (Les Moore 2002, 89), originated by Rene Caisse and based, she said, on a formula used by an Ojibwa medicine man. All the ingredients except *Ulmus* are native to Europe, so this is ultimately not Native American in origin. Sheep sorrel has a long non-Native use in cancer.

Echinacea —with *Calendula, Trifolium, Galium,* and other herbs, according to the case, to ease exhaustion during chemotherapy. I call this "chemo companion." Contraindicated in leukemia.

Trifolium pretense —slowly boil red clover blossoms down into a paste, attending carefully and stirring regularly. This is a time-consuming process, but it yields a famous cancer salve for the skin, and an internal remedy for prostate and other cancers. (Evidently the active ingredients are not heat-sensitive.)

CHAGA *(INONOTUS OBLIQUUS)*

If there is a single remedy that might be called a "miracle remedy" in the treatment of cancer, it would be the chaga mushroom, traditionally used by northern people in Finland, Russia, Siberia, and North America for cancer. In the north woods of Minnesota, it is known by the Native people as "the mushroom that grows in the birch tree." I have seen it remove diagnosed cancer in less than thirty days; I have seen it hold dangerous cancers in check for years; and I have many herbalist friends who could give more testimonials. Margi Flint told me that she has used it successfully in melanoma "many times." It can also be used as a preventive.

5. Acute Conditions

For ease of use, it may be desirable for the reader to color the page edges of this section red or another bright color, in order to be able to find it quickly in acute and first-aid situations. (This can be done with different colors for any section where easy access is desired.)

Fever

Fever with Little or No Sweat (warming, stimulating, and relaxing diaphoretics): • Anagallis • ANGELICA (incipient fevers, coughs, and colds; warm decoction or tincture) • Aralia spinosa • ARCTIUM (skin dry or profusely oily) • Borago • Carthamus (fever in infants, with constipation; exanthema, chicken pox; tincture or oil) • CHAMOMILLA (tension, pain, complains; one cheek red, the other pale; skin dry) • Cnicus • Dioscorea (dry skin) • Echinacea (exhaustion) • Ephedra • EUPATORIUM PERFOLIATUM (hard to break a sweat) • Fumaria • Glechoma (antiviral; inflammation of middle ear and facial mucosa) • HEDEOMA (full, pungent heat of skin, face, and neck; hot infusion) • HYSSOPUS (dry skin; sore throat; respiratory inflammation; deep heat in organs) • Inula (checked perspiration, sudden onset of cold; incipient bronchitis, cough; warm decoction or tincture) • LIGUSTICUM • Majorana • Mentha piperita • MENTHA PULEGIUM • NEPETA (infantile fever; infantile constipation) • Ocimum • Origanum • Polemonium (skin cold, dry, torpid, with languor, internal venous congestion) • Polygonum hydropiperoides, punctatum (stimulant for cold, dry, inactive skin; heart action suppressed by internal congestion) • Rosmarinus (colds, fevers) • SALVIA (colds, fevers, sore throat, lungs) • Sassafras (promotes circulation, thins the blood; root bark) • Satureja (warm infusion in the early stages of fever, inflammation, colds, catarrh) • Scrophularia (lymphatic assistance) • THYMUS (incomplete sweat; contagious fever; cough, lungs) • Vinca minor • Zanthoxylum (inactive skin, depressed nervous function) • ZINGIBERIS (sudden cold, checked perspiration; fresh rhizome; bath or hot tea).

Fever (cooling agents): • ACHILLEA (incomplete, somewhat oily sweat; red, flushed face; rapid, nonresistant, full pulse; red tongue, blue in center) • Agastache • AMYGDALUS (hot, dry skin) • ASCLEPIAS TUBEROSA (harsh, dry skin; softens and moistens gently) • Borago (exhaustion) • BUPLEURUM • Chrysanthemum • Citrus limonum (juice, in water) • ECHI-NACEA • Hibiscus • Lonicera • Melilotus (blood congestion, mild perspiration; cools by thinning the blood) • MELISSA (specific for most acute children's fevers) • MENTHA PIPER-ITA (fever with chills) • MENTHA SPICATA (incipient fever, with nausea and vomiting) • Papaver somnifera (dry skin with nervousness, restlessness, constipation; poppy seed tea) • Rehmannia (uncooked root) • SAMBUCUS (parched, dry, red skin; blue swollen skin, or both) • Selenicereus (excited heart activity) • Tilia (early stages of influenza, colds, and fevers, especially in children; excessive immune response) • Tussilago (respiratory; cool infusion) • Verbena (hard to break a sweat; flooding pulse).

Fever with Sweat: • ACHILLEA (incomplete sweat) • ARC-TIUM (excessive oily sweat) • Asclepias tuberosa (profuse sweat) • CINNAMOMUM CASSIA (thin, fair, firm, moist skin; spontaneous sweating and low fever—Huang) • Lobelia (high fever with profuse sweat) • MELISSA (almost specific for clammy palms) • MONARDA FISTULOSA (specific for generalized cool, clammy skin) • Platanus (twig, bark, or heartwood) • SAMBUCUS (blue, pale, clammy skin) • SALVIA (relaxed skin and nervous system, night sweats) • Verbena (profuse sweating) • Veronica (drowsiness; hot tea).

Intermittent Fever (Chills and Fever, Influenza, Malaria):
• ACHILLEA (sudden intense fever with chills; irregular chills) • Acorus (sudden flush of heat; chills with exhaustion) • AGRIMONIA (with pain) • ANGELICA (influenza, often with respiratory involvement; at beginning or end) • Aralia racemosa • Aristolochia (homeopathic; septic tendency) • Artemisia absinthium • ARTEMISIA ANNUA (specific for malaria) • Asclepias tuberosa • Betonica • BUPLEURUM • CAPSICUM (stimulant; use at the start) • Ceanothus (spleen congestion and pain; glandular fever) • Centaurium • Centella (fatigue) • Chamomilla (one cheek red, the other pale; complains, whines) • Chelidonium • Chimaphila • Chionanthus • Cinnamomum spp. (fever/chills; bark in hot wine) • CINCHONA (tonic for debility following chills and fever) • CNICUS (intermittent chills; may originate in serious inflammation of organs) • Cornus florida • Dipsacus • ECHINACEA (malaria; continue for three weeks afterward to prevent relapse) • Eryngium (with upper respiratory infection) • Eucalyptus (malaria) • EUPATORIUM PERFOLIATUM (influenza, chills, crushing pain in bones, "aching all over") • Filipendula (slowly developing) • Geum urbanum (chills and catarrh, initial onset, sore throat — Grieve) • Hypericum • Juglans cinerea • Ledum (cold, shivery conditions with chattering teeth) • Liriodendron • Marrubium (cold; constipation) • Menyanthes • Petroselinum • Populus tremuloides • Potentilla • Salix alba (gouty, rheumatic) • SAMBUCUS (beginning of influenza, with dry skin) • Taraxacum (disturbed sleep) • Tilia (nervous tension associated with flu) • Verbena (severe chills; skin won't open; convulsions in children).

Fever, Low-grade, Prolonged, Septic (stimulants and antiseptics): • Acacia • ACHILLEA (phlebitis, boils, abscesses;

nonresistant pulse of febrile exhaustion) • Aesculus hip. (phlebitis) • ALLIUM SATIVA (external; mixed with egg white or other preparation, on sepsis) • Anthemis cotula (stimulant for low-grade fever, depressed vital powers, congestion of internal organs; cold, shrunken, shriveled skin surface) • Aralia racemosa (needs confirmation) • Aristolochia serpentaria (low-grade, septic, exhausted; skin atonic, circulation feeble; confirmed in flesh-eating bacterial fever; small or homeopathic doses) • AVENA (nervous exhaustion) • BAPTISIA (low-grade fever with putrid, sticky discharges, swollen glands, lack of circulation) • CALENDULA (infections, boils; external) • CARBO VEGETABILIS (homeopathic; never fully recovered from previous illness) • Carthamus (low-grade fever with skin eruptions; brings out eruptions) • Dicentra (general malaise and indisposition to exertion after protracted disease; with sluggishness of digestion, glands, kidneys, skin, circulation) • ECHINACEA (low immunity, exhaustion, low-grade fever, swollen veins, infected wounds, boils, abscesses) • Eupatorium perfoliatum • Eleutherococcus • Eupatorium purpureum (abscesses, purulent matter in system) • Hyssopus (low-grade infection and fever, dry skin) • Lycii (with fluid loss) • Phytolacca • PLANTAGO (draws out pus, infection; "digests" putrid tissue and "reincarnates" new tissue; infected roots of teeth; external, on boils and infected wounds) • Rehmannia (low-grade fever, wasting diseases, heat in the blood, hemorrhage during high fever, thirst, mouth/tongue sores, sore throat, restless and irritable mind; uncooked root) • Scrophularia (combines well with Rehmannia in the above conditions; clears lymphatic stagnation) • Solidago (low-grade fever, sores, tired kidneys following fever; relapse as waste tries to pass through kidneys).

Fever, Systemic: • Achillea (Weiss) • Baptisia (sepsis) • Echinacea (sepsis) • Polemonium.

Fever, Eruptive: See "Skin."

Rash (to bring out): • Carthamus (tea or tincture of the flower tops; even cooking oil will do) • Cimicifuga • Pulsatilla.

Post-Febrile Symptoms: • Achillea (exhausting, long-term fever, post-febrile weakness) • Agropyron repens (heavy urine during and after fever; cold infusion with lemon) • Amygdalus (reddish, irritable skin, heat) • Arctium (dry skin) • Arnica (shock; choppy pulse) • Baptisia • Bupleurum ("diseases that tend to begin externally as an acute syndrome and linger for a prolonged period"—Tierra) • Carthamus (shock) • Cichorium (long, lingering, intermittent) • Cinchona (bitter astringent for exhaustion, indigestion, lack of appetite) • Echinacea (builds white blood cells; keeps the system clean) • Eupatorium perfoliatum (edema after scarlet fever) • Galium (dark urine) • Gentiana (lack of appetite after prolonged fever) • Geum (post-influenza) • Lactuca • Leonurus (heart palpitations and nervousness) • Lycopus (exhaustion; rapid, very irregular pulse) • Melissa (nervousness) • Monarda fistulosa (clammy skin from pores not closing) • Ocimum (recovery from debilitating chills that wear out nervous system and gall-bladder reflex) • Panax quinquefolius (restores dried-out fluids) • Prunus serotina (reddish, irritable skin; rapid, irregular pulse) • Rosmarinus (exhaustion following hepatitis, influenza, low-grade fevers—Weiss) • Salvia (trembling) • Solidago (kidneys can't handle waste products; dark, heavy or light, thin urine) • Tilia (nervousness following colds) • Ulmus (emaciation after long fever) • Verbena (convulsions) • Veratrum viride (heart overstimulated, exhausted by strong pulse; homeopathic dose).

Agents Acting on the Sebaceous Glands (Oily Sweat, Excessive or Deficient): • ARCTIUM (seed and root) • Celastrus • Helianthus (seed).

Note: Above information derived from William Cook (1869).

Chickenpox: • CARTHAMUS • CIMICIFUGA • Echinacea • PULSATILLA.

Delirium: • Belladonna (homeopathic; as if possessed by a violent animal) • Hyoscyamus (homeopathic; as if possessed by an evil spirit).

Hectic Fever: • Lycium (night sweats) • Panax quinquefolius • Prunus serotina • Pulsatilla.

Note: Hectic fever occurs in exhausted febrile states, where the fluids are driven off by heat and there is weakness and lack of resistance; TCM calls this "yin-deficiency fever." The cheeks are often red with a "hectic flush" in the afternoon, with night sweats at night.

Lyme Disease: • ANDROGRAPHIS (chills and fever, chronic and acute) • Cimicifuga (muscular pain) • DIPSACUS (chills and fever, brain fog, many symptoms; at onset and chronic) • Quercus (with Dipsacus—Krekow) • Polygonum japonica • Sida acuta (co-infection) • Smilax • VERBENA (co-infection with stiff, painful neck).

Malaria: • Andrographis • ARTEMISIA ANNUA (specific) • Ceanothus (swollen spleen) • Cinchona (debilitated states after the main fever has passed—Scudder) • Dipsacus • Euonymus • Eupatorium perfoliatum.

Note: All the remedies under the "Intermittent" heading may have some application here as well.

Measles: • Asclepias tuberosa (catarrhal manifestation; high fever; brings out eruptions) • Borago • Carthamus (brings out eruptions) • Drosera • Echinacea • Eupatorium perfoliatum • Euphrasia (with eye complications) • Trifolium.

Meningitis, Encephalitis, Brain Fever: • CIMICIFUGA (meningitis; never well since, or during) • Echinacea (with underlying sepsis; profound prostration) • Leonurus (tick-borne — Rogers) • SALVIA (fever with unconsciousness, trembling) • Scutellaria (spinal) • Verbena.

Mononucleosis, Glandular Fever: • Astragalus • BAPTISIA • Calendula • Ceanothus (spleen complications) • Codonopsis • Commiphora myrrha • Echinacea • HELIANTHEMUM (often available only in homeopathic form as Cistus canadensis) • Iris • Isatis • Phytolacca • Scrophularia.

Chronic Fatigue Syndrome: This is so often due to lingering effects of mononucleosis — "never been well since mono" — that one should strongly consider using the above mononucleosis remedies.

Mumps: • Asclepias tuberosa • Phytolacca • Trifolium.

Bacterial (antibacterial remedies): • Achillea (full, nonresistant, rapid pulse) • Baptisia (typhoid fever) • Berberis (hard, rapid pulse) • Echinacea (septic, exhaustive fever) • Lomatium.

Note: Use large doses of Capsicum, Armoracia, Angelica, Ligusticum, *and* Myrica *("Fire Cider"-type formulae) to bring blood to the head and expel microbes.*

Virus (antiviral remedies): • Astragalus • Baptisia (exhaustion) • Calendula • GNAPHALIUM • HELICHRYSUM (essential oil) • Hypericum • SAMBUCUS (flower or berry) • Urtica (tea).

Viruses have a sedative or depressing effect on the organism, so they produce chills, while bacteria have a stimulating effect and produce heat.

FORMULARY

Cinchona —with *Achillea, Mentha piperita, Asclepias tuberosa* (influenza). BHP 1983, 67.

Eupatorium perfoliatum —with *Achillea, Sambucus, Asclepias, Angelica,* and *Capsicum* or *Zingiberis* (influenza).

Liriodendron —with *Cornus florida, Prunus serotina* (malaria, influenza, intermittent fever). This Cherokee malaria remedy became famous during the Civil War, when quinine was difficult to get in the Confederacy, due to the blockades. It is from Richard Foreman, quoted by Porcher.

Hyssopus —with *Calendula, Arctium, Hypericum* (fever with dry skin). Expanded from BHP 1983, 117.

Hyssopus —with *Verbena, Rubus canadensis, Centaurium erythraea,* and a pinch of *Capsicum* (fever with dry skin, dark urine). Les Moore 2002, 17.

Sambucus flower —*Achillea* flower, *Mentha piperita* (influenza). Traditional.

Sambucus flower —with *Mentha piperita, Tilia europaea, Verbascum* spp. (rhinitis, influenza, throat, ear). Les Moore 2002, 10.

Sambucus —with *Fumaria* and *Borago* (diaphoretic in fever). "But none are equal to the elder, fumitory, and borage"—Tilke.

Agni, the Inner Fire

Ayurvedic medicine has gifted the world with a beautiful metaphor for describing the inner fire of the body. The inner digestive/metabolic fire is located in the center of the body, in the pyloric sphincter of the stomach. It is called the *agni* in Sanskrit, a word related to our terms "igneous" and "ignition."

From there the *agni* radiates outward in all directions, to the periphery of the organism, keeping everything warm and cozy. With it the *agni* brings water and nutrition —as in Chinese medicine, fire is associated with transformation, transportation, spreading, and movement. The *agni* is blocked by *ama,* which has the properties of unhealthy dampness, stickiness, thickness, impurity, coldness, and sluggishness. It is likened to a phlegm that covers, dampness, and suppress the fire anywhere from the center to the periphery.

We have similar traditions in the West; we speak of "fire in the belly," now meaning just a psychological quality—the gumption to keep going, no matter what. However, in traditional Western herbalism we have a very close analog in the teachings of Samuel Thomson. This self-taught farmer-cum-herbalist, who popularized herbalism in the early nineteenth century, taught that the stomach was like a stove: all that was needed to maintain health was to clean out the ashes (oops, I think my wood stove needs some of that attention!) and keep the fire stoked with fuel. The fire can then radiate outwards to the periphery and keep the organism warm, moist, and nourished.

The enemy of this fire is, first of all, cold. When external cold enters, it closes the pores in the periphery and keeps the heat from its natural movement outwards onto the surface of the skin. On the other hand, if the fire in the center dies down, the fire cannot radiate to the surface, and cold can flow in from outside. The ash blocking the stove was likened by Thomson to phlegm or "canker," as he called it, adhering to the walls of the stomach and impeding outward flow. The properties of canker are basically the same as those of *ama.*

Thomson likened the fire in the stomach to a fountain: if it is dammed up around the periphery, the water becomes still, and stillness is the attribute of death, not life. On the other hand, if the fountain itself dies down, it becomes a stagnant little puddle, also still. The flow of the fountain is the flow of life.

While it might be most appropriate to put this discussion under the stomach and small intestine, where it is often placed in Ayurveda, it equally belongs under the discussion of fever. Thomson himself saw the inner fire as requiring attention at the center, to remove canker; in the circulation, to move warmth, water, and food to the periphery; and in the pores of the skin, to keep them open. His follower, Dr. Cook (1869) therefore separated the diaphoretics for opening the skin and releasing the hear of the fever, or the chill of cold, into two categories: the relaxing diaphoretics that open the pores and release chill, and the warming diaphoretics that warm the center and open the pores from increased internal heat.

Injuries, First Aid

Very often we see first-aid salves and ointments that simply combine the top vulneraries (calendula, plantain, St. John's wort, comfrey, etc.) without a thought as to the nature of the wound. These products are fine for first aid, but deny us the opportunity to treat more expertly by combining for broad-spectrum effects rather than specific wound qualities. Formulas work well in first aid, and we should try to identify a specific formula that matches the specific wound in every case. To this end, I have included in my discussion of injuries and first aid a section on tissue states and the skin surface.

Heat/Excitation: The surface overreacts to injury, resulting in histaminic activity; carmine-red color; use cooling herbs: *Amygdalus, Hypericum, Prunus serotina, Rosa, Tilia.* Some cooling power is also to be had from demulcents: *Althaea, Chondrus, Lilium candidum* (petal; much-used in France in the past) or *L. longiflorum, Ulmus.* Most carrier oils are warming and stimulating, so for cooling we prefer a lotion or coconut oil. Hemorrhages are bright-red, and difficult to stop; use *Achillea.*

Cold/Depression: This is a common condition when a poison or bacteria has gotten into a wound, or there is poor peripheral circulation and the body cannot defend itself, which invites bacteria to invade. This requires the healing stimulants, warming remedies, and antiseptics. Warming and stimulating remedies include: *Angelica, Arnica, Calendula, Capsella, Capsicum, Commiphora myrrha, Hydrastis, Hypericum, Inula, Ruta, Sassafras, Solidago, Stachys palustris, Trillium, Urtica, Zanthoxylum.* Warming oils to combine with these include peanut (warm) and olive (mildly warming). Antiseptics include: *Arnica, Baptisia, Capsicum, Inula, Isatis,* and the conifers used by the American

Indian people, including *Pinus*, *Thuja*, *Tsuga*, and *Abies*. Snakebite and venom remedies include: *Achillea* (spider), *Cimicifuga*, *Echinacea*, *Eryngium*, *Eupatorium rugosum*, *Goodyeara*, *Lavandula*, *Plantago*, *Polygala senega*.

Dry/Atrophy: If the wounded area is poorly nourished, dry, wasted, etc., we should think of demulcents and nutritives: *Calendula*, *Chondrus*, *Lilium candidum*, *Lilium longiflorum*, *Polygonatum*, *Symphytum*, *Trigonella*, *Ulmus*. Stimulants also help by getting nutrition to the area: *Hydrastis* is both nutritive and stimulating. To stimulate tissue regrowth: *Arctium* (leaf), *Centella*, *Symphytum* (leaf), externally.

Damp/Stagnation: This tissue state occurs when the matrix in the area of the wound is not clean, and there is a need for both local and systemic cleansing. Drawing agents (usually astringents) are needed, and possibly systemic alteratives, as well as local cleansing. Use: *Centella*, *Helianthemum*, *Plantago*, *Scrophularia*, *Stellaria*.

Tension: This is a factor when the nerves are involved. Pain causes a person to hold the injured part tense, or hold the breath. Holding the breath releases endorphins (the body's natural opiates), which reduce the pain. *Agrimony* is specific for pain that causes one to hold the breath. Add these agents for relieving tension to other remedies used for the wound itself: *Agrimonia* (stoic), *Chamomilla* (very sensitive and tender; whines and complains), *Hypericum* (severe pain), *Potentilla* (holds the breath), *Verbascum*, *Withania* (compensatory tension in nearby muscles), *Zanthoxylum* (tortured feeling).

Relaxation: The more free the bleeding, the more we think of an astringent to help close the lips of the wound and staunch the blood (astringents are contraindicated if the wound is *not* bleeding): *Achillea*, *Ajuga*, *Alchemilla*, *Rubus*, *Rumex crispus*, *Sanguisorba*, *Symphytum* (may cause tissue overgrowth). Astringents also act as drawing agents to draw out splinters, infected material, pus. Drawing agents: *Allium sativa* (infected wounds), *Plantago* (open, infected wounds), *Pinus* (pine sap keeps the wound clean while drawing out metal, bullets, etc.—Navajo; confirmed), *Symphytum* (wounded cartilage).

Abrasions, Cuts, Wounds: • ACHILLEA (active bleeding, bruises with bleeding, painful cuts; internal bleeding and blood blisters) • Ajuga • Alchemilla (torn skin, passive hemorrhage; rinse after dental surgery) • ALLIUM CEPA (cut a red onion in half, place over wound to draw; very old folk remedy with many confirmations) • ALLIUM SATIVA (local dressing) • ALTHAEA (external) • Amygdalus (histaminic irritation; red around wound) • Angelica • Arctium (gaping wounds, missing tissue; fill the wound with fresh root or leaf—LeSassier; confirmed) • CALENDULA (red, sore, infected cuts, cat scratches, cuts that are worse from exposure to water; purulent, infected) • CAPSELLA (oozing, passive hemorrhage; fresh plant or tincture best) • CAPSICUM (to stop bleeding; external) • Ceanothus (delayed coagulation; old bruises and contusions; external) • Centella • Chamomilla (complains about the pain) • Commiphora myrrha (abrasion) • Cnicus (indolent, infected) • Equisetum (especially for weak connective tissue, slow-healing wounds) • Geum (stimulating astringent) • Hydrastis (excessive bleeding, clean cuts; contraindicated for dirty, infected wounds because it will seal in dirt and pus) • HYPERICUM (cuts with nerve damage, inflammation and pain, loss of parts; heals slowly and closes the flesh from the inside; believed to reconnect nerves) • Ledum (puncture wounds; surface mottled pale and blue, poor oxidation, spasm from wound; prevents tetanus, according to homeopathy) • LILIUM CANDIDUM (drawing agent; flowers preserved in oil; place on cut, bruise, pus, splinter—French folk remedy) • Lycopus (bleeding) • PLANTAGO (drawing agent; dirty, infected cuts, puncture wounds without much bleeding) • Prunella (draws out heat of infection) • Prunus serotina (histaminic irritation) • Rubia (bleeding from a fresh, green wound) • Rubus canadensis (mild bleeding; external) • Rumex crispus (cuts and wounds; poultice)

• Salvia (infected cut) • SANGUISORBA (all types of bleeding) • Sanicula • SOLIDAGO (bruises, old wounds) • STACHYS PALUSTRIS ("woundwort"; severe lacerations and bleeding; severed tissues) • Stellaria (external) • Symphytum (old wounds that are slow to heal; gaping wounds; generates flesh from the outside inwards; can cause overgrowth of tissue; external, combines well with Calendula) • Trillium (bleeding) • Ulmus • VINCA MINOR (bleeding from nose, mouth, after tooth extraction).

Bruises: • ACHILLEA (red and blue; bruise with bleeding; blood blister; works better than Arnica when the origin of the bruise is violent) • ANGELICA (blue, green, gray, yellow color) • ARNICA (red and blue; without bleeding; strain, sprain) • Bellis perennis (bruises to deep tissues; obstetric injury) • CALENDULA (general remedy; compress for blow to the eye) • Carbo vegetabilis (homeopathic or powder of charcoal; blue and yellow color of bruise, old stagnant bruises) • CARTHAMUS (red and blue color; toxic undertone) • CHELIDONIUM (beat-up feeling; "thought by some to be superior to Arnica"—French; external) • Collinsonia (leaf poultice) • Hamamelis (subconjunctival hemorrhage) • Heracleum (compress) • Humulus • Hypericum (areas rich in nerves) • POLYGONATUM • Polygonum multiflorum (prepared root; external) • RUTA (nerve, bone, tendon; with swelling) • Sambucus (blue and swollen ankles, wrists) • SASSAFRAS (black and blue; in older persons; external) • SOLIDAGO (bruises, cuts, sores; especially good for spine, back; external) • Stellaria (external) • Symphytum (black eye) • Thymus (compress, pillow).

Burns: • Abies balsamea (fir sap, from bubbles on the bark; external—Keewaydinoquay) • Achillea (deep burns) • AGRIMONIA (holding breath due to pain; "this is my favorite burn medicine"—Wood) • ALOE VERA (fresh gel) • Arctium (crushed leaf, with egg white; old Amish remedy)

• ASTRAGALUS (increases circulation, nutrition to surface; removes heat and toxins) • CALENDULA (chemical burns to eyes; ulcerative burns; immediate dressing can prevent blisters) • CENTELLA (lessens scar tissue, prevents ulceration, speeds recovery; external, internal) • Chamomilla (external) • HAMA-MELIS (pain, scalds, burnt lips, tongue, mouth, eyes, cornea; external) • HYPERICUM (sunburn, radiation burns, pain; oil, externally) • Iris versicolor (scalds, sunburn) • LAVANDULA (reduces pain, prevents infection, increases circulation, supports blood-vessel recovery; oil, externally—old folk remedy; often confirmed) • Linum (flaxseed oil) • Lycopodium (spores; not commercially available) • Melaleuca (prevents infection) • Mentha piperita (pain, burning; lessens hypersensitivity) • MONARDA FISTULOSA (with cold sweat; lessens scar tis-sue—Crow; confirmed) • Passiflora (recent burns; external) • Plantago (herpes, shingles, blisters, burns; external) • Polygo-natum (external) • POTENTILLA (analogous to Agrimonia) • Prunella (external) • Sambucus • Symphytum (indolent burns, slow recovery; "do not use where there is redness, puffi-ness or oozing"—Hershoff and Rotelli) • Ulmus (paste to pro-tect and heal burns) • Urtica (burning, stinging pain; kidney congestion from burn's waste products) • Zingiberis (fresh juice of rhizome on first- and second-degree burns; lessens inflamma-tion and pain).

Blisters: See "Skin."

Bones, Broken: • Achillea (bruising, bleeding, pain) • Ajuga • Calendula (lymphatic congestion with broken collarbone) • Dipsacus (Chinese, European) • EUPATORIUM PERFOLI-ATUM (crushed and broken bones) • Eupatorium purpureum (when the former is unavailable) • EQUISETUM (weak skin, hair, nails; poor bone-healing from silica deficiency; chronic swelling after broken bone; internal, or bath) • Hieracium pilo-sella • Medicago • Piscidia (pain) • Polygonatum (removes bruising, sets bones in the right place, heals quickly) • Rehmannia (cooked root) • Spikenard (Occom) • SYMPHYTUM (old, difficult, slow-healing broken bones; heals quickly but causes callous and overgrowth; can join the bones when incorrectly set; external) • Trigonella • URTICA • VERBASCUM (use externally on broken ribs and toes that cannot be set; especially good for digits; sets the bones in the right place).

Note: For the first three or four days, use Achillea, Arnica, *or* Ledum *to remove clotted blood; then switch to bone-healing with* Eupatorium perfoliatum *or* Symphytum *for a month. Bone-healing could be very precise in Native American medicine. The Mohegan medicine man Samuel Occom (1754) gave one formula for breaks around the fingers, feet, and hands, and another for the thighs, arms, and limbs. Unfortunately, except for spikenard in the second recipe, he didn't use names we understand today.*

Chilblains: • Acorus calamus (wash) • Arnica (external) • Calendula (ointment) • CAPSICUM • Juglans nigra (leaf wash) • Krameria (external) • Viscum (berry ointment).

Frostbite: • Acorus calamus (wash) • Equisetum (bath) • Quercus (bath) • Verbascum • Viscum (wash).

Insect Bite: • Achillea (brown recluse spider) • Cimicifuga (external) • Eupatorium cannabinum (smoke smudge, to keep away insects) • Eupatorium perfoliatum, E. purpurea (substitute for the following) • Eupatorium rugosum (spider) • Gentiana (anaphylaxis, bee sting) • Hypericum • Nicotiana (tobacco poultice) • OCIMUM (dried leaves, remoistened with water) • Opuntia (pad poultice) • PLANTAGO • Salvia.

Nerve Injury: • ACHILLEA (after cerebrospinal injuries and surgery; to prevent blood stagnation from pressing on spinal and cerebral injury) • Acorus (oil, external) • Agrimonia (pain, tension, holding the breath) • Betonica (pain, hysteria, frenzy, head injury)

• Chamomilla (irritability) • Eschscholzia (nerve damage; sharp, shooting pain) • Heracleum • HYPERICUM (tortured, painful, inflamed nerves) • Lactuca (blow to the testicles) • Osmorhiza (numbness, pain, peripheral neuralgia, debility) • Valeriana ("wonderful for chronic marauding pain when taken at sub-sedative doses"—Sedlacek) • WITHANIA (nourishing; external, in ghee) • ZANTHOXYLUM (tortured, painful).

Poison Ivy/Oak (for external application): • Alnus • Ampelopsis (leaf and twig) • COMPTONIA • Echinacea • GRINDELIA • IMPATIENS (wipe on immediately) • Lithospermum (wash) • Lobelia (vinegar tincture) • Lycium (combine with Lithospermum) • Monarda fistulosa • Plantago • Polygonatum • Quercus • Rosmarinus (in vinegar).

Scorpion Sting: • Artemisia ludoviciana (external; apply a cloth saturated in the tincture) • Opuntia (pad poultice) • Populus (leaf poultice).

Severe Fluid or Blood Loss: • Cinchona • Gelsemium (exhaustion, lethargy; after sweating) • Panax ginseng (collapse with feeble, minute pulse, dry tongue).

Shock: • ACONITUM (homeopathic; for animal fear) • ARNICA • CARTHAMUS (tincture; or even safflower cooking oil, if nothing else is available) • Panax ginseng (feeble pulse, shallow respiration, shortness of breath, cold extremities, cold sweat) • Rosmarinus.

Snakebite: • Allium cepa (sliced onion; put on bite—Doyle) • Baptisia (sepsis) • Cimicifuga (neurological symptoms; tea or tincture, every hour) • ECHINACEA (stops spread and sepsis) • Eupatorium rugosum • Eryngium yuccifolium ("rattlesnake master"—the most important snakebite remedy of the Southeastern Indian people) • Fraxinus (root bark tea—Native

American) • Iris (wear for protection against—Native American) • Juglans nigra (bark and leaf tea) • Monarda fistulosa (bite burns like fire—Olson) • Opuntia (split open the prickly pear pad, poultice on the site, moist side down, if available; change every hour) • Plantago (immediate application, if available) • Polygonum bistorta (root tea) • Populus (aspen or cottonwood-leaf poultice) • Vitis (wild grape leaf tea).

Spider Bite: • Achillea (brown recluse) • Calendula • ECHINACEA • EUPATORIUM RUGOSUM (if not available, use cousin E. perfoliatum or E. purpureum) • HYPERICUM (red streak up arm) • PLANTAGO.

Note: Also see snakebite remedies, above.

Sunburn (external treatment): • ALOE (fresh gel) • CALENDULA (external) • Cucurbita citrullus (internal) • HYPERICUM (external) • IRIS (external) • Potentilla (internal) • Rosa (petals in vinegar; external).

Sunstroke: • Echinacea • Melilotus (for sunstroke—Lakota usage) • Melissa • Primula.

Unconsciousness (to revive): • Achillea (for head injury; smell) • Betonica • CARBO VEGETABILIS (homeopathic) • Lobelia • Symphytum (apparent brain death; no brain activity; has revived unconscious patients).

Drawing Agents: • Allium cepa (cut a red onion in half, and use cut half on skin or ear to draw out object, venom, or matter; onion syrup on chest to draw out mucus) • Agrimonia (splinters) • Amygdalus (draw out abscess—Graf; parasites—Grieve) • GLECHOMA (footbath with Plantago for heavy metals—Dowling) • Monarda fistulosa ("draw out fire" from a burn – Crow; confirmed, Wood) • Pinus strobus • PLANTAGO (draw out splinter, pus, infection, abscess) • Prunella (infection, pus, heat—LeSassier; pieces of metal—Keewaydinoquay • Sinapis alba (mustard pack on chest to loosen mucus).

Note: Green leaves in general are cooling and drawing.

FORMULARY

Acorus—"Sweet flag good for Cloted Blood"—Samson Occom, Mohegan medicine man, 1754.

Achillea—in safflower oil, for bleeding, contusion with bleeding.

Arnica—always contraindicated with an open wound.

Calendula—dried flowers: fill jar, then fill with mineral oil; let sit 6 weeks; strain and use oil.

Calendula—with Chondrus and Ulmus (nutritive, slightly warming). BHP 1983, 45.

Calendula—with Hydrastis and Commiphora myrrha (stimulating). BHP 1983, 45.

Calendula—with Symphytum leaves in mineral oil (for gaping wounds).Carthamus—always use safflower oil, if possible, when making oils for bruises. Even by itself it is helpful.

Hypericum—always include St. John's wort oil when the nerves are involved. Pick on a dry, sunny day, more than twenty-four hours after rain.

Lilium candidum—petals in oil or alcohol; a very widespread French folk remedy until after WWII. Use Lilium longiflorum if *L. candidum* is not available.

Ocimum—dried leaves; remoisten with a few drops of water to make a small poultice to put on a sting; it temporarily increases the sting as it pulls out poison, but prevents further pain and swelling. Can use any kind of basil—Doyle.

Plantago—My favorite salve is made from fresh plantain leaves chopped fine and added to coconut oil, which reinforces the cooling property of plantain and turns a beautiful green color.

THE CONSOLIDA

The established wound-healing remedies of the Middle Ages and Renaissance were called "consolida," meaning that they "consolidated" the wound, brought the lips of the wound together, or strengthened the tissue. Here is a list from Olaf Rippe and Margret Madejsky's *Die Kräuterkunde des Paracelsus* (2013, 182):

- Consolida minor (*Symphytum officinale*)
- Consolida media (*Ajuga reptans*)
- Consolida mediana (*Vinca minor*)
- Consolida minor (*Prunella vulgaris, Menyanthes trifoliata, Bellis perennis, Sanicula europaea*)
- Consolida mucilaginosa (*Symphytum officinale*)
- Consolida regalis (*Delphinium regalis*)
- Consolida rubea (*Potentilla tormentilla*)
- Consolida aurea (*Hypericum perfoliatum*)
- Solidago (*Solidago virga-aurea*)

URTICA

"When in doubt, give Nettles."

—DAVID HOFFMAN

Therapeutic Index of Clinical Conditions and Diseases

About the Authors

MATTHEW WOOD has been a practicing herbalist for over thirty-five years and is an internationally known teacher on the subject. Wood has an MS degree from the Scottish School of Herbal Medicine (accredited by the University of Wales) and is a registered herbalist in the American Herbalist Guild. He is the author of eight books on herbal medicine, including *The Book of Herbal Wisdom, The Practice of Traditional Western Herbalism,* and *The Earthwise Herbal.* For more information, please visit www.matthewwoodherbs.com.

DAVID RYAN C Ac, C Hom, CMT is a Northern California healer, teacher, and practitioner of Tai Ji and Qi Gong. He is currently working on a book on the Gurdjieff meditations and Qi Gong for the five elements and seven centers, *In Search of the True Self.*

TITLES BY MATTHEW WOOD

available from North Atlantic Books

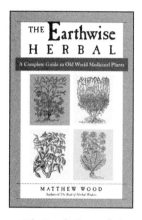

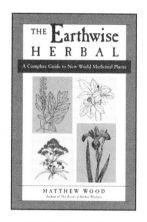

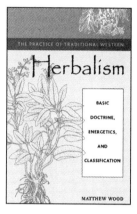

*The Earthwise Herbal
(Old World)*
978-1-55643-692-5

*The Earthwise Herbal
(New World)*
978-1-55643-779-3

*The Practice of Traditional
Western Herbalism*
978-1-55643-503-4

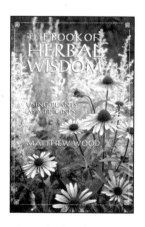

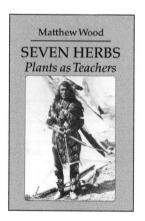

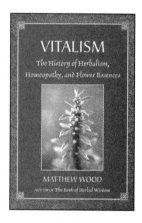

The Book of Herbal Wisdom
978-1-55643-232-3

Seven Herbs
978-0-93819-091-2

Vitalism
978-1-55643-340-5

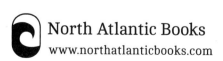

North Atlantic Books
www.northatlanticbooks.com

North Atlantic Books is an independent, nonprofit publisher committed to a bold exploration of the relationships between mind, body, spirit, and nature.

About North Atlantic Books

North Atlantic Books (NAB) is a 501(c)(3) nonprofit publisher committed to a bold exploration of the relationships between mind, body, spirit, culture, and nature. Founded in 1974, NAB aims to nurture a holistic view of the arts, sciences, humanities, and healing. To make a donation or to learn more about our books, authors, events, and newsletter, please visit www.northatlanticbooks.com.